Obstetrics and Gynaecology

For UKMLA and Medical Exams

First edition authors:

Nick Panay

Ruma Dutta

Audrey Ryan

J A Mark Broadbent

Second edition authors:

Maryam Parisaei

Archana Shailendra

Ruma Dutta

J A Mark Broadbent

Third edition authors:

Chidimma Onwere

Hemant N. Vakharia

Fourth edition authors:

Sophie Eleanor Kay

Charlotte Jean Sandhu

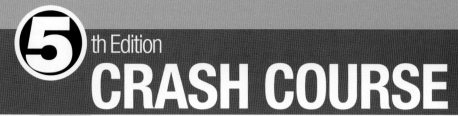

CRASH COURSE
5th Edition

SERIES EDITOR

Philip Xiu

MA (Cantab), MB BChir, MRCP, MRCGP, MScClinEd, FHEA, MAcadMEd, RCPathME
Honorary Senior Lecturer
Leeds University School of Medicine
PCN Educational Lead
Medical Examiner
Leeds Teaching Hospital Trust
Leeds, UK

FACULTY ADVISOR

Fevzi Shakir

MBBS, BSc (Hons), MRCOG, MSc
Consultant Obstetrician and Advanced Gynaecological Endoscopic Surgeon
Royal Free London NHS Foundation Trust
London, UK

Obstetrics and Gynaecology

Dila Zengin
MD, MRCOG, PgCert (epidemiology)
Specialty Registrar in Obstetrics & Gynaecology
Cambridge University Hospitals NHS Foundation Trust
Cambridge, UK

Sophie Strong
MBBS, BSc (Hons), MRCOG
Specialty Registrar in Obstetrics & Gynaecology
Barts Health NHS Trust
London, UK

Jacqueline Sia
MBChB, BSc (Hons), MRCOG
Specialty Registrar in Obstetrics & Gynaecology
Barts Health NHS Trust
London, UK

ELSEVIER

First edition 1999
Second edition 2004
Third edition 2008
Fourth edition 2013
Updated Fourth edition 2015
Fifth edition 2025

Notices

Practitioners and researchers must always rely on their own experience and knowledge in evaluating and using any information, methods, compounds or experiments described herein. Because of rapid advances in the medical sciences, in particular, independent verification of diagnoses and drug dosages should be made. To the fullest extent of the law, no responsibility is assumed by Elsevier, authors, editors or contributors for any injury and/or damage to persons or property as a matter of products liability, negligence or otherwise, or from any use or operation of any methods, products, instructions, or ideas contained in the material herein.

ISBN: 978-0-443-11536-3

Content Strategist: Trinity Hutton
Content Project Manager: Shivani Pal
Design: Miles Hitchen
Marketing Manager: Deborah Watkins

Printed in India

Last digit is the print number: 9   8   7   6   5   4   3   2   1

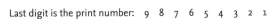

Working together
to grow libraries in
developing countries

www.elsevier.com • www.bookaid.org

Series editor's foreword

With great honour and pride, we present the latest edition of the *Crash Course* series. This series has traversed a journey of nearly a quarter-century, stemming from the vision of Dr. Dan Horton-Szar, and his legacy continues to walk with us on this pathway of knowledge.

The series has been popular with students worldwide, selling over **1 million copies** and being translated into more than **8 languages**, reinforcing our commitment to global learning.

We remain extremely grateful for your unwavering trust. The series has once again been refreshed and fully upgraded in accordance with the rapidly changing medical guidelines, ensuring the content is comprehensive, accurate and fully up-to-date.

This latest series continues our tradition of integrating clinical practice with basic medical sciences, tailored meticulously for today's medical undergraduate curriculum. A central highlight of this instalment is our emphasis on high-yield exam content designed specifically for the UKMLA curriculum.

The addition of the **Rapid UKMLA Index** at the beginning of the book enhances this offering, serving as a valuable aid to students to track their exam preparation efficiently. We have also revised all self-assessment questions to align with the single best answer format in line with the latest UKMLA examination style. We have also added *High-Yield Association Tables*. These are essential tools designed to aid students in recognizing clinical patterns and acing vignette-style exam questions. By condensing complex medical scenarios into digestible, manageable insights, these tables ensure efficient learning. They connect symptoms, diagnosis and treatment, bolstering understanding and confidence in tackling the rigorous UKMLA exams. This comprehensive approach makes these tables an indispensable asset in your exam preparations.

Utilizing student feedback, we have strived to maintain the core principles of this series: delivering precise and readable text that brings together depth and clarity. The authors are experienced junior doctors who successfully navigated these exams recently, ensuring practical and tested guidance. A team of expert faculty advisors from across the United Kingdom ensures the content's accuracy, making it resilient and reliable.

As we turn a new chapter with the latest edition, we honour the past, cherish the present, and embrace the promise of the future. We wish you every success in your journey of learning and growth and hope that this series adds value to your life, both as students and as future medical professionals.

Philip Xiu

Prefaces

Author and Faculty Advisor

The field of medicine is continually evolving, with new discoveries and treatments constantly being developed and introduced at a tremendous pace. Keeping abreast of clinical advances is a challenge in any branch of medicine, but especially so in a specialty as diverse as Obstetrics and Gynaecology - From advances in gynaecological cancer treatment, to new technologies in laparoscopic/robotic gynaecological surgery and assisted reproductive techniques.

True to the spirit of the Crash Course series, this fifth edition aims to serve as an essential guide to the contemporary medical student seeking to gain a sound knowledge and understanding of this unique specialty. It has been revised and updated to reflect the latest clinical guidelines and evidence-based practices, with information presented succinctly through the use of choice figures, and carefully designed flowcharts and tables. New chapter summaries at the end of each chapter have been added to prompt you on key take-away points when revising. The popular self-assessment section has been fully revised with new "single best answer" questions to test your understanding and aid exam preparation.

Despite significant advancements in reproductive healthcare and international efforts to improve women's health worldwide, thousands of women continue to die every day due to complications in pregnancy and childbirth, the majority of which are largely preventable. Multiple barriers persist in improving outcomes; the lack of education, unsafe abortion, and above all a lack of access to sexual and reproductive healthcare being major factors.

This piece of work is the distillation of our cumulative years of experience. Regardless of where you find yourself in your medical career, we hope this book will provide a solid foundation in Obstetrics and Gynaecology, enabling you to make a difference in women's health wherever you may practice.

Jacqueline Sia, Dila Zengin, Sophie Strong, and Fevzi Shakir

Series editor's acknowledgement

We would like to express our sincere gratitude to those who have provided their support and expertise in preparing this sixth edition of the *Crash Course* series. Our junior doctor contributors' participation in crafting the manuscript has been indispensable. Their first-hand experience and current medical knowledge have infused realism and practicality into our content.

Our faculty editors deserve a special note of thanks. They have extensively validated the correctness of the information, ensuring that the content is not just accurate but also contemporaneous, credible, and aligns with the latest medical standards.

We extend our heartfelt thanks to our publisher, Elsevier. Their staff have demonstrated an unwavering commitment to quality, maintaining the high standards set since the first edition. Their insights have routinely enriched the content and process alike.

Our Commissioning Editor, Jeremy Bowes, deserves a special mention for his consistent support and guiding hand throughout the development process. His directions and advice have bettered this edition and spurred us on our quest for excellence.

We are greatly indebted to Alex Mortimer for her wisdom, practical insights and valuable guidance. A big thank you to our Content Strategists, Trinity Hutton and Cloe Holland-Borosh, who need special acknowledgement for meticulously outlining the direction and scope of the content. They've managed to mix details with a strategic plan, keeping our readers in mind.

Lastly, much gratitude is owed to our Content Project Managers, Taranpreet Kaur, Ayan Dhar, Shivani Pal and Tapajyoti Chaudhuri, who have juggled the numerous day-to-day tasks with utmost dedication and perseverance. Despite the ever-approaching deadlines, they have shown remarkable patience and steadfast determination, ensuring that each step of the book's development was accomplished seamlessly.

In conclusion, we sincerely thank each of these wonderful people for their outstanding contributions and support, without which this work wouldn't have been achieved. Their passion, commitment and collaborative effort have helped us bring this edition together.

Philip Xiu

Dedications

To my mother, who has walked every step of this journey with me. And to Jon, who read every word, and dragged me across the finishing line. Most of all to the patients, who continue to teach us, and whose stories inspire the pages of this book.

Jacqueline Sia

To my wonderful family and friends.

Dila Zengin

With thanks and eternal gratitude to my wonderfully supportive family who have always been my biggest cheerleaders. And to Villanelle, who spent countless hours by my side, through every page written. To the medical students reading this book - do your reading(!), get to know your patients not just their diagnoses and be the best version of a holistic clinician you can be, to help support those through some of their most vulnerable moments.

Sophie Strong

To all my family who continue to support me throughout my life and career, giving me the foundation to which I have built from and continue to do so. In addition thank you to all our patients who trust us and give us the privilege of looking after them.

Fevzi Shakir

Rapid UKMLA Index

The UKMLA Curriculum Conditions Priority levels have been based on the below:

Level 1: Conditions that a newly qualified doctor should have a good knowledge of and be able to recognise and manage.
Level 2: Conditions requiring knowledge for recognising and confirming diagnosis and planning first-line management in straightforward cases.
Level 3: Conditions where recognition of clinical presentation and describing principles of management are important.

Continued

Contents

Contents

Contents

Basic anatomy and examination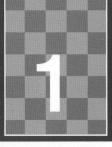

BASIC ANATOMY

Basic anatomical knowledge of the female pelvis is essential for obstetrics and gynaecology. It enables one to understand the mechanisms of normal function and facilitates an appreciation of the processes of labour and reproduction. It lays the foundation for understanding gynaecological pathology and its influence on women's health.

THE BONY PELVIS

The bony pelvis functions to support the weight of the upper body and provide attachments for muscles of the pelvic floor. It is formed by the sacrum and a pair of innominate bones (Fig. 1.1) and is divided into the 'true' and 'false' pelvis by the pelvic brim. The innominate bones articulate posteriorly with the sacrum at the sacroiliac joints and are joined anteriorly at the symphysis pubis. The true pelvis lies below the pelvic brim and forms the bony margins of the birth canal, which accommodates the passage of the foetus during childbirth.

CLINICAL NOTES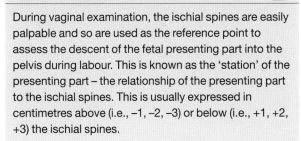

During vaginal examination, the ischial spines are easily palpable and so are used as the reference point to assess the descent of the fetal presenting part into the pelvis during labour. This is known as the 'station' of the presenting part – the relationship of the presenting part to the ischial spines. This is usually expressed in centimetres above (i.e., −1, −2, −3) or below (i.e., +1, +2, +3) the ischial spines.

The bony pelvis also functions to protect the female reproductive organs – the uterus, fallopian tubes and ovaries. These organs lie in close proximity to the urinary bladder anteriorly and the rectum posteriorly (Fig. 1.2). The vagina, urethra and anal canal, all traverse the pelvic floor, of which the levator ani muscles provide principal support. Pathology in one tract can thus easily affect adjacent tracts.

THE VULVA

The term 'vulva' is used to describe all of the external female genitalia – the mons pubis, labia majora and minora, clitoris, external urinary meatus, vaginal vestibule, vaginal orifice (introitus) and hymen (Fig. 1.3). The surface of the vulva up to the inner aspect of the labia minora is covered by stratified keratinized squamous epithelium. The vaginal mucosa is made up of non-keratinizing stratified squamous epithelium. Structures opening into the vaginal vestibule are the external urinary meatus, vaginal orifice, Bartholin glands and Skene ducts.

CLINICAL NOTES

The Bartholin's glands are a pair of mucus-secreting glands located on either side of the vaginal introitus. Their ducts drain into the vestibule and the secretions from these glands function to provide lubrication during sexual intercourse. Bartholin cysts may form if the ducts become occluded and can develop into a painful and swollen abscess in the presence of infection. Smaller cysts/abscesses can be managed conservatively with antibiotics, while larger ones tend to undergo incision and drainage. Marsupialization, where the edges of the cyst wall are sutured to the surrounding skin, helps to prevent the cyst from reforming. Use of a balloon catheter (word catheter) is an alternative that allows continual drainage of the cyst over a period of 3 to 4 weeks. The word catheter is now becoming the norm, as it allows more for an ambulatory procedure to take place.

THE UTERUS

The uterus is a hollow, pear-shaped, muscular organ that measures 7.5 cm × 5.0 cm × 2.5 cm on average. It consists of a body (corpus uteri), fundus, cornua, isthmus and cervix (Fig. 1.4). The terms 'anteversion' and 'retroversion' are often used to describe the position of the uterus (Fig. 1.5). The uterus may

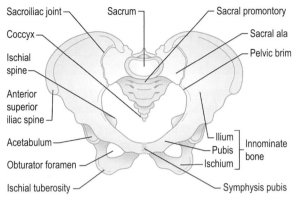

Fig. 1.1 The bony pelvis. (From de Costa C. *Essential Obstetrics and Gynaecology.* 5th ed. pp. 2–11. © 2020.)

also be folded anteriorly or posteriorly along its longitudinal axis ('anteflexion' or 'retroflexion').

The wall of the uterus is comprised of three layers:

(a) The perimetrium (serosa): The outer serous layer derived from overlying peritoneum.
(b) The myometrium: The middle, muscular layer comprising of smooth muscle fibres.
(c) The endometrium: The innermost layer which is the epithelial lining of the uterine cavity. This layer is under hormonal regulation and undergoes cyclical changes during the menstrual cycle in response to fluctuation levels of oestrogen and progesterone. The endometrium is made up of two layers:

- *Stratum functionalis*: A superficial functional layer consisting of mucus-secreting columnar cells. This layer

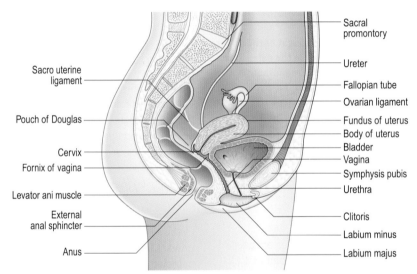

Fig. 1.2 Sagittal view of female pelvic anatomy. (From Young O, Duncan C. *Macleod's Clinical Examination.* pp. 211–236. © 2018.)

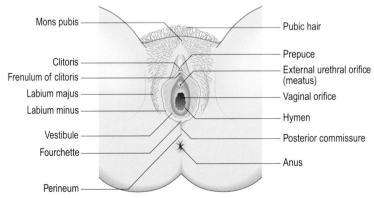

Fig. 1.3 External female genitalia. (From Young O, Duncan C. *Macleod's Clinical Examination.* 14th ed. pp. 211–236. © 2018.)

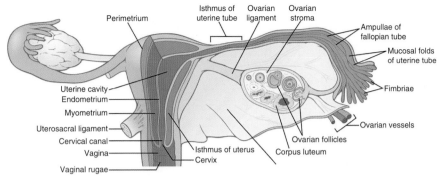

Fig. 1.4 The female reproductive system. (From *Guyton and Hall Textbook of Medical Physiology.* Hall JE, Hall ME. 14th ed. pp. 1027–1044. © 2021.)

is shed during menstruation, approximately every 28 days.

- *Stratum basalis*: A basal layer that is not shed, consisting of stem cells which help to regenerate the functional layer.

THE CERVIX

The cervix is joined to the corpus uteri by the isthmus of the uterus and connects the uterus and vagina. It is approximately 2.5 cm long and consists of an external cervical os (opening into the vagina), an internal cervical os (opening into the uterine cavity), and the endocervical canal running between the external and internal os (Fig. 1.6). The ectocervix (outer part of the cervix exposed to the vagina) is covered by non-keratinized stratified squamous epithelium, similar to that of the vagina, while the endocervix (endocervical canal) is lined by a single layer of mucin-secreting simple columnar (glandular) epithelium.

The squamocolumnar junction (SCJ) is the histological junction between the stratified squamous epithelium of the ectocervix and the simple columnar (glandular) epithelium of the endocervix. The location of the SCJ in relation to the external cervical os changes over the course of a woman's lifetime and is dependent on age and oestrogen exposure (Fig. 1.6).

Pre-puberty, the SCJ is located close to the external cervical os. Under the influence of oestrogen, in women of reproductive age, columnar epithelial cells at the lower part of the endocervical canal evert onto the ectocervix, exposing delicate columnar epithelial cells to the acidic environment of the vagina, and pushing the original SCJ outwards away from the external cervical os. Columnar epithelial cells react by transforming into squamous epithelium, a process known as squamous metaplasia. This takes place from the original SCJ, resulting in a 'new' SCJ being formed between the remaining everted columnar epithelium and the newly formed metaplastic squamous epithelium. The new SCJ progressively 'migrates' across the ectocervix towards the external os during the reproductive years. It often recedes within the endocervical canal following menopause and is not visible on speculum examination.

The 'transformation zone' refers to the area of metaplastic squamous epithelium formed between the ectocervix and the endocervix, and extends from the original SCJ to the new SCJ. It is the commonest place on the cervix for precancerous changes to develop as it is a dynamic area where columnar cells are continuously undergoing squamous metaplasia. Cells can be sampled from this area and examined for cellular abnormalities suggestive of premalignant lesions or cancer. This forms the basis of cervical cancer screening (see Chapter 12).

CLINICAL NOTES

Eversion of columnar epithelium onto the ectocervix is known as an ectropion, often visible on speculum examination as a reddish, raw-looking area on the outer surface of the cervix. Ectropions become more pronounced during puberty, pregnancy and with COCP use. As columnar epithelial cells are delicate, they are easily prone to injury. PCB or IMB secondary to an ectropion are common presentations, especially in women of reproductive age.

THE FALLOPIAN TUBES

The fallopian tubes extend outwards on each side from the cornua of the uterus, enclosed within the mesosalpinx (a superior fold of the broad ligament). Each tube is made up of four sections (Fig. 1.4):

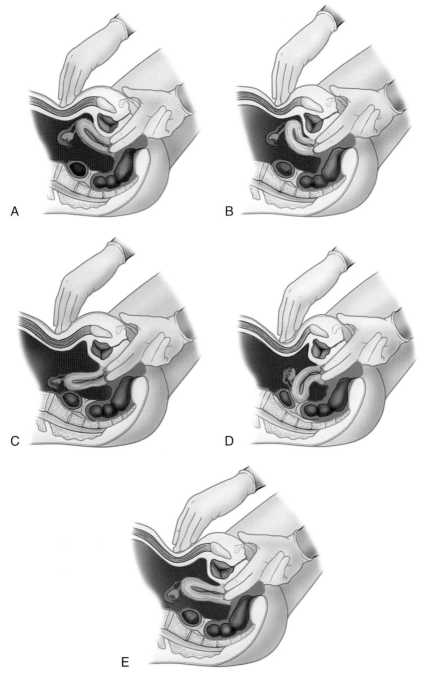

Fig. 1.5 Positions of the uterus. The uterus may be found in one of several positions: (A) Anteverted: Commonest uterine position; entire uterus is tilted forward such that the uterine fundus is anterior to the cervix. (B) Anteflexed: Body of the uterus is folded anteriorly in its longitudinal axis, angled forwards towards the bladder. (C) Retroverted: Entire uterus is tilted backwards such that the cervix is anterior and the uterine fundus is posterior. (D) Retroflexed: Body of the uterus is folded posteriorly in its longitudinal axis angled backwards towards the Pouch of Douglas. (E) Axial: Uterus lies in the mid-position. (From Ball JW, Dains JE, Flynn JA. Solomon BS, Stewart RW. *Seidel's Guide to Physical Examination*. 10th ed. pp. 448–498. © 2023.)

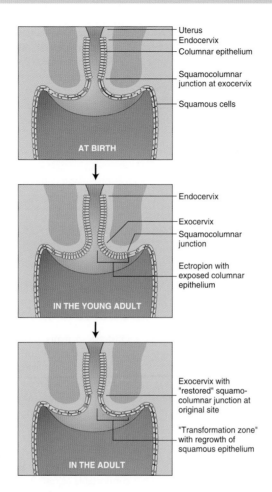

Transformation zone: columnar epithelium replaced by
stratified squamous epithelium (metaplasia)

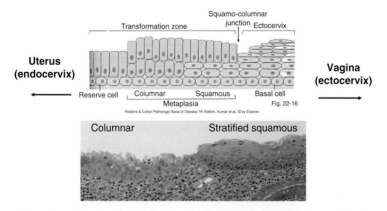

• Transformation zone is the site where most cervical cancers originate

Fig. 1.6 The squamocolumnar junction and transformation zone. (From John
A. Damianos, Matthew J. Christensen, Hubert Huang, Ted O'Connell, Katie P.
Carsky, Ryan A. Pedigo. *USMLE Step 1 Secrets in Color*, 5th ed. 2022.)

(a) The interstitium: The narrowest part of the tube leading out from the uterine cavity.

(b) The isthmus: A narrow section of the tube extending from the interstitium.

(c) The ampulla: A wider section of the tube that is the site of fertilization.

(d) The infundibulum: A funnel-shaped expansion of the tube surrounded by a fringe of finger-like projections called fimbriae. Here, the tube opens into the peritoneal cavity in close proximity to the ovary.

At the time of ovulation, fimbriae at the infundibulum collect the released ovum, which is then wafted through the tube by tubal peristalsis. The fallopian tubes are also lined by ciliated columnar epithelial cells, which function to aid the movement of the ovum through the tube.

CLINICAL NOTES

Sterilization is performed by occluding both fallopian tubes with the use of clips or sutures. A salpingectomy can also be performed for this purpose. A 'lap-and-dye' test is a laparoscopic procedure that tests for tubal patency. It is performed by injecting a watery dye (methylene blue) through the cervix and observing for spillage from the infundibulum. A hysterosalpingogram (HSG) is a radiological procedure which utilizes radio-opaque dye to visualize the shape of the uterine cavity and test for tubal patency.

THE OVARIES

The ovaries are paired organs with both reproductive and endocrine functions. They are attached on each side of the uterus to the posterior surface of the broad ligament, and lie within a shallow depression known as the ovarian fossa. Each ovary is made up of an outer cortex, comprised of connective tissue stroma and numerous ovarian follicles, each containing an oocyte at different stages of development, and an inner medulla, through which ovarian blood vessels and nerves enter the ovary (Fig. 1.4). The ovarian arteries are direct branches of the abdominal aorta.

GENERAL EXAMINATION

A general examination should always be performed as gynaecological signs of disease are not limited to the pelvis and/or genitalia. The following general assessment should be made:

- Clinical observations: Heart rate, blood pressure, temperature, respiratory rate and oxygen saturations
- Body mass index (BMI)
- Cardiovascular examination: Cardiac murmurs, signs of anaemia or oedema
- Respiratory examination
- Distribution of facial and body hair

HINTS AND TIPS

Both obstetric and gynaecological examinations follow the logical steps of:
- Inspection
- Palpation
- Percussion
- Auscultation

Obstetric examination

Obstetric patients should be examined in a semi-recumbent position and not flat on their backs. This is due to *supine hypotensive syndrome,* where the gravid uterus compresses the inferior vena cava and reduces venous return to the heart, resulting in postural hypotension and syncope. If prolonged, fetal compromise may occur due to reduced uteroplacental circulation.

Inspection

On general observation, assess whether the patient appears comfortable at rest. Is there any indication of pain or distress? Does the patient look systemically well or unwell?

Abdominal masses: A gravid uterus can often be seen per abdomen from approximately 12 to 14 weeks' gestation. The shape and size of the abdomen should be noted. Are there any additional masses visualized, for example, an umbilical hernia or fibroid?

Stigmata of pregnancy: *Striae gravidarum* (stretch marks) are caused by pregnancy hormones that stimulate the splitting of the dermis and can occur relatively early in pregnancy. New striae appear red and sometimes inflamed and can be sore and itchy; old striae from previous pregnancies appear pale and silvery. Striae are commonly found over the abdomen, upper thighs, buttocks and breasts. Increased skin pigmentation can occur in pregnancy. The *linea nigra* is a dark vertical line of hyperpigmentation running from the xiphisternum to the symphysis pubis. Other areas that can undergo pigmentation in pregnancy include the areola, vulva and cheeks (*chloasma*).

Surgical scars: Examine carefully for surgical scars as they can often be well healed. Previous caesarean section scars are transverse suprapubic scars often hidden in the pubic hairline. Laparoscopic surgery scars will usually have an umbilical scar site and additional small abdominal sites.

Palpation

Before palpating the abdomen always enquire about areas of tenderness and palpate these areas last. On obstetric palpation, the following features are being assessed:

- Uterine size
- Fetal lie
- Fetal presentation
- Fetal position
- Engagement and station

Uterine size

The uterus first becomes palpable abdominally at around 12 weeks' gestation. An approximation of the gestation (and therefore uterine size) can be made by assessing the fundal height in relation to the following anatomical landmarks: Symphysis pubis (12 weeks), umbilicus (20 weeks) and xiphisternum (36 weeks; Fig. 1.7). Towards term, as the presenting part enters the pelvis, the level of the uterine fundus may drop slightly.

The distance between the uterine fundus and symphysis pubis, known as symphysial-fundal height (SFH), is a more objective method of assessing uterine size and gestation. Using the medial border of the left hand, start at the xiphisternum and palpate down the abdomen until the fundus is reached. Ensure that this is the highest point of the uterus and take note that this may not be in the midline. Place the end of a tape measure at the fundus, marking side faced down (to minimize observer bias), and measure the distance from the fundus to the upper border of the symphysis pubis. Turn the tape measure over to reveal the distance in centimetres. At 20 weeks' gestation, the SFH is approximately 20 cm and increases by 1cm per week. The SFH measurement ± 2 cm should equal the gestation (e.g., at 34 weeks' gestation the SFH should be between 32 and 36 cm). While SFH is a crude measurement technique and varies in precision between measures, it can be used to identify patients measuring large- or small-for-dates (e.g., growth-restricted babies).

Clinical assessment of liquor volume is not as accurate as objective assessment using ultrasound. However, it can alert the examiner to the possibility of reduced or increased liquor volume, leading to appropriate management. Reduced liquor volume (oligohydramnios) is suggestive when the uterus measures small-for-dates, with easily palpable fetal parts. With increased liquor volume (polyhydramnios), the uterus is abnormally large, tense to touch and fetal parts are almost impossible to distinguish. In these situations, an ultrasound scan should be ordered to objectively assess foetus growth and liquor volume.

Fetal lie

Fetal parts are usually palpable from around 24 weeks' gestation. In a singleton pregnancy, there are two fetal 'poles', the head and the buttocks. The fetal 'lie' is the relationship between the long axis of the foetus and the long axis of the uterus. This is usually longitudinal but can be transverse or oblique (Fig. 1.8). To determine the lie, first palpate for the head and buttocks. The head feels bony, round and hard, and can be balloted. The buttocks tend to be softer and less distinctly round. Next, locate the fetal back (usually curved and smooth) and limbs (usually irregular and knobbly) (Fig. 1.9). In some situations, the fetal parts may be difficult to palpate (Table 1.1).

In a longitudinal lie, the fetal poles will be palpable at the fundus and suprapubic region. In a transverse lie, the foetus is lying at right angles to the mother and the fetal poles will be palpable in both flanks. In an oblique lie, the foetus is lying at 45 degrees to the long axis of the uterus, and one of the fetal poles will be palpable in the iliac fossa.

Fetal presentation

The fetal 'presentation' is the part of the foetus that presents to the maternal pelvis. This is most commonly the head or 'vertex' (cephalic presentation) but can also be the buttocks (breech presentation), shoulder, brow or face (Fig. 1.10). Any presentation other than a cephalic presentation is called a 'malpresentation'.

Fetal position

The fetal 'position' is defined as the relationship of the denominator of the presenting part to the maternal pelvis. The denominator changes according to the presenting part: the occiput in a vertex presentation, the mentum (chin) in a face presentation and the sacrum in a breech presentation. Knowing the fetal position is more relevant during labour and delivery, and is assessed more accurately by vaginal examination (see Chapter 26).

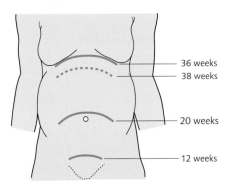

Fig. 1.7 Fundal height in relation to abdominal landmarks. (From Kay SE, Sandhu CJ. *Crash Course Obstetrics and Gynaecology*. 4th ed. pp. 1–9. © 2019.)

- 36 weeks
- 38 weeks
- 20 weeks
- 12 weeks

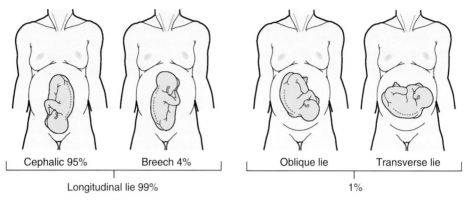

Cephalic 95%   Breech 4%   Oblique lie   Transverse lie

Longitudinal lie 99%   1%

Fig. 1.8 Fetal lie at term. (From Hutchison L. *Clinical Obstetrics and Gynaecology.* pp. 401–417. © 2023.)

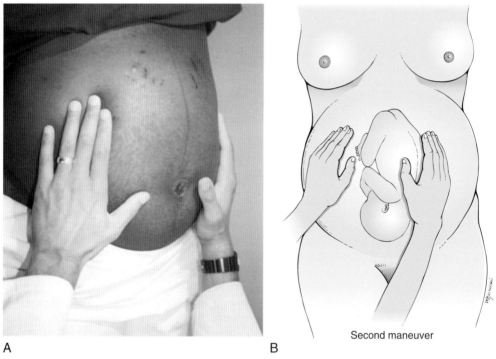

Second maneuver

A   B

Fig. 1.9 Palpating the fetal lie and presentation. (A) Position of clinician's hands on mother's abdomen. (B) Illustration of relationship of clinician's hands and foetus. (From Swartz MH, Deli B. *Textbook of Physical Diagnosis: History and Examination.* 8th ed. pp. 520–534. © 2021.)

Engagement and station

The presenting part of the foetus (usually the head) is said to be engaged when the widest diameter of the head (the biparietal diameter) has passed through the pelvic brim (Fig. 1.11).

Engagement is expressed in terms of the number of 'fifths palpable' and is assessed abdominally by attempting to ballot the head suprapubically between the thumb and fingers of the right hand (Fig. 1.12). When three-fifths or more of the fetal

Table 1.1 Situations where fetal parts may be difficult to palpate

Types of reason	Description
Maternal reasons	Maternal obesity Muscular anterior abdominal wall
Uterine reasons	Anterior uterine wall fibroids Uterine contraction/Braxton Hicks contraction
Fetoplacental reasons	Anterior placenta Increased liquor volume

head is palpable abdominally, the head is not engaged because the widest diameter of the head has not passed the pelvic brim. When two-fifths or less of the head is palpable, the head is clinically engaged.

During labour, as the fetal presenting part descends into the pelvis, a vaginal examination should be performed to determine the 'station' of the presenting part – The relationship of the presenting part to the ischial spines (Fig. 1.11). This is usually expressed in centimetres above (i.e., −1, −2, −3) or below (i.e., +1, +2, +3) the ischial spines. The engagement of the presenting part should correlate with the station. When the presenting part is engaged (two-fifths palpable), the leading edge of the presenting part will be at the level of the ischial spines (station 0).

AUSCULTATION

The fetal heart should be auscultated using a Pinard stethoscope or more commonly, a hand-held Doppler ultrasound device (Sonicaid). First establish the fetal lie and presentation, and feel for the back of the foetus. In cephalic presentations, the fetal heart is best heard over the anterior fetal shoulder, approximately halfway between the umbilicus and the anterior superior iliac spine. In breech presentations, it is best heard at the level of the umbilicus. The fetal heart rate usually sits between 110 and 160 beats per minute and should be clearly differentiated from the maternal pulse.

Obstetric pelvic examination

Obstetric pelvic examination (speculum and vaginal examination) is not routinely performed at antenatal appointments. Indications for examination include cervical assessment and progress in labour, suspected rupture of membranes and vaginal bleeding. Intrapartum vaginal examination is discussed in Chapter 26.

CLINICAL NOTES

An antenatal obstetric examination is incomplete without a blood pressure check and urinalysis assessing for protein, blood and the presence of infection.

GYNAECOLOGICAL EXAMINATION

ETHICS

The intimate nature of the gynaecological examination makes it essential for you to fully explain what the examination will involve in order to obtain informed consent. This should be documented clearly in the medical notes. Every effort should be made to ensure that dignity is maintained. The patient should be given privacy to und ress and provided with a modesty sheet to cover themselves. They should be covered as much as possible during the examination. A chaperone should ideally always be present, regardless of the gender of the healthcare professional.

ABDOMINAL EXAMINATION

Inspection

Abdominal distension: Is the abdomen distended? Can you see an obvious mass? A gravid uterus, pelvic tumour, organomegaly, hernia and ascites are all possible causes.

Surgical scars: Their site and number inform you of previous laparoscopic or open operations. For example, umbilical scars in laparoscopy, suprapubic transverse incisions from Caesarean sections. Asking the patient, or checking their medical records, can confirm these.

Palpation

Is the patient comfortable or in pain? Ask if the pain can be localized (*'Can you point with a finger where your pain is?'*) and palpate these areas last.

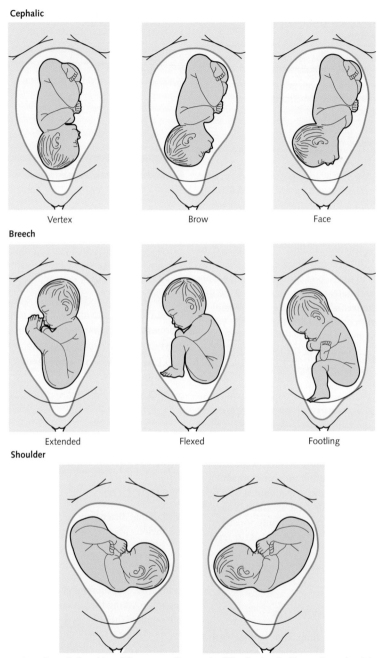

Cephalic

Vertex | Brow | Face

Breech

Extended | Flexed | Footling

Shoulder

Fig. 1.10 The fetal presentation: the relationship of the presenting part of the foetus to the maternal pelvis. (From Kay SE, Sandhu CJ. *Crash Course Obstetrics and Gynaecology*. 4th ed. pp. 1–9. © 2019.)

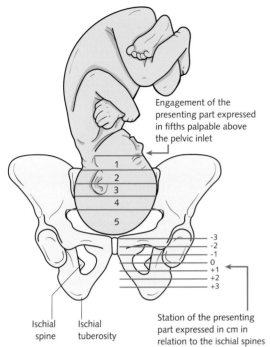

Engagement of the presenting part expressed in fifths palpable above the pelvic inlet

1
2
3
4
5

-3
-2
-1
0
+1
+2
+3

Ischial spine   Ischial tuberosity

Station of the presenting part expressed in cm in relation to the ischial spines

Fig. 1.11 Engagement and station of the fetal head. (From Kay SE, Sandhu CJ. *Crash Course Obstetrics and Gynaecology*. 4th ed. pp. 1–9. © 2019.)

Be systematic in your technique: Choose a 4-quadrant or 9-sector approach when palpating the abdomen and examine each area in sequence. Use the flat of the hand and flexor surfaces of the fingers, first superficially, then deeper. Is there abdominal guarding? Is there rebound tenderness? These suggest peritonism.

If there is a mass, assess if it is fixed or mobile, its size and shape, where it arises from, its consistency, regularity and tenderness. Fibroids can be palpated as a mobile, non-tender, enlarged, firm and irregular mass arising from the pelvis (if the lower border cannot be felt beneath the pubic bone, it is probably arising from the pelvis). The size of a pelvic mass can be described as similar to a pregnant abdomen (e.g., '20-week size' is equivalent to umbilical level). Palpate for lymphadenopathy in the groin, and any organomegaly (liver, spleen, kidneys).

Percussion and auscultation

Differences in dullness and resonance in percussion allow you to delineate masses and identify anatomy beneath (e.g., dullness of a full bladder, resonance of tympanic bowel loops). Auscultate for bowel sounds to inform you of their activity or absence.

In postoperative patients with abdominal distension, absence of bowel sounds may suggest ileus or obstruction.

Pelvic examination

A pelvic examination has several components:

- Inspection of the external genitalia
- Internal inspection of the vagina and cervix using a speculum
- Bimanual examination

The most common position for carrying out a pelvic examination is the dorsal position with the patient lying on their back. Ask the patient to lie back, bend their knees, put their ankles together and let their knees fall apart. Ensure that the patient is covered appropriately, and that you have lubricating gel and a speculum open and to hand. Note that if the patient has an intact hymen (commonly someone who has never had penetrative vaginal intercourse), speculum and bimanual examination is usually not performed unless under anaesthesia.

Inspection of the external genitalia

Inspect the vulva for inflammation, ulceration, erythema, swellings, lesions, atrophic changes, discolouration and old scars. Examine the hair distribution, as hirsutism may be a sign of androgen excess and other endocrine disorders. Dermatological conditions such as eczema and psoriasis can affect vulval skin and cause significant itching – excoriation marks are often a tell-tale sign. Patchy white discolouration may point to conditions such as lichen sclerosis while the swelling of a Bartholin's cyst or abscess is easily noticeable at the introitus. Ulceration may be a sign of malignancy or sexually transmitted infections such as herpes. A deficient or scarred perineum is usually secondary to trauma from previous vaginal delivery. The degree of bulge of a uterovaginal prolapse through the introitus can be assessed by asking the patient to bear down, and stress incontinence might be demonstrated when the patient coughs.

Speculum examination

A Cusco (bivalve) speculum is commonly used to inspect the vagina and cervix, and these come in a variety of sizes. Select an appropriate size and ensure that it is well lubricated. Part the labia and gently introduce the speculum into the vagina, rotating it upwards or downwards until the blades are horizontal (Fig. 1.13). The speculum should be inserted angled posteriorly (i.e., into the bed) as most uteri are anteverted. When the speculum is fully inserted, slowly open the blades to visualize the cervix.

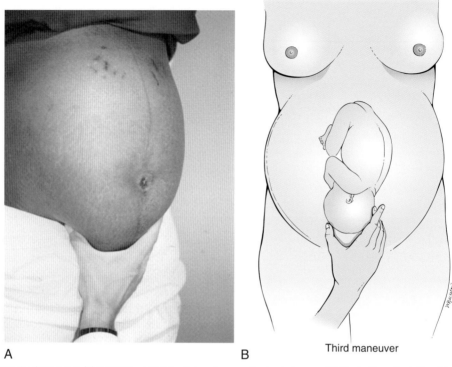

A   B   Third maneuver

Fig. 1.12 Ballotting the fetal head. (A) Position of clinician's hand on mother's abdomen. (B) Illustration of relationship of clinician's hand and foetus. (From Swartz MH, Deli B. *Textbook of Physical Diagnosis: History and Examination*. 8th ed. pp. 520–534. © 2021.)

Inspect the vaginal mucosa for signs of atrophy or inflammation. Note the presence of any abnormal discharge, e.g., White with a thick cottage-cheese appearance (candidiasis), yellowish green (*Trichomonas vaginalis*), greyish with a fishy odour (bacterial vaginosis) or yellowish and purulent (chlamydia/gonorrhoea).

Inspect the appearance of the cervix, looking for visible growths, ulceration, polyps, inflammation and erythema. An ulcerated cervix with an irregular punctate surface may suggest malignancy and prompt urgent referral for colposcopy. Small, transparent Nabothian follicles are a common and benign finding. In patients who are pregnant or on the combined oral contraception pill (COCP), a cervical ectropion may be seen. The appearance of the cervical os changes with childbirth – from small and round to more irregular and slit-like. You may also notice threads from an intrauterine device protruding from the os.

A vaginal speculum is a more useful tool for assessing uterovaginal prolapse (Fig. 1.14). With the patient in the left lateral position, the speculum is gently inserted into the vagina and used to retract the anterior and posterior vaginal walls in turn. A cystocoele or rectocoele (bulge of the anterior and posterior walls, respectively) can then be assessed by asking the patient to bear down or cough.

CLINICAL NOTES

When infection is suspected (e.g., from the history, symptoms of vaginal discharge or irregular bleeding), swabs may be taken from the posterior vaginal fornix (high vaginal swab) or the cervical canal (endocervical swab). In asymptomatic patients, swabs may also be taken to screen for sexually transmitted infections.

High vaginal swab (HVS) – This is used to test for organisms such as *Candida*, *Trichomonas vaginalis* and bacterial vaginosis.

Endocervical swab – This is sent for polymerase chain reaction nucleic acid amplification testing (PCR NAAT) to identify *Chlamydia trachomatis* and *Neisseria Gonorrhoea*.

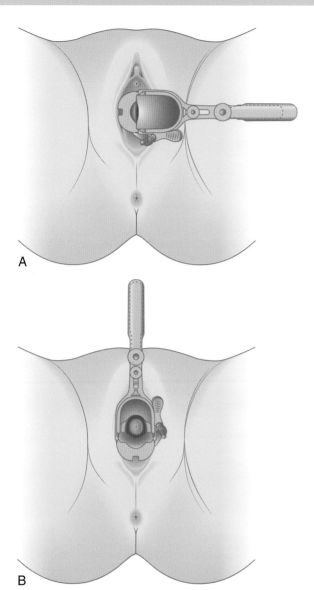

A

B

Fig. 1.13 Bivalve speculum examination. (A) Insertion of the speculum. (B) Visualization of the cervix after rotation through 90 degrees. (From Yip C, Duncan C. *Macleod's Clinical Examination.* 15th ed. pp. 239–269. © 2024.)

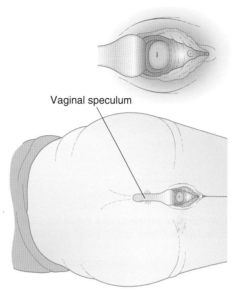

Vaginal speculum

Fig. 1.14 Examination in the lateral semiprone positions with a vaginal speculum. (From Symonds EM, Symonds IM. *Essential Obstetrics and Gynaecology*, 4th ed. Churchill Livingstone, 2004.) (From Carseldine W, Symonds I. *Talley & O'Connor's Clinical Examination.* 9th ed. pp. 778–796. © 2022.)

Bimanual examination

A bimanual examination is performed to further elicit any pelvic masses or tenderness and assess the uterus. With lubricating gel, gently insert the index finger into the vagina, followed by the middle finger if this is tolerated. Palpation of the vaginal walls and fornices is important to exclude scarring, cysts and masses that can easily be missed on inspection. The presence of thickening of vaginal nodules in the Pouch of Douglas is suggestive of endometriosis.

The cervix feels like the tip of the nose and its size, shape, position, consistency, angle and mobility should be assessed. Take note of any irregularities or tenderness. Severe pain when moving the cervix is known as 'cervical excitation' or 'cervical motion tenderness' and is suggestive of pelvic pathology, often associated with pelvic inflammatory disease, ectopic pregnancy and ovarian torsion.

The fingers of the right hand are then used to elevate and steady the uterus while the left hand palpates for the fundus abdominally (reverse if left handed) (Fig. 1.15). An anteverted uterus is usually palpable between the two hands and feels like a plum. A retroverted uterus (around 10% of women) is usually felt as a swelling in the posterior vaginal fornix. The size, position, consistency, regularity and mobility of the uterus should be noted. A fixed immobile uterus is usually the result of adhesions caused by endometriosis, surgery or infection. An irregular bulky uterus is suggestive of fibroids.

To examine the adnexa, the fingers of the right hand should be positioned in each of the lateral vaginal fornices while the left hand palpates the corresponding iliac fossa abdominally (reverse if left handed) (Fig. 1.15). Normal premenopausal

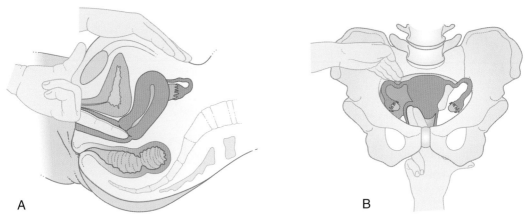

A   B

Fig. 1.15 (A) Bimanual examination of the pelvis. (B) Examination of the lateral fornix. (From Symonds IM, Arulkumaran S. *Essential Obstetrics and Gynaecology*. pp. 232–241. © 2020.)

ovaries are not always palpable depending on the size of the patient. Fallopian tubes and postmenopausal ovaries should not be palpable. If an adnexal mass is discovered, then its size, shape, consistency, mobility and whether it is fixed to the uterus or not should all be noted. The presence and degree of tenderness should also be noted.

● Chapter Summary

Knowledge of basic pelvic anatomy and examination techniques is essential in obstetrics and gynaecology to identify, diagnose and manage both normal and pathological presentations.

UKMLA Conditions
Cervical screening (HPV)
Chlamydia
Gonorrhoea
Trichomonas vaginalis

UKMLA Presentations
Abdominal distension
Abdominal mass
Bleeding antepartum
Pelvic mass
Vaginal discharge
Vaginal prolapse
Vulval itching/lesion

It is often said in medicine that 80% of diagnoses can be made by history alone. A comprehensive and accurately taken history allows one to home in on a diagnosis, corroborated by a focused physical examination and relevant investigations. History-taking in obstetrics and gynaecology builds on the general schema you would have learnt in medicine (Figs 2.1 and 2.2). One should appreciate that questions asked may involve confidential and often very personal information, which patients may find embarrassing. Establishing a good rapport with the patient and developing a sensitive and non-judgemental manner is essential. Always ask who has accompanied the patient (do not assume it is their partner) and ascertain whether they are comfortable having them present during the consultation.

History-taking is a skill that is easy to learn but difficult to master. Do not worry about seemingly taking longer than your seniors at this important task. Speed will follow with practice, and your questioning will become more succinct. Skilful is the student who manages to turn detective work into a flowing conversation.

THE PATIENT'S DETAILS

Before starting any consultation, always introduce yourself, giving your name and role. Check that you have the correct patient in front of you (a not uncommon error often made in busy A&E settings!) and obtain appropriate consent. Establish the patient's gender identity and preferred pronouns. These are key details of a contemporaneous medical record:

- The patient's name, date of birth, hospital number, NHS number and address (check if labels/identifying tags with this information are available!).
- Preferred pronouns.
- Time and date of consultation.
- Source of referral (e.g., General Practitioner, A&E, Fetal Medicine Unit).
- Your signature, printed name, role and bleep number.

COMMUNICATION

GENDER IDENTITY

Refers to an individual's personal sense, and subjective experience, of their own gender. This concept is not a dichotomy with 'male' or 'female' as the only possibilities, but rather a spectrum of gender identity.

GENDER DIVERSITY

A term used to refer to gender-diverse people, it is an umbrella term encompassing all those individuals whose gender identity does not align with the sex they were assigned at birth. 'Trans' or 'transgender' are still commonly used terms to refer to gender-diverse people.

Healthcare professionals should be aware of the many barriers preventing transgender and gender-diverse (TGD) people from accessing healthcare. TGD people often face discrimination and social exclusion and as a result are at increased risk of healthcare inequalities and mental health illness.

In line with the GMC's guidance on Good Medical Practice, we should endeavour to treat patients as individuals in order to deliver patient-centred care. All patients should be treated with respect and dignity. The following are some tips to help make your practice more inclusive:

- Always ask about a patient's gender identity if you are unsure. Never guess or assume.
- Use your patient's preferred name, title and pronouns (e.g., he/she/they).
- Avoid labels such as 'husband' and 'wife' and opt for the word 'partner' instead.

Note: The terminology used to describe gender identity and gender diversity has undergone much change over time and is continuing to evolve. As our communities grow, so do the words we use in describing ourselves. Definitions stated here follow common usage in the UK in 2023.

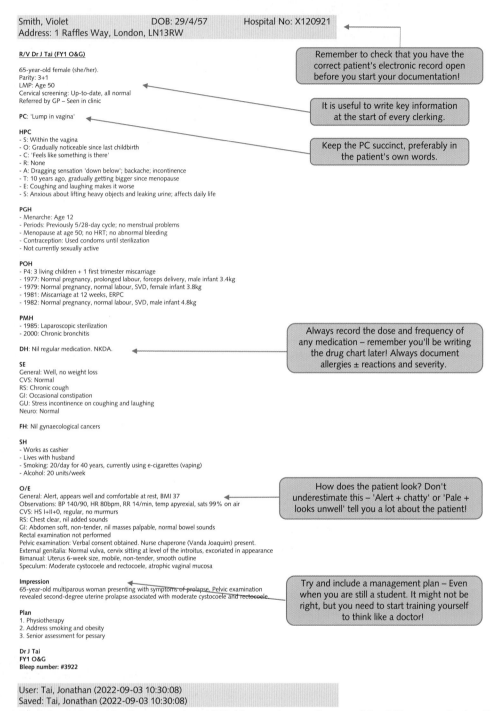

Smith, Violet   DOB: 29/4/57   Hospital No: X120921
Address: 1 Raffles Way, London, LN13RW

R/V Dr J Tai (FY1 O&G)

65-year-old female (she/her).
Parity: 3+1
LMP: Age 50
Cervical screening: Up-to-date, all normal
Referred by GP – Seen in clinic

PC: 'Lump in vagina'

HPC
- S: Within the vagina
- O: Gradually noticeable since last childbirth
- C: 'Feels like something is there'
- R: None
- A: Dragging sensation 'down below'; backache; incontinence
- T: 10 years ago, gradually getting bigger since menopause
- E: Coughing and laughing makes it worse
- S: Anxious about lifting heavy objects and leaking urine; affects daily life

PGH
- Menarche: Age 12
- Periods: Previously 5/28-day cycle; no menstrual problems
- Menopause at age 50; no HRT; no abnormal bleeding
- Contraception: Used condoms until sterilization
- Not currently sexually active

POH
- P4: 3 living children + 1 first trimester miscarriage
- 1977: Normal pregnancy, prolonged labour, forceps delivery, male infant 3.4kg
- 1979: Normal pregnancy, normal labour, SVD, female infant 3.8kg
- 1981: Miscarriage at 12 weeks, ERPC
- 1982: Normal pregnancy, normal labour, SVD, male infant 4.8kg

PMH
- 1985: Laparoscopic sterilization
- 2000: Chronic bronchitis

DH: Nil regular medication. NKDA.

SE
General: Well, no weight loss
CVS: Normal
RS: Chronic cough
GI: Occasional constipation
GU: Stress incontinence on coughing and laughing
Neuro: Normal

FH: Nil gynaecological cancers

SH
- Works as cashier
- Lives with husband
- Smoking: 20/day for 40 years, currently using e-cigarettes (vaping)
- Alcohol: 20 units/week

O/E
General: Alert, appears well and comfortable at rest, BMI 37
Observations: BP 140/90, HR 80bpm, RR 14/min, temp apyrexial, sats 99% on air
CVS: HS I+II+0, regular, no murmurs
RS: Chest clear, nil added sounds
GI: Abdomen soft, non-tender, nil masses palpable, normal bowel sounds
Rectal examination not performed
Pelvic examination: Verbal consent obtained. Nurse chaperone (Vanda Joaquim) present.
External genitalia: Normal vulva, cervix sitting at level of the introitus, excoriated in appearance
Bimanual: Uterus 6-week size, mobile, non-tender, smooth outline
Speculum: Moderate cystocoele and rectocoele, atrophic vaginal mucosa

Impression
65-year-old multiparous woman presenting with symptoms of prolapse. Pelvic examination revealed second-degree uterine prolapse associated with moderate cystocoele and rectocoele.

Plan
1. Physiotherapy
2. Address smoking and obesity
3. Senior assessment for pessary

Dr J Tai
FY1 O&G
Bleep number: #3922

User: Tai, Jonathan (2022-09-03 10:30:08)
Saved: Tai, Jonathan (2022-09-03 10:30:08)

Remember to check that you have the correct patient's electronic record open before you start your documentation!

It is useful to write key information at the start of every clerking.

Keep the PC succinct, preferably in the patient's own words.

Always record the dose and frequency of any medication – remember you'll be writing the drug chart later! Always document allergies ± reactions and severity.

How does the patient look? Don't underestimate this – 'Alert + chatty' or 'Pale + looks unwell' tell you a lot about the patient!

Try and include a management plan – Even when you are still a student. It might not be right, but you need to start training yourself to think like a doctor!

Fig. 2.1 Example of electronic clerking for gynaecology. HPC, *History of presenting complaint*; O/E, *on examination*; PGH, *previous gynaecological history*; PMH, *past medical history*; POH, *previous obstetric history*; SE, *systemic enquiry*; SH, *social history*.

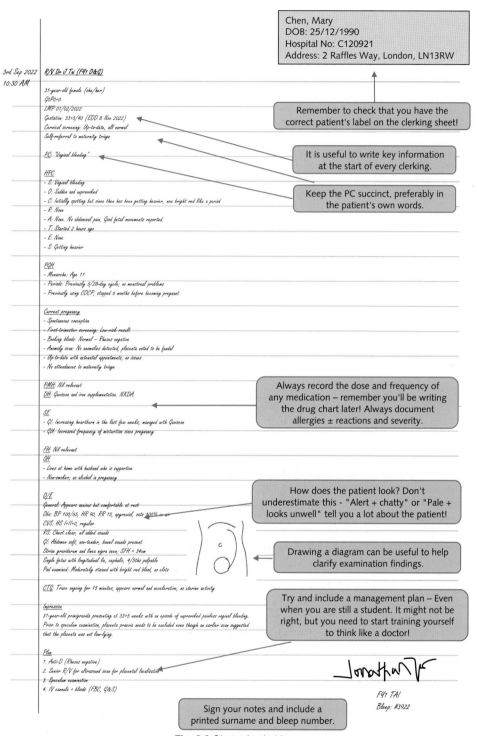

Chen, Mary
DOB: 25/12/1990
Hospital No: C120921
Address: 2 Raffles Way, London, LN13RW

3rd Sep 2022
10:30 AM

R/V Dr J Tai (F4t O&G)

31-year-old female (she/her)
G0P0+0
LMP 01/02/2022
Gestation: 33+5/40 (EDD 8 Nov 2022)
Cervical screening: Up-to-date, all normal
Self-referral to maternity triage

PC: "Vaginal bleeding"

HPC
- S: Vaginal bleeding
- O: Sudden and unprovoked
- C: Initially spotting but since then has been getting heavier, now bright red like a period
- R: None
- A: None. No abdominal pain. Good fetal movements reported.
- T: Started 2 hours ago
- E: None
- S: Getting heavier

PGH
- Menarche: Age 11
- Periods: Previously 5/28-day cycle; no menstrual problems
- Previously using COCP, stopped 6 months before becoming pregnant

Current pregnancy
- Spontaneous conception
- First-trimester screening: Low-risk result
- Booking bloods: Normal - Rhesus negative
- Anomaly scan: No anomalies detected; placenta noted to be fundal
- Up-to-date with antenatal appointments, no issues
- No attendances to maternity triage

PMH: Nil relevant
DH: Gaviscon and iron supplementation. NKDA.

SE
- GI: Increasing heartburn in the last few weeks, managed with Gaviscon
- GU: Increased frequency of micturition since pregnancy

FH: Nil relevant
SH
- Lives at home with husband who is supportive
- Non-smoker; no alcohol in pregnancy

O/E
General: Appears anxious but comfortable at rest
Obs: BP 100/65, HR 90, RR 15, apyrexial, sats 100% on air
CVS: HS I+II+0, regular
RS: Chest clear, nil added sounds
GI: Abdomen soft, non-tender, bowel sounds present
Striae gravidarum and linea nigra seen; SFH = 34cm
Single fetus with longitudinal lie, cephalic, 4/5ths palpable
Pad examined: Moderately stained with bright red blood, no clots

CTG: Trace ongoing for 15 minutes, appears normal and accelerative, no uterine activity

Impression
31-year-old primigravida presenting at 33+5 weeks with an episode of unprovoked painless vaginal bleeding. Prior to speculum examination, placenta praevia needs to be excluded even though an earlier scan suggested that the placenta was not low-lying.

Plan
1. Anti-D (Rhesus negative)
2. Senior R/V for ultrasound scan for placental localisation
3. Speculum examination
4. IV cannula + bloods (FBC, G&S)

[signature]

F4t TAI
Bleep: #3922

Callout boxes:

Remember to check that you have the correct patient's label on the clerking sheet!

It is useful to write key information at the start of every clerking.

Keep the PC succinct, preferably in the patient's own words.

Always record the dose and frequency of any medication – remember you'll be writing the drug chart later! Always document allergies ± reactions and severity.

How does the patient look? Don't underestimate this - "Alert + chatty" or "Pale + looks unwell" tell you a lot about the patient!

Drawing a diagram can be useful to help clarify examination findings.

Try and include a management plan – Even when you are still a student. It might not be right, but you need to start training yourself to think like a doctor!

Sign your notes and include a printed surname and bleep number.

Fig. 2.2 Obstetric clerking.

PRESENTING COMPLAINT

The presenting complaint (PC) is often documented in the referral letter or A&E clerking; however, this may not necessarily reflect what the patient is concerned about. It is often worthwhile to open with a general question such as *'What brings you in today?'* or *'How may I help you today?'* in order to establish what the patient sees as their PC in their own words.

When there are multiple problems, list them in order of importance (i.e., which concerns the patient most). This would help you prioritize investigations and guide management. Throughout the consultation, consider that there may be a hidden agenda, especially when the patient seems hesitant to discuss an issue or if there are incongruous findings. For example, the patient may complain about vaginal discharge, although their main concern is pain during intercourse. Always ask if there is anything else bothering the patient that they wish to discuss – You will often find that their most pertinent concern is revealed only towards the end of the consultation.

HISTORY OF PRESENTING COMPLAINT

After establishing the PC, you should explore the patient's presenting symptoms in greater detail. A useful mnemonic for this is 'SOCRATES'. Often used to assess pain, it is also applicable to most other symptoms. SOCRATES can provide a structured framework for the history of presenting complaint (HPC), helping you to remember important questions to ask in order to take a comprehensive history.

'SOCRATES'

Site	Ask about **where** the symptom is located: • *'Where is the pain?'* • *'Can you point to where the pain is?'*
Onset	Ask about **when** and **how** the symptom developed: • *'When did all this first start?'* • *'Did the pain come on suddenly or gradually?'* E.g., Ovarian torsion typically presents with pain that is sudden in onset; hirsutism of rapid onset is more likely to be due to an androgen-producing tumour.
Character	Ask the patient to **describe** the symptom: • *'How would you describe the pain?'* • *'Is it sharp, stabbing, dull, heavy, dragging, colicky, twisting, spasming, period-like?'* E.g., Uterine prolapse is often described as a dragging pain/sensation; onset of labour may be likened to period-like pain.
Radiation	Ask if the symptom **moves** anywhere else: • *'Does the pain radiate anywhere?'* E.g., Pain due to endometriosis can radiate to the back or into the upper thighs.

Associated symptoms	Ask if anything else seems **related** to the main symptom: • *'Do you notice anything else that seems related?'* E.g., Nausea and vomiting (may be associated with peritonitis), weight loss (may be associated with malignancy) and deep dyspareunia (associated with endometriosis).
Time course	Ask about **how long** the symptom has been present for: • *'How long has this problem been going on for?'* • *'Is the pain constant or does it come and go? How long does it last for?'* • *'How has the problem changed over time? Is it getting worse?'*
Exacerbating and relieving factors	Ask if anything makes the symptom **better** or **worse**: • *'Does the symptom seem related to your periods/diet/recent sexual encounter?'* E.g., Endometriosis and PMS-related symptoms tend to be cyclical; IBS symptoms tend to be exacerbated by certain foods; prolapse symptoms tend to be worse on standing and better on lying down. • *'Have you tried any over-the-counter medication?'* • *'What have you found helps with the problem?'*
Severity	Assess the **severity** of the symptom using a numerical scale or impact on quality of life: • *'On a scale of 0 to 10, with 0 being no pain and 10 being the worst pain you have ever experienced, how severe is the pain?'* • *'How does this affect your quality of life?'* E.g., Severe dysmenorrhoea may necessitate regular time off work; urinary incontinence may cause a patient to be reluctant to leave their home.

IBS, Irritable bowel syndrome; *PMS,* premenstrual syndrome.

GYNAECOLOGICAL HISTORY

Menstrual history

The following characteristics of the patient's menstrual cycle should always be noted:

- **Last menstrual period (LMP)**
  - Date of the first day of the last menstrual period.
- **Age at menarche**
  - The average age is around 12 years in the UK.
- **Pattern of bleeding**
  - Length of cycle: The time between the first day of one period (i.e., the first day of menstruation) to the first day of the next period. This is commonly around 28 days but may vary between 21 and 42 days.
  - Regularity: Establish whether periods are regular or irregular. Irregular periods are suggestive of anovulation or irregular ovulation.
  - Duration of bleeding: A normal period usually lasts between 4 and 7 days.
  - Bleeding pattern is usually expressed as a fraction, where the numerator is the length of the period in days and the denominator is the length of the cycle in days, e.g., a cycle of length of 4–6/28–35 means that a patient bleeds for 4 to 6 days every 28 to 35 days.
- **Menstrual flow**
  - The average menstrual blood loss is around 30 to 40 mL during each period.
  - Determining the heaviness of bleeding is inherently very subjective. Some women with heavy menstrual bleeding will find this normal, while others will complain of heavy periods with average menstrual blood loss.
  - In practice, heavy menstrual bleeding can be assessed based on the number of sanitary pads or tampons used in a day, the presence of blood clots, 'flooding' (when menstrual blood soaks through sanitary ware, clothing or bedsheets) and symptoms of anaemia.
- **Dysmenorrhoea**
  - How severe is the pain? Is the pain relieved with simple analgesia?
  - Have periods always been painful (primary dysmenorrhoea) or only recently (secondary dysmenorrhoea)?
- **Abnormal uterine bleeding**
  - Includes heavy menstrual bleeding, intermenstrual bleeding and postcoital bleeding.
  - Should always be investigated as it may be the first symptom of underlying disease.
- **Associated symptoms**
  - E.g., Urinary or bowel symptoms, nausea and vomiting, migraines, mood swings.

- **Menopause**
  - Age at menopause.
  - Menopausal symptoms, e.g., hot flushes, mood swings, vaginal dryness.
  - Postmenopausal bleeding.
  - Use of hormone replacement therapy (HRT).

TERMINOLOGY

Menarche	Age of onset of the first menstrual period.
Amenorrhoea	The absence of menstruation. • **Primary amenorrhoea**: The absence of menstruation by the age of 16 in the presence of normal growth and secondary sexual characteristics. • **Secondary amenorrhoea**: The absence of menstruation for more than 6 months in a patient who is not pregnant and who has previously had periods.
Oligomenorrhoea	Irregular menstruation defined by a cycle length between 6 weeks and 6 months.
Dysmenorrhoea ('Period pain')	Pain during menstruation. • **Primary dysmenorrhoea**: Pain occurring just before or during menstruation, in the absence of any identifiable underlying pelvic pathology. • **Secondary dysmenorrhoea**: New onset pain during menstruation occurring when menstruation has previously not been painful, more likely to indicate underlying pelvic pathology.
Climacteric ('Perimenopause')	The time prior to the menopause when periods become increasingly irregular and are associated with menopausal symptoms.
Menopause	The cessation of menstruation or last ever menstrual period. This diagnosis is a retrospective one and is only made after 12 months of absent menstruation.

Abnormal uterine bleeding (AUB)	Defined as any unscheduled vaginal bleeding occurring outside of usual menstruation, or menstrual bleeding that is excessive or irregular.
Heavy menstrual bleeding (HMB)	Defined as excessive menstrual blood loss greater than 80 mL during each period.
Postmenopausal bleeding (PMB)	Vaginal bleeding occurring more than 12 months after the menopause.
Intermenstrual bleeding (IMB)	Nonmenstrual vaginal bleeding occurring between periods.
Postcoital bleeding (PCB)	Nonmenstrual vaginal bleeding occurring during or shortly after sexual intercourse.

SEXUAL ACTIVITY AND CONTRACEPTION

- **Sexual activity**
  - Establish whether the patient has ever been sexually active. If so, is the patient currently sexually active? Further questioning into sexual practices and risk assessment for sexually transmitted infections may be required depending on the PC (see Chapter 8).
- **Dyspareunia**
  - Refers to pain during sexual intercourse and can be superficial or deep.
  - Superficial dyspareunia
    - Pain localized to the vulva or introitus of the vagina.
    - Causes: Inadequate lubrication, vaginal atrophy, genital infection, female genital mutilation, vulvodynia, vaginismus (involuntary contraction of the pelvic floor muscles).
  - Deep dyspareunia
    - Pain perceived inside the vagina or pelvis, often associated with deep penetration.
    - Causes: Endometriosis, adhesions, fibroids, pelvic inflammatory disease, vaginismus.
    - Contraception.
  - Establish whether the patient is currently using any method of contraception.
  - If relevant, ask about previous methods of contraception, duration of use, and why they were stopped. Note whether they were prescribed for contraceptive purposes or menstrual disorders.

CERVICAL SCREENING

The NHS cervical screening programme invites women and anyone with a cervix (i.e., trans men and nonbinary individuals assigned female at birth) aged 25 to 64 for cervical screening. In England and Northern Ireland, patients receive an invite every 3 years between the ages of 25 and 49, and then every 5 years until the age of 64. In Wales and Scotland, patients receive an invite every 5 years between the ages of 25 and 64. This may vary in other countries and healthcare settings.

Establish whether the patient is up-to-date with cervical screening. Ask about previous abnormalities along with any colposcopic investigation or treatment received (e.g., cone biopsy, LLETZ – large loop excision of the transformation zone – procedures). Has the patient received the human papillomavirus (HPV) vaccine?

VAGINAL DISCHARGE

Note if there has been any abnormal vaginal discharge which is unexpected (not physiological) by the patient. Determine its consistency (e.g., thin vs. thick), characteristics (e.g., colour, smell), associated symptoms (e.g., dysuria, abdominal pain, rash, ulcer) and recent events (e.g., new sexual partner, contraception).

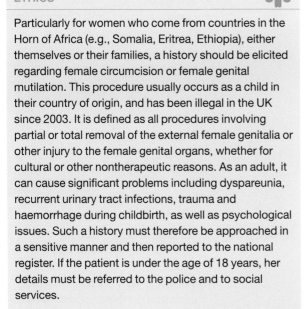

ETHICS

Particularly for women who come from countries in the Horn of Africa (e.g., Somalia, Eritrea, Ethiopia), either themselves or their families, a history should be elicited regarding female circumcision or female genital mutilation. This procedure usually occurs as a child in their country of origin, and has been illegal in the UK since 2003. It is defined as all procedures involving partial or total removal of the external female genitalia or other injury to the female genital organs, whether for cultural or other nontherapeutic reasons. As an adult, it can cause significant problems including dyspareunia, recurrent urinary tract infections, trauma and haemorrhage during childbirth, as well as psychological issues. Such a history must therefore be approached in a sensitive manner and then reported to the national register. If the patient is under the age of 18 years, her details must be referred to the police and to social services.

OBSTETRIC HISTORY

Gravidity: Refers to the total number of pregnancies a patient has had, including any current pregnancy, and irrespective of pregnancy outcome.

Parity: Often documented as X+Y. The first number 'X' refers to the number of livebirths and stillbirths after 24 weeks of gestation. The second number 'Y' refers to the number of pregnancies ending before 24 weeks.

Primigravida: A person who is pregnant for the first time.

Multigravida: A person who has been pregnant two or more times.

HINTS AND TIPS

G0P0: A patient who has never been pregnant before.

G1P0+1: A patient who has had one pregnancy which turned out to be an ectopic pregnancy.

G3P1+1: A patient who is currently pregnant and has had two previous pregnancies including one child born after 24 weeks gestation and one miscarriage at 9 weeks.

G2P2: A patient who is currently pregnant and has previously delivered twins at 36 weeks gestation. Note that in a multiple pregnancy, gravidity counts as one and if delivered after 24 weeks, then parity would be two (if twins) or three (in the case of triplets).

HISTORY OF CURRENT PREGNANCY

Gestation of pregnancy is usually recorded as the number of weeks + days out of 40 completed weeks of pregnancy, i.e., a patient at 36 + 4 weeks of gestation would be documented as 36 + 4/40. The following should be enquired about:

- Results of screening for genetic anomalies (if accepted by the patient).
- Outcome of ultrasound scans, including dating and anomaly scans and any additional growth scans.
- Antenatal appointments and scheduled investigations.
- Any problems such as bleeding, reduced fetal movements or abdominal pain.
- Any new diagnoses in pregnancy or initiation of medication (e.g., insulin for gestational diabetes, low-molecular-weight heparin for deep vein thrombosis).

PAST OBSTETRIC HISTORY

In chronological order, document each pregnancy, detailing the following:

- Year, duration of gestation and outcome (i.e., livebirth, miscarriage, termination, ectopic).
- Need for assisted reproductive techniques.
- For miscarriages and terminations of pregnancy: Any complications or operative procedures required.
- Complications of pregnancy
  - Antenatal, e.g., gestational diabetes, pre-eclampsia, deep vein thrombosis.
  - Labour and delivery, e.g., postpartum haemorrhage, third-degree perineal tears.
  - Postpartum, e.g., postpartum depression, caesarean section wound infection.
- Mode of delivery and reasons for any operative delivery.
- Birthweight, method of feeding, condition of the baby at birth and admission to the neonatal unit.

PAST MEDICAL AND SURGICAL HISTORY (PMH/PSH)

This section should detail pre-existing medical conditions (e.g., hypertension, diabetes, autoimmune disease) and previous surgery, especially those gynaecology related (e.g., laparoscopy for endometriosis or ectopic pregnancy). These may have implications on management, such as assessing suitability for surgery, and may be risk factors for complications antenatally and intrapartum. Previous psychiatric history is particularly relevant in obstetrics due to the risk of postnatal depression (see Chapter 31).

DRUG HISTORY (DH) AND ALLERGIES

List clearly the patient's regular medication (remember to include hormonal contraception and HRT), over-the-counter medication and any other herbal remedies or supplements (some have significant drug interactions). Reviewing drug concordance is good practice. Clarify why a drug is taken, if it is unclear from the history given (e.g., metformin for polycystic ovary syndrome (PCOS) or diabetes, beta-blockers). Certain medications are contraindicated in pregnancy due to teratogenic effects (e.g., antiepileptics and neural tube defects, doxycycline) and will need to be discontinued or switched. Check for allergies (known and suspected) and document associated reactions and their severity.

SYSTEMIC ENQUIRY

This section consists of screening questions for symptoms in other main systems of the human body. These may or may not be related to the PC. It is also an opportunity to identify forgotten symptoms or 'red flag' symptoms of other possibly related illnesses. Proximity of neighbouring systems like the

System	Symptoms
General	• Fever • Weight loss/gain • Night sweats • Loss of appetite • Fatigue • Rash
Cardio-respiratory	• Chest pain especially pleuritic • Palpitations • Peripheral oedema • Shortness of breath • Palpitations • Cough • Haemoptysis
Gastrointestinal	• Nausea and vomiting • Abdominal pain • Bloating • Jaundice • Change in bowel habit: Constipation, diarrhoea, melaena, dyschezia
Genitourinary	• Urinary incontinence: Urgency, frequency, nocturia, incontinence after exercise/coughing/laughing • Dysuria • Haematuria • Discharge • Vaginal bleeding • Genital pain/dragging/the feeling of 'something coming down' • Need for digital manipulation for defecation or micturition
Neurological	• Visual disturbance: Blurring, 'flashing', floaters, visual loss • Headache • Motor or sensory disturbance: Muscle weakness, numbness, paraesthesia • Syncope • Seizures

gastrointestinal and genitourinary tracts to the reproductive organs suggests their relative importance. Remember that certain symptoms are more common in pregnancy, including shortness of breath, fatigue and urinary frequency.

FAMILY HISTORY (FH)

Conditions and diseases affecting related family members may often provide clues of potential diagnoses or inform of risks regarding a patient's health or genetics. Individuals with a strong family history of breast, ovarian or uterine cancers may be carriers of DNA mismatch repair genes (i.e., Lynch syndrome) or BRCA1/BRCA2 gene mutations. Genetic conditions may prompt a referral to a geneticist. Certain autosomal recessive conditions (e.g., beta thalassaemia, cystic fibrosis) are more common in communities with higher levels of consanguineous marriages. In obstetrics, a family history of diabetes, hypertension and pre-eclampsia may confer increased risk to the current pregnancy.

SOCIAL HISTORY (SH)

Occupation, smoking habits, alcohol consumption and recreational drug use should be noted. This is also an opportunity for health promotion (e.g., smoking cessation, dietary advice, exercise) in a nonjudgemental manner. Consider what kind of support network a patient has at home for postsurgical care or a newborn baby. Keep an open mind about the possibility of

domestic violence. The risk of this increases during pregnancy and healthcare professionals should be aware of local safeguarding procedures and avenues for support.

COMMUNICATION

Presenting your findings can seem like a daunting task at first. This may not have been taught to you at medical school, but don't panic. Aim to present your history in a logical, structured way. Avoid skipping back and forth, and present only relevant negative points in the history. Here is an example of how to present a typical history (see clerking notes in Fig. 2.1):

'ST is a 27-year-old primip at 34 weeks and 2 days gestation, who was referred by her GP due to vaginal bleeding that started 2 hours ago and was unprovoked. Since then, the bleeding has gradually become heavier and is now like a period. She is otherwise fit and well, with no relevant past medical or past surgical history. Her cervical smears are up to date, and previously normal. Her antenatal course has been uneventful. The placenta was noted to be fundal at her last ultrasound. She is only on iron supplementation and has no known drug allergies. She currently smokes 20 cigarettes a day'.

● Chapter Summary

- History-taking in O&G is similar to what you would have learnt initially in medicine as a student, with the addition of specific questions to ask, often involving confidential and very personal information.
- Ensure key details are included in a clerking, including the patient's details, date and time, as this forms a contemporaneous medical record (remember this is a legal document).
- Be aware of gender identity and diversity, treating all patients with respect and dignity.
- Ask open questions. Be alert for a hidden agenda.
- Use the mnemonic 'SOCRATES' to explore the patient's presenting symptom(s).
- In a gynaecology history, remember to ask about cervical screening and contraception.
- In an obstetric history, gravidity refers to the total number of pregnancies and parity refers to the number of livebirths and stillbirths after 24 weeks' gestation.
- Practice presenting a succinct history!

FURTHER READING

Royal College of Obstetricians and Gynaecologists (RCOG): Female genital mutilation management: RCOG green top guideline no. 53. UK, 2009, RCOG London.

Royal College of Obstetricians and Gynaecologists (RCOG): Care of Transgender and Gender Diverse Adults within Obstetrics and Gynaecology: Consultation document July–August 2022. London, UK, 2022, RCOG.

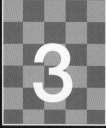

INTRODUCTION

Following taking a history, there are several investigations that you can perform alongside and after your examination; when considering which studies to request, always start with the basic bedside tests first, working your way to the more invasive and complex investigations when necessary.

GYNAECOLOGY BEDSIDE TESTS

Urine

Female patients of childbearing age presenting with abdominal pain or vaginal bleeding need to have a urinary pregnancy test to guide their differential diagnoses. Urine dipstick should be performed to assess for a urinary tract infection and haematuria. If positive for leucocytes and nitrates, this should be sent for microscopy, sensitivity and culture. This confirms if an infection is present and which antibiotics are sensitive to it.

CLINICAL NOTES

Urine pregnancy tests can detect a pregnancy from 3 to 4 days after implantation. By day 7, 98% will be positive. These kits can detect levels of human chorionic gonadotropin (HCG) as low as 10–25 mIU/mL.

BLOOD TESTS

Specific blood tests can be helpful in the diagnosis of different gynaecological disorders (Table 3.1).

SWABS

Patients presenting with abnormal vaginal discharge and/or abdominal pain with pyrexia, where infection is suspected, should have a swab taken (Table 3.2).

SMEARS

The UK National Screening in Cervical Cytology Programme was designed to detect early abnormal changes in the cells of the cervix, which, if left untreated, could progress to cancer.

- Age 25 to 49 years require one smear every 3 years
- Age 50 to 64 years require one smear every 5 years

Using a Cusco's speculum to visualize the cervix, a Cytobrush is used to perform a 360° sweep (10 complete rotations) of the cervical os (Fig. 3.1). The sample is placed into a medium and sent to the laboratory. Samples are first screened for the presence of the human papilloma virus (HPV), which has been linked to >95% of cervical cancers. Only if this virus is detected are the cells analysed with cytology.

Table 3.1 Indications for blood tests performed for gynaecological presentations

Blood test	When useful:
Full blood count (FBC) – haemoglobin	Acute or chronic anaemia secondary to menorrhagia, per vaginal bleeding or malignancy
Full blood count (FBC) – white cell count	Infection
Clotting screen	Suspected clotting disorder with menorrhagia
Follicle-stimulating hormone, luteinizing hormone, oestradiol, testosterone, sex hormone-binding globulin, progesterone	Subfertility, polycystic ovarian syndrome and menopause
CA-125	Ovarian cancer tumour marker
C-reactive protein (CRP)	Acute or chronic infection and inflammatory diseases
Serum human chorionic gonadotropin (HCG), progesterone	Helpful when assessing ectopic pregnancy, pregnancy of unknown location and molar pregnancy

Table 3.2 Indication and type of swabs used in gynaecology

Type of swab	Site	Common organisms
High vaginal	Posterior fornix of the vagina	- *Candida albicans* - Bacterial vaginosis
Endocervical (nucleic acid amplification test, NAAT)	From the cervical os	- *Chlamydia trachomatis* - *Neisseria gonorrhoeae*
Wound	Recent surgical wound	- *Staphylococcus aureus* - Methicillin-resistant *Staphylococcus aureus* - Anaerobes
Viral	Genital vesicles	- Herpes simplex virus 1 and 2

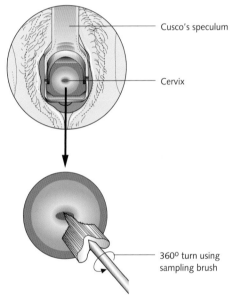

Cusco's speculum

Cervix

360° turn using sampling brush

Fig. 3.1 A smear test.

GYNAECOLOGY PROCEDURES

Imaging

A range of imaging techniques can be used in gynaecology depending on the pathology you are trying to exclude or identify.

Ultrasound

The ultrasound machine has long been described as the gynaecologists' 'third eye'. Ultrasonography is a safe and easily accessible method of investigating pelvic organs. It can either be performed via the transabdominal or transvaginal route. Transvaginal scans, although more invasive, give excellent higher quality images (compared with transabdominal scans) of the adnexa (fallopian tubes and ovaries) and allow you to detect very early pregnancies (Fig. 3.2). Transabdominal ultrasound is a noninvasive alternative; however, images obtained are often limited (as the ultrasound waves must travel further, so lower frequencies have to be used, which results in poorer quality images), especially in patients with a high body mass index.

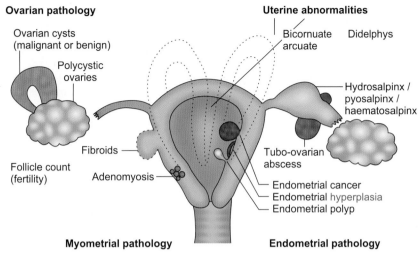

Ovarian pathology

Ovarian cysts
(malignant or benign)

Polycystic
ovaries

Follicle count
(fertility)

Uterine abnormalities

Bicornuate   Didelphys
arcuate

Hydrosalpinx /
pyosalpinx /
haematosalpinx

Tubo-ovarian
abscess

Fibroids

Adenomyosis

Endometrial cancer
Endometrial hyperplasia
Endometrial polyp

Myometrial pathology   **Endometrial pathology**

Fig. 3.2 Identifiable pathology on ultrasound scan.

MRI can be used to assess for deep infiltrating endometriosis (more in Chapter 7) or for assisting with characterizing ovarian cysts. CT scans are generally reserved for cancer staging or post-operative unwell patients where an abdominal collection needs to be excluded.

HYSTEROSCOPY

A hysteroscopy is an investigation using an endoscope (fine camera) inserted through the cervix to inspect the uterine cavity (Fig. 3.3). Distension medium such as normal saline is commonly used. It is the gold standard investigation of abnormal uterine bleeding and can identify endometrial polyps, a uterine cavity septum, adhesions, submucosal fibroids and endometrial carcinoma. During operative hysteroscopy, procedures such as polypectomy, endometrial biopsy and transcervical resection of fibroids can be performed. Hysteroscopy can be performed under general anaesthetic or as an outpatient procedure. Complications of the procedure include infection, bleeding and uterine perforation (therefore, potential damage to the surrounding bowel, bladder and ureters).

CYSTOSCOPY

A cystoscopy is like a hysteroscopy, although the endoscope is inserted through the urethra and into the bladder. It can identify bladder polyps, cancer, stones, diverticulum, signs of chronic inflammation and filling abnormalities. It can be performed under general anaesthetic or as an outpatient procedure.

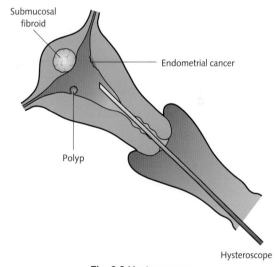

Submucosal
fibroid

Endometrial cancer

Polyp

Hysteroscope

Fig. 3.3 Hysteroscopy.

LAPAROSCOPY

Laparoscopy is the mainstay of investigating pelvic pain. It is used to diagnose and treat pelvic diseases such as endometriosis, adhesions and adnexal cysts.

Laparoscopy is performed under general anaesthetic. After emptying the bladder and instrumenting the uterus, if manipulation is required, entry is gained into the peritoneal cavity. This can be achieved with a Veress needle or through direct trocar entry using various techniques. A pneumoperitoneum using carbon dioxide to achieve a pressure of 20 mmHg is initially used to allow the safe insertion of laparoscopic ports. The laparoscope can then be passed through the port into the pelvis, and the organs can be visualized. The operating pressure is then commonly reduced to 12 to 15 mmHg or lower (Fig. 3.4).

Risks of laparoscopy include bowel, bladder, ureteric and vascular injury (<1%). If laparoscopy is not possible, there are complications, or a large specimen needs to be removed, the laparoscopic procedure may need to be converted to a laparotomy.

HINTS AND TIPS

Laparoscopy, when compared with open surgery, is associated with less pain and blood loss, better visualization of organs and pathology, a shorter hospital stay and better cosmetic results.

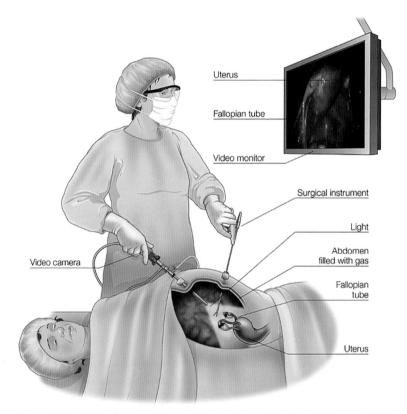

Fig. 3.4 Laparoscopy. (From: Hartman CJ, Kavoussi LR. *Handbook of Surgical Technique*. 1st Edition. pp 63–77. 2018.)

Chapter Summary

- It is essential to use investigations and a thorough history and examination to aid diagnosis.
- Always remember to check the patient's pregnancy status.
- Ensure the basics are performed before requesting more invasive investigations, which are associated with more risks.
- Hysteroscopy, cystoscopy and laparoscopy can all be used as diagnostic and operative procedures.

UKMLA Conditions
Anaemia
Bacterial vaginosis
Cervical screening (HPV)
Chlamydia
Gonorrhoea

UKMLA Presentations
Abnormal urine analysis
Acute abdominal pain
Gonorrhoea
Subfertility
Urinary discharge

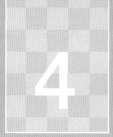

Abnormal uterine bleeding

THE MENSTRUAL CYCLE

Abnormal uterine bleeding (AUB) is a common problem experienced by women and a common presentation to primary and secondary care. Knowledge of the normal menstrual cycle is essential to understanding the patho-aetiology of gynaecological disease. Within the normal menstrual cycle, the following are necessary:

- An intact hypothalamic–pituitary–ovarian (HPO) axis.
- A functioning ovarian cycle: The presence of responsive follicles in the ovaries.
- A functioning uterine/endometrial cycle: The presence of a responsive endometrium.
- A functioning and structurally normal uterus, cervix and vagina.

AUB can be caused by malfunction or disease at any of these levels. Causes can be physiological or pathological and may not require investigation or treatment as long as serious pathology can be excluded.

THE HYPOTHALAMIC–PITUITARY–OVARIAN AXIS

The average menstrual cycle lasts around 28 days, with day 1 being the first day of menstruation and ovulation occurring on approximately day 14. The menstrual cycle is controlled by the endocrine system via the HPO axis (Fig. 4.1). The hypothalamus acts on the pituitary gland by secreting gonadotrophin-releasing hormone (GnRH), a decapeptide, in a pulsatile manner. GnRH travels and binds to receptors on the anterior pituitary gland, stimulating synthesis and release of follicle-stimulating hormone (FSH) and luteinizing hormone (LH). FSH and LH travel through the bloodstream to act on the ovaries.

FSH stimulates growth and development of the ovarian follicles, with a single dominant follicle eventually maturing to become the Graafian follicle. It also stimulates the production of oestradiol by granulosa cells of the Graafian follicle.

LH plays an essential role in ovulation. A mid-cycle surge of LH triggers the rupture of the Graafian follicle with release

of the oocyte (Fig. 4.2). LH also stimulates sex hormone production, mainly testosterone, which is converted by FSH into oestradiol.

Increased levels of oestrogen and progesterone exert a negative feedback effect on both the pituitary gland and hypothalamus, resulting in decreased production of GnRH, LH and FSH.

THE OVARIAN CYCLE

Follicular phase: Days 1 to 8

At the beginning of the cycle, a rise in FSH and LH (in response to falling oestradiol and progesterone levels at menstruation) stimulates follicle growth and development. A single dominant follicle reaches full maturation, becoming the Graafian follicle within which lies the developing oocyte. The remaining ovarian follicles undergo atresia. Increasing levels of oestradiol produced by the Graafian follicle inhibit the release of FSH and LH by negative feedback, preventing hyperstimulation of the ovary and the maturation of multiple follicles.

Ovulation: Day 14

Oestrogen exerts negative feedback at relatively lower levels and positive feedback at higher levels. Rising oestradiol levels eventually peak, surpassing a threshold level and stimulating a mid-cycle surge of LH by positive feedback. Within 18 hours, the mature Graafian follicle ruptures with release of the oocyte.

Luteal phase: Days 15–28

Following ovulation, the Graafian follicle regresses to become the corpus luteum, which produces progesterone to prepare the endometrium for implantation of a fertilized ovum. Increasing levels of progesterone and oestradiol produced by the corpus luteum exert negative feedback on LH and FSH production. The corpus luteum later degenerates, resulting in a fall in progesterone levels which triggers menstruation, initiating the next cycle. If fertilization occurs, human chorionic gonadotrophin (hCG) secreted by the trophoblast serves to maintain the corpus luteum and ensure continued production of progesterone, preventing menstruation.

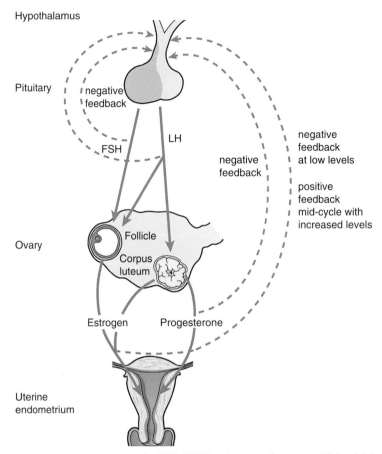

Hypothalamus

Pituitary

negative
feedback

FSH

LH

negative
feedback

negative
feedback
at low levels

positive
feedback
mid-cycle with
increased levels

Ovary

Follicle

Corpus
luteum

Estrogen   Progesterone

Uterine
endometrium

Fig. 4.1 The hypothalamic–pituitary–ovarian–uterine axis. *FSH*, Follicle stimulating hormone; *LH*, luteinizing hormone. (From Cameron S. *Clinical Obstetrics and Gynaecology.* Elsevier, 2023: 48–60. © 2023.)

CLINICAL NOTES

Some women can experience brief iliac fossa pain associated with ovulation. This is known as mid-cycle pain or 'mittelschmerz' (German for 'middle pain' or 'pain in the middle of the month').

Progesterone levels peak 1 week after ovulation (day 21 of a typical 28-day cycle) and are used in the investigation of subfertility. A serum progesterone level >30 nmol/L confirms that ovulation has taken place.

In women who experience prolonged cycles beyond 28 days, take note that it is the follicular phase that lengthens. The luteal phase remains constant at 14 days. Hence, ovulation always occurs 14 days before the first day of the LMP.

THE UTERINE/ENDOMETRIAL CYCLE

The endometrium of the uterus undergoes changes in response to the cyclical production of hormones by the ovaries. It is composed of two layers:

- Superficial/functional layer: This layer responds to hormonal stimulation and is shed during menstruation. It is made up of spiral arteries.
- Basal layer: This layer regenerates the superficial layer after menstruation and is made up of straight arteries.

Proliferative phase

This phase coincides with the follicular phase of the ovarian cycle. Exposure of the endometrium to high levels of oestradiol produced by the ovary stimulates repair and regeneration of the endometrium following menstruation, with progressive

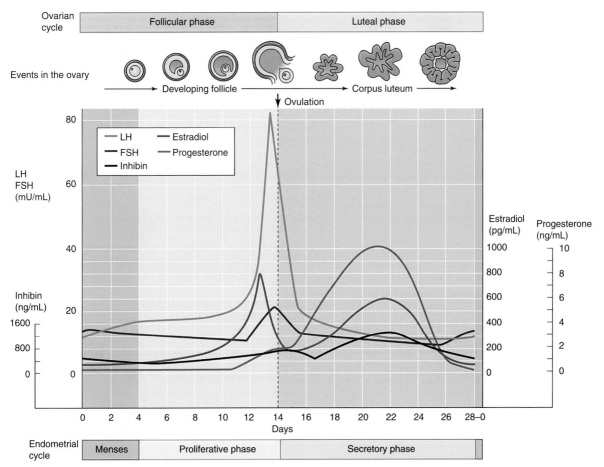

Fig. 4.2 The menstrual cycle. *FSH*, Follicle stimulating hormone; *LH*, luteinizing hormone. (From Mesiano S, Jones EE. *Medical Physiology.* Elsevier, 2017: 1108–1128.e1. © 2017.)

endometrial thickness, vascularity and proliferation of endometrial glands and blood vessels.

Secretory phase

This phase coincides with the luteal phase of the ovarian cycle. Following ovulation, progesterone produced by the corpus luteum induces secretory changes in the endometrial glands, creating a more favourable environment in the endometrium and facilitating implantation.

Menstrual phase

At the end of the luteal phase, degeneration of the corpus luteum occurs in the absence of fertilization, with a decline in oestradiol and progesterone levels. This is associated with prostaglandin-induced vasospasm of the uterus with spasmodic contraction of the spiral arteries, leading to ischaemic necrosis and shedding of the functional layer of the endometrium (menstruation).

ABNORMAL UTERINE BLEEDING

AUB is an overarching term used to describe any kind of bleeding disturbance that is excessive, irregular, unscheduled or occurring outside of normal menstruation. It includes irregular bleeding, intermenstrual bleeding (IMB), postcoital bleeding (PCB), postmenopausal bleeding (PMB) and heavy menstrual bleeding (HMB). The International Federation of Gynaecology and Obstetrics (FIGO) has described a classification system for the causes of AUB. These are grouped under categories using the acronym PALM-COEIN (see Table 4.1).

HEAVY MENSTRUAL BLEEDING

HMB is defined in a clinical setting as 'excessive menstrual blood loss that has an adverse impact on a woman's physical, social, emotional and/or material quality of life, and which

Table 4.1 FIGO PALM-COEIN classification system for causes of abnormal uterine bleeding

Structural causes (PALM)	
P – Polyps (endometrial, endocervical)	
A – Adenomyosis	
L – Leiomyomas (uterine fibroids)	
M – Malignancy and hyperplasia	
Nonstructural causes (COEIN)	
C – Coagulopathy	• Platelet dysfunction • Thrombocytopaenia • von Willebrand disease
O – Ovulatory dysfunction	• Thyroid disease • Polycystic ovarian syndrome (PCOS) • Anovulatory cycles or other disturbances to ovulation
E – Endometrial causes	• Disturbances to local vascular function • Dysfunctional uterine bleeding
I – Iatrogenic	• Contraceptive use, e.g., copper intrauterine contraceptive device, combined oral contraceptive pill (COCP), depot injections, progesterone-only pill (POP) • Anticoagulants
N – Not classified	• Other causes not otherwise classified • Caesarean section niche

occurs alone or in combination with other symptoms'. It is common, affecting up to 25% of women in Western Europe. While the cause of HMB is usually benign, HMB frequently leads to iron-deficiency anaemia, which can make activities of daily living a struggle. The practical difficulties of managing excessive bleeding can also negatively impact on family, social and working life.

Average menstrual blood loss is typically between 30 and 40 mL per cycle, although in research studies, HMB is defined as a total menstrual blood loss of >80 mL per month. It is important to note that a diagnosis of HMB should be made on a woman's own subjective evaluation of bleeding and the impact of this on her quality of life. Only around 50% of women who report heavy periods actually experience menstrual blood loss of >80 mL per month. Two-thirds of women with genuine HMB will suffer from iron-deficiency anaemia.

Aetiology

Causes of HMB include most of the overall causes of AUB as listed in the PALM-COEIN classification system.

Structural causes

Any pathology that enlarges/distorts the uterine cavity or increases endometrial tissue will increase the surface area of menstruating endometrium, leading to HMB. Uterine fibroids (leiomyomas) are the commonest structural lesions to cause heavy periods, and produce prostaglandins implicated in the aetiology of HMB (Chapter 5). They may also cause IMB and PCB depending on their location.

Adenomyosis is associated with HMB and dysmenorrhoea and is characterized by invasion of the endometrial glands into the smooth muscle of the uterine myometrium. The diagnosis is usually made on ultrasound or MRI, and a diffusely enlarged uterus with a whorl-like trabeculated appearance is characteristic.

Endometrial polyps are benign localized outgrowths arising from the endometrium. They can appear at any age and are usually asymptomatic though they can cause IMB, HMB and PMB. Protrusion of a polyp through the cervix may cause PCB. Occasionally, a polyp may develop simple or complex hyperplasia, or rarely, undergo malignant transformation.

Endometrial hyperplasia is a premalignant condition that can progress to cancer if left untreated. It is often associated with irregular, anovulatory cycles. Although rare, malignancy should always be excluded especially in patients experiencing AUB, or who have pre-existing endometrial hyperplasia, or the presence of risk factors.

Systemic conditions

Around 90% of women with coagulation disorders such as von Willebrand disease, clotting factor deficiencies and thrombocytopaenia will experience HMB. Anovulatory cycles or other disturbances to ovulation may cause irregular cycles with prolonged, heavy or erratic bleeding. This is due to inadequate progesterone production in the luteal phase of the menstrual cycle, leading to erratic shedding of the endometrium. Examples include PCOS and hypothyroidism. Anovulatory cycles are more common in adolescence and in the peri-menopausal period.

Iatrogenic causes

Use of the copper intrauterine contraceptive device (IUCD) is the most common iatrogenic cause of HMB. Other hormonal contraceptives may also be associated with heavy or irregular bleeding. Around 50% of women on anticoagulants will experience heavy periods.

Dysfunctional uterine bleeding

Dysfunctional uterine bleeding is the most common cause of HMB and is the term used in the absence of recognizable pelvic pathology or systemic causes for HMB. It is therefore a diagnosis of exclusion. The precise cause for this is unknown although mechanisms regulating haemostasis at the level of the endometrium appear to be implicated. Altered endometrial prostaglandin metabolism may also play a role. In such cases, women may simply be seeking reassurance and not necessarily want treatment.

Assessment of heavy menstrual bleeding (HMB)

History taking

Establish the date of the last menstrual period (LMP), the regularity, pattern and duration of menstrual bleeding, along with associated symptoms such as pain. A recent change in the pattern of menstruation is more likely to indicate underlying pelvic pathology. Dysmenorrhoea is often associated with HMB, usually during the first few days of a period. Chronic pelvic pain may indicate the presence of endometriosis, adenomyosis or pelvic inflammatory disease (PID). Structural lesions may be associated with PMB and IMB.

An attempt should be made to quantify the volume of bleeding. Estimation of the degree of menstrual blood loss is inherently subjective, and the amount of sanitary protection and duration of bleeding often do not correlate with the actual volume of blood lost. Nevertheless, the following features are more likely to indicate significant HMB:

- Passage of large clots
- Need for double sanitary protection (pads and tampons)
- Flooding through clothes or onto bedding
- Need for frequent changes of sanitary protection (2 hours or less)
- Adverse impact on quality of life: Inability to work or attend school, fear of leaving the house during menstruation
- Presence of symptoms of anaemia: Fatigue, lethargy, shortness of breath, light-headedness

A thorough medical and surgical history, and general systemic enquiry should be undertaken. Women with unopposed oestrogenic stimulation of the endometrium by exogenous or endogenous oestrogen (e.g., obesity, PCOS, oestrogen-only hormone replacement therapy (HRT), oestrogen-secreting tumours of the ovary), tamoxifen use, nulliparity, obesity and type II diabetes are at increased risk of endometrial hyperplasia and cancer. A family history of endometrial, breast, ovarian or colorectal cancer is also significant.

Symptoms such as dry skin, hair loss and easy bruising would indicate further investigation for thyroid disease and coagulation disorders. Confirm the date and result of the last cervical screen, as well as a history of IMB or PCB, which may be associated with malignancy. Enquire about the use of contraception and whether this correlates with any change in bleeding pattern. A drug history including prescribed and over-the-counter medication should be elicited.

Examination

A general examination should be performed, looking for signs of systemic conditions such as anaemia and thyroid disease. Fibroids may be palpated on abdominal examination, classically as an enlarged, firm and irregular pelvic mass. Abdominal distension with ascites is suggestive of malignancy.

Speculum examination may reveal vaginal discharge and cervical pathology including cervicitis, cervical polyps or frank malignancy. Endometrial polyps and pedunculated fibroids can sometimes be seen prolapsing through the cervical os. A bimanual examination should be performed, and the adnexa palpated for the presence of any masses. An enlarged, 'bulky' uterus is suggestive of fibroids, while a uniformly enlarged, soft, tender ('boggy') uterus is typically associated with adenomyosis. Endometriosis is indicative in the presence of a fixed, immobile uterus with palpable nodules in the posterior vaginal fornix.

Investigations

Investigations are aimed at excluding systemic and local causes of HMB.

Blood tests

A full blood count to assess for anaemia should be carried out for all women presenting with HMB. Iron studies are not routinely indicated. Thyroid function tests should only be performed if clinically suspected from the history and examination findings. Coagulation studies should be considered for women with HMB since menarche, or those with a personal and/or family history suggestive of a bleeding disorder.

Imaging

Ultrasound is the first-line imaging modality used in the identification and assessment of pelvic structural pathology. A transvaginal approach is preferred as this provides better visualization, especially in obese women. Transabdominal ultrasound should be performed if the transvaginal route is not appropriate. Pelvic ultrasound can confirm the presence, location and size of any uterine fibroids, endometrial polyps, adenomyosis and adnexal masses. Uterine size and endometrial thickness can also be determined, along with the nature of any cysts (e.g., simple, multiloculated, solid).

Cervical screening

Cervical screening should be performed when due, or sooner if there is a history of IMB or PCB. A referral to colposcopy should be made if the cervix looks suspicious on examination.

Endometrial assessment

Assessment of the endometrium in the form of endometrial biopsy should be performed in all women over the age of 40, as well as in younger women with HMB refractory to treatment, persistent IMB or irregular bleeding, or risk factors for endometrial hyperplasia/cancer. Endometrial biopsy can be performed in the outpatient setting, as a stand-alone procedure (pipelle biopsy) or in conjunction with hysteroscopy. A pipelle biopsy has high levels of patient acceptability and lower complication rates, without the need for inpatient admission or general anaesthesia. It is, however, limited in its assessment as it only samples <5% of the endometrium, and may miss both benign and malignant endometrial pathology.

Hysteroscopy allows direct visualization of the uterine cavity and is therefore the gold standard for assessing intrauterine pathology. It can be performed under general anaesthesia or in the outpatient setting (with the option of local anaesthetic). A hysteroscope is a narrow, rigid telescope that is passed through the cervix and into the uterine cavity. Water is used to distend the uterine cavity, allowing visualization. Hysteroscopy can generally identify endometrial/cervical polyps, submucous fibroids, endometritis and endometrial hyperplasia/cancer. Endometrial biopsy and polypectomy can be performed during the same procedure. Outpatient hysteroscopy with concurrent endometrial biopsy and polypectomy can be undertaken so long as this is tolerated by the patient.

Management

Treatment of HMB should be tailored to the patient's preferences and fertility wishes, and take into account medical comorbidities, associated symptoms such as pain, and the presence of structural lesions (e.g., fibroids, polyps, adenomyosis). It is important to note that side effects and efficacy of different treatment options may vary between individuals, and hormonal therapy may be contraindicated in certain conditions such as thromboembolic disease.

Treatment of endometrial cancer will be considered in Chapter 12. The management of HMB secondary to fibroids will be addressed in Chapter 5.

Medical – nonhormonal treatment

Nonsteroidal antiinflammatory drugs (NSAIDs) including ibuprofen and mefenamic acid inhibit the cyclooxygenase enzyme system which controls the production of cyclic endoperoxides from arachidonic acid. NSAIDs reduce menstrual blood loss by around 30% and confer analgesic benefit. The main side effect is gastrointestinal irritation although this can be mitigated with the use of proton-pump inhibitors such as omeprazole.

Tranexamic acid is an antifibrinolytic agent that inhibits the activation of plasminogen to plasmin, reducing excessive fibrinolytic activity in the endometrium. This promotes the formation of clots and reduces blood loss by around 50%. Tranexamic acid may cause gastrointestinal side effects including nausea. They should be avoided in patients with previous thromboembolic disease.

Both NSAIDs and antifibrinolytics only need to be taken during menstruation, and are best suited for women wishing to conceive or who decline hormonal therapy.

Medical – hormonal treatment

The levonorgestrel intrauterine system (LNG-IUS) dramatically reduces menstrual blood loss by around 95% and is widely recommended as first-line management for HMB. Amenorrhoea occurs in up to 50% of long-term users due to endometrial atrophy. It also serves as a highly effective long-acting reversible contraceptive method, although fertility returns almost immediately upon removal. Unlike other synthetic long-acting progestogens (see below), the LNG-IUS exerts its effects locally with minimal systemic absorption. Side effects are usually limited to breakthrough bleeding in the initial year of use. Women should be counselled on anticipated changes in their menstrual bleeding pattern, particularly in the first few cycles. They should be advised to persevere for at least six cycles to see the benefits of the treatment.

When taken in a cyclical fashion, the combined oral contraceptive pill (COCP) inhibits ovulation and produces regular shedding of a thin endometrium. It is associated with a 50% reduction in menstrual blood loss. Use of the COCP is contraindicated in women ≥35 years who smoke ≥15 cigarettes/day, BMI ≥35, and those with a history of breast cancer, cardiovascular disease (e.g., diabetes mellitus, hypertension, stroke), migraines with aura, thromboembolic disease and prothrombotic conditions (e.g., factor V Leiden, antiphospholipid syndrome).

Synthetic oral progestogens such as norethisterone and medroxyprogesterone acetate can be used to treat HMB and are sometimes used in high doses to arrest heavy bleeding. They tend to be more effective at regulating cycles and controlling bleeding when taken long term, and women should be advised to persist with treatment for at least 3 months. Synthetic long-acting progestogens may also be administered via depot injection and the implant. Side effects include weight gain, breast tenderness, acne, bloating and headaches, although women tend to be most bothered by breakthrough bleeding that can be erratic and heavy.

Additional medical therapies such as ulipristal acetate and gonadotrophin-releasing hormone (GnRH) analogues are available to women with HMB secondary to fibroids. These will be discussed in Chapter 5.

Surgical

Surgical management of HMB depends on the underlying diagnosis:

Hysteroscopy

Endometrial polyps and submucous fibroids are usually surgically excised under hysteroscopic guidance.

Myomectomy or uterine artery embolization

These are options in the management of fibroids with conservation of the uterus (see Chapter 5).

Endometrial ablation

Endometrial ablation is a day-case procedure that reduces menstrual blood loss by producing an 'iatrogenic' Asherman syndrome. The endometrium is destroyed down to the endomyometrial border, and the ensuing intrauterine adhesions prevent regeneration. Menstrual blood loss is reduced by up to 90%, and around 50% of patients will become amenorrhoeic. Earlier techniques involved laser or diathermy resection of the endometrium under a hysteroscopic procedure. Newer devices have been developed, including thermal balloon, microwave ablation and bipolar radiofrequency impedance-controlled ablative techniques. These place less emphasis on hysteroscopy and carry fewer risks. Although endometrial ablation does not guarantee amenorrhoea as hysterectomy does, advantages include speed of surgery and quicker recovery time. Some procedures can even be performed under local anaesthetic in an outpatient setting. Success rates of various ablative techniques are similar, and the procedure is associated with high patient satisfaction rates.

Endometrial ablation is not suitable for women wishing to preserve fertility. Uterine perforation is a rare complication that could lead to damage to surrounding organs and major blood vessels, requiring laparoscopic or open repair. Fluid overload is a more common complication that occurs with the absorption of large quantities of irrigation fluid, resulting in hyponatraemia due to dilutional effects. In extreme overload, congestive cardiac failure, hypertension, neurological symptoms, haemolysis and coma can occur.

Hysterectomy

Hysterectomy is the only definitive treatment for HMB and may be considered when other treatment options have failed, are contraindicated, or are declined by the woman. Hysterectomy is a commonly performed procedure in the UK with 1 in 5 women having a hysterectomy before the age of 60. HMB was found to be the primary reason in approximately 40% of cases. However, the number of hysterectomies performed due to HMB has fallen in recent years due to better diagnostic abilities, improved medical treatment options and the development of effective endometrial ablative techniques.

Hysterectomy can be performed by an abdominal, vaginal or laparoscopic approach. This is dependent on operator skill and experience, uterine size, previous abdominal surgery, the need for ovarian conservation, the size, number and location of any uterine fibroids, and other co-existing pelvic pathology such as endometriosis. Total abdominal hysterectomy tends to be performed in women with large uteri, multiple large fibroids, adenomyosis, pelvic adhesions, endometriosis, or in cases where morcellation should not be performed (such as in suspected malignancy). A subtotal abdominal hysterectomy involves removal of the body of the uterus while the cervix is left behind, however, cervical screening must be continued.

The decision on whether to remove the ovaries is dependent on several factors such as the age of the woman, a family history of breast or ovarian cancer, and personal preference. The average age of natural menopause in most industrialized countries is 51 years. Consequently, oophorectomy in premenopausal women leads to premature iatrogenic menopause, with detrimental short- and long-term health sequelae. Examples of short-term effects include vasomotor symptoms (hot flushes, night sweats), mood changes, sexual dysfunction (dyspareunia, reduced libido, vaginal dryness) and sleep disturbance. Oestrogen also has a protective effect on bone strength, cardiovascular health and neurocognitive function. A wealth of evidence exists, demonstrating the association between premenopausal oophorectomy and an increased risk of stroke, osteopenia and osteoporosis, neurocognitive decline, dementia and coronary heart disease. These tend to occur in women for whom HRT is contraindicated. Current clinical practice recommends the use of HRT up to the age of natural menopause for symptomatic relief and to mitigate the adverse long-term health consequences of premature menopause. HRT can be continued beyond this as long as the patient is comfortable with the associated risks. Alternative pharmacological, nonpharmacological and complementary therapies may be considered for women unable or unwilling to take HRT, although the evidence for these is limited. For women who choose ovarian conservation, the benefit of this needs to be weighed up against the possible risk of future ovarian cancer.

Abdominal hysterectomy is associated with longer postoperative recovery times and higher complication rates compared to both vaginal and laparoscopic approaches. Around 50% of women undergoing abdominal hysterectomy and 25% of those undergoing vaginal hysterectomy will experience a complication. These include bleeding, infection (urinary tract, respiratory, wound), damage to the urinary tract or bowel, venous thromboembolism and pelvic floor prolapse with associated bladder and bowel dysfunction. The mortality rate following hysterectomy for benign disease is very low, approximately 6 per 10,000, and is usually a consequence of cardiovascular disease or sepsis.

COMMUNICATION

The provision of information and patient education is an extremely important part of the management process. Treatment recommendations for HMB should take into account the woman's fertility plans, as many treatments temporarily or permanently inhibit fertility. The decision to remove the ovaries at the time of hysterectomy requires informed discussion with the woman regarding the health consequences of premature menopause, impact on quality of life, as well as the risks, benefits and limitations of HRT.

INTERMENSTRUAL BLEEDING AND POSTCOITAL BLEEDING

IMB refers to spontaneous vaginal bleeding occurring at any time during the menstrual cycle other than during normal menstruation. It can sometimes be difficult to differentiate true IMB from irregularly frequent periods. IMB may be cyclical or completely random and is commonly associated with the use of hormonal contraception (referred to as unscheduled or breakthrough bleeding). PCB refers to nonmenstrual vaginal bleeding that is immediately precipitated by penetrative sexual intercourse. Many women will present with a combination of PCB and IMB.

It is important to note that both IMB and PCB are not diagnoses but symptoms that necessitate further investigation as they may indicate serious underlying pathology. Although malignancy is an uncommon cause of bleeding in younger women, it must be considered and excluded in all patients.

Aetiology

Causes of IMB and PCB are similar, and can be of vaginal, cervical and endometrial origin (see Table 4.2). Always perform a pregnancy test as pregnancy-related bleeding such as ectopic pregnancy and gestational trophoblast disease may mimic IMB.

Assessment of intermenstrual/postmenopausal bleeding

History and examination is similar to that in HMB. It is important to ask additional questions regarding the presenting complaint of IMB or PCB, and include a sexual health and cervical screening history. In summary:

- Systemic history
  - Unexplained weight loss
  - Night sweats or fever
  - Fatigue/malaise/lethargy
- Menstrual history
  - Last menstrual period
  - Regularity, cycle length and volume
  - Duration, pattern and volume of PCB/IMB
  - Timing of PCB/IMB in the menstrual cycle
  - Associated symptoms: Pain, fever, discharge, dyspareunia, menopausal symptoms
- Obstetric history
- Gynaecological history
  - Contraceptive use
  - Cervical screening: Whether this is up-to-date, the most recent result, previous abnormalities
  - Previous gynaecological surgery or investigations
- Sexual history: Risk factors for sexually transmitted infections (STIs)
- Medical history: Especially bleeding disorders, diabetes mellitus and previous malignancy
- Drug history: Prescribed and over-the-counter medication
- Family history: Especially endometrial, colon, ovarian and breast cancer

All women presenting with IMB or PCB should have a full examination including:

- Abdominal examination: Note the presence of any ascites or pelvic masses.
- Pelvic examination (speculum and bimanual). Note the presence of any:
  - Contact bleeding
  - Friable tissue or ulceration
  - Cervical excitation or tenderness
  - Endometrial or cervical polyps
  - Vaginal discharge

Table 4.2 Causes of intermenstrual bleeding and postcoital bleeding

Causes of IMB and PCB	
Physiological	• Spotting around the time of ovulation (1%–2% of women) • Hormonal fluctuation during the peri-menopausal period
Vaginal	• Infection (vaginitis) including sexually transmitted infections (STIs) such as *Chlamydia trachomatis* and *Neisseria gonorrhoea* • Trauma or sexual abuse • Atrophy • Malignancy
Cervical	• Infection (cervicitis) including STIs such as *Chlamydia trachomatis* and *Neisseria gonorrhoea* • Cervical polyps • Ectropion (more common in pregnancy and with combined oral contraceptive pill (COCP) use) • Malignancy
Uterine	• Leiomyomas (uterine fibroids): Especially submucous • Endometrial polyps • Infection (endometritis) • Adenomyosis • Endometrial hyperplasia and malignancy
Iatrogenic	• Tamoxifen and use of hormone replacement therapy (HRT) • Following a cervical smear or treatment to the cervix • Drugs altering coagulation: Anticoagulants, selective serotonin reuptake inhibitors (SSRIs), corticosteroids • Alternative remedies when taken with hormonal contraceptives: Ginseng, ginkgo, soy supplements and St. John's wort • Hormonal contraception: Levonorgestrel intrauterine system (LNG-IUS), progesterone-only pill (POP), COCP (especially missed pills), depot injection, implant

• Calculation of BMI: High BMI is an independent risk factor for endometrial cancer

Investigations

Urine test
A urine pregnancy test should be performed to exclude the possibility of pregnancy. A midstream urine sample should be sent to exclude a urinary tract infection.

Microbiology swabs/STI screen
Microbiology swabs and a screen for STIs (if applicable), including high and low vaginal swabs, endocervical swabs and urethral swabs, should be performed. *Chlamydia trachomatis* infection can be tested by an endocervical swab or a urine sample.

Pelvic ultrasound
Transvaginal ultrasound may identify pathology such as a thickened endometrium, uterine fibroids or endometrial/cervical polyps.

Specialist tests
If abnormalities are noted on the cervix, or cervical screening is due, a cervical screen or biopsy may be taken. A referral to colposcopy should be made if the cervix looks suspicious on examination or if there is persistent PCB even if the cervical screen is normal.

Endometrial biopsy should be performed in all women over the age of 45 presenting with IMB or PCB, as well as in younger women with persistent IMB/PCB or risk factors for endometrial hyperplasia/cancer. Hysteroscopy with endometrial biopsy should be considered in women whose history is suggestive of submucous fibroids, polyps or endometrial pathology.

Management

There is a high rate of spontaneous resolution of IMB (up to 37%) and PCB (up to 51%) and so management will depend on the cause of IMB or PCB:

Infection
Treat as per microbiology guidelines for the specific organism cultured and its sensitivities. In the case of STIs, women should be referred or advised to self-refer to a sexual health clinic for a full sexual health screen and contact tracing.

Vaginal atrophy
Advise a trial of a vaginal moisturizing cream or topical oestrogen.

Cervical polyps

Cervical polyps are benign pedunculated outgrowths arising from the endocervical epithelium and can protrude through the external os into the vagina. Smaller polyps may be avulsed in the outpatient setting while larger polyps may require ligation of the base followed by excision under general anaesthesia.

Endometrial polyps and submucous fibroids

Endometrial polyps and submucous fibroids are usually surgically excised under hysteroscopic guidance.

Cervical ectropion

This may resolve spontaneously following pregnancy or if the COCP is stopped. Smaller ones may be cauterized with silver nitrate in the outpatient setting. For larger ectropions, referral to colposcopy for cryocautery or diathermy may be considered.

Malignancy

The management of gynaecological malignancies will be discussed in Chapter 12.

Hormonal contraception

Unscheduled/breakthrough bleeding in the first 3 months of starting a new hormonal contraceptive and up to 6 months for the LNG-IUS or progesterone-only implant is considered normal. If bleeding persists beyond the first 6 months or is of new onset, investigation is required.

POSTMENOPAUSAL BLEEDING

Menopause is a retrospective diagnosis made 1 year after the LMP. PMB therefore refers to vaginal bleeding occurring more than 1 year after the menopause.

Aetiology

Atrophic changes to the lower genital tract such as atrophic vaginitis are the most common cause of PMB. PMB is the cardinal symptom of endometrial cancer in postmenopausal women and should be investigated promptly until proven otherwise. Approximately 10% of women in the UK presenting with PMB will be found to have a gynaecological malignancy. Other causes of PMB include infection (e.g., STIs), endometrial and cervical polyps, submucous fibroids, foreign bodies such as pessaries used to treat pelvic organ prolapse, endometrial hyperplasia and other malignancies of the genital tract (cervical, vaginal, vulval, ovarian).

Assessment of postmenopausal bleeding

A full medical and gynaecological history should be taken as per HMB and IMB/PCB. A focused history of the nature of the PMB is useful for considering the differential diagnosis. Atrophic changes to the genital tract usually present with recurrent small amounts of bleeding, whereas profuse vaginal bleeding or the presence of a bloodstained offensive discharge is an ominous sign and can indicate cervical or endometrial malignancy. Local symptoms of oestrogen deficiency include vaginal dryness, soreness and superficial dyspareunia. Enquire about vulval itching (pruritus vulvae), pain and the presence of lesions ('lumps or bumps'). These may indicate benign vulvar dermatoses such as lichen sclerosis and planus although malignancy should always be excluded. Establish the use of HRT and risk factors for endometrial hyperplasia and cancer. Medical comorbidities such as obesity, diabetes mellitus and coagulation disorders should be noted.

Investigations

Microbiology swabs/STI screen

Microbiology swabs and a screen for STIs (if applicable), including high and low vaginal swabs, endocervical swabs and urethral swabs, should be performed.

Pelvic ultrasound

Transvaginal ultrasound is the preferred imaging modality and should be performed in all women presenting with PMB. A postmenopausal endometrial thickness (ET) of >4 mm is considered abnormal and warrants further investigation with hysteroscopy and endometrial biopsy.

Hysteroscopy and endometrial biopsy

Hysteroscopic assessment of the uterine cavity with endometrial biopsy should be performed in women with:

- ET >4 mm
- Risk factors for endometrial hyperplasia/cancer
- Normal ET but persistent episodes of PMB
- A previously normal endometrial biopsy but persistent episodes of PMB

Management

Treatment depends on the underlying pathology. Endometrial polyps and submucous fibroids are usually surgically excised under hysteroscopic guidance. Topical oestrogen therapy is indicated for atrophic vaginitis and will help to alleviate symptoms associated with local oestrogen deficiency such as vaginal dryness and dyspareunia. Low-dose vaginal oestrogen preparations (e.g., creams, pessaries, tablets) are safe and effective, with minimal systemic absorption, and can be continued indefinitely. Women prescribed systemic HRT who have a uterus should receive oestrogen supplementation combined with a progestogen in order to minimize the risk of endometrial hyperplasia and cancer associated with unopposed oestrogenic stimulation of the endometrium.

The management of gynaecological malignancies will be discussed in Chapter 12.

● Chapter Summary

- The topics covered in this chapter are common presentations to gynaecology outpatients.
- The key to management of heavy menstrual bleeding, intermenstrual bleeding, postcoital bleeding and postmenopausal bleeding is identifying the underlying cause, as this will guide treatment.
- Investigations should be initiated promptly, particularly with postmenopausal bleeding, as a differential diagnosis we must consider is malignancy.
- It is crucial that as healthcare providers we emphasize the importance of screening programmes such as the cervical screening programme to reduce incidence of malignancy diagnoses.

UKMLA Presentations
Menstrual problems

BACKGROUND

Uterine fibroids (leiomyomas) are common, benign, smooth muscle tumours of the myometrium, occurring in around 25% of women of reproductive age (and increasing thereafter). At hysterectomy, 70% of all uteruses have been found to contain microscopic fibroids. Fibroids tend to have a higher incidence in women of African and Afro-Caribbean descent. Other risk factors include nulliparity and obesity. Fibroid growth is hormone-dependent and influenced by oestrogen exposure – fibroids tend to enlarge with increasing age and during pregnancy (hyper-oestrogenic state), and shrink after the menopause (but do not disappear). They are generally slow-growing tumours. Malignancy in the form of sarcomatous change (leiomyosarcoma) can occur, although rare (1:1000).

Histologically, uterine fibroids are not only composed of well-circumscribed whorled bundles of smooth muscle cells that resemble the architecture of normal myometrium but also contain fibrous and connective tissue. Fibroids receive their blood supply from the capsule surrounding the main muscle mass. Size may vary from microscopic growths to extremely large masses occupying the entire abdominal cavity. Fibroids may be single or multiple, and are categorized according to their location within the myometrium (Fig. 5.1):

- **Intramural**: Located within the myometrium, contained within the uterus wall.
- **Subserosal**: Located on the serosa (outer surface) of the uterus, projecting into the abdominal cavity.
- **Submucosal**: Located close to the endometrium. Growth extending into the endometrial cavity results in distortion of the endometrium (and increased bleeding).
- **Cervical**: Arise from the cervix.
- **Pedunculated**: Refer to fibroids attached to the uterus by a stalk. Subserosal, submucosal and cervical fibroids can all be pedunculated.

CLINICAL NOTES

Risk factors for fibroids	Protective factors for fibroids
African and Afro-Caribbean ethnicities	Cigarette smoking
Increasing age	Use of the COCP
Nulliparity	Menopause
Obesity	

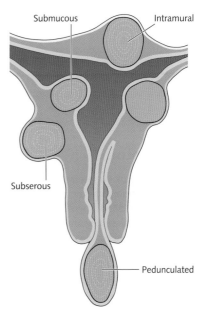

Fig. 5.1 Categorization of fibroids: submucosal fibroids impact on the endometrial cavity, intramural fibroids lie within the uterus wall, subserosal fibroids lie on the outer surface of the womb. Pedunculated fibroids are attached to the uterus through a stalk. (Source: Kay SE, Sandhu CJ. *Crash Course Obstetrics and Gynaecology*. Elsevier; 2019:33–36.)

CLINICAL PRESENTATION

Around 50% of women with fibroids are asymptomatic, and the condition is only diagnosed incidentally, such as during pregnancy or on abdominal examination. Symptoms often correlate with the size and location of any fibroids present.

Abnormal uterine bleeding

The most common presenting symptom of fibroids is abnormal uterine bleeding (AUB), particularly HMB, which occurs in approximately one-third of women with fibroids. Fibroids may cause enlargement/distortion of the uterine cavity, resulting in increased endometrial blood supply and increasing the surface area of menstruating endometrium, leading to HMB. Women may present with symptoms of iron-deficiency anaemia. Submucous fibroids may be associated with IMB and PCB, and can sometimes prolapse through the cervix, causing pain and heavy bleeding.

Pain and discomfort

Chronic pelvic pain and dysmenorrhoea can occur alongside HMB. Acute pain may result from fibroid degeneration (breakdown), torsion of a pedunculated fibroid and prolapse of a submucous fibroid through the cervix. Abdominal swelling and distension, pelvic varicosities, and pressure effects on the bladder, kidneys and rectum may cause general discomfort.

Pressure symptoms

Women may present with symptoms secondary to pressure effects on surrounding abdominal organs. Pelvic pressure results from the growth of large fibroids within the abdominal/pelvic cavity causing abdominal swelling and distension. Pressure on the bladder leads to reduced bladder capacity and symptoms of urinary frequency, urgency and nocturia. Extensive fibroids can cause ureteric compression and hydronephrosis, affecting renal function. Posterior fibroids pressing on the rectum may cause tenesmus, constipation and dyschezia.

Pregnancy complications

It is important to note that many women with fibroids will have uncomplicated pregnancies. Nevertheless, fibroids tend to increase in size due to the hyper-oestrogenic state of pregnancy, and large fibroids can mechanically obstruct labour, prevent vaginal delivery and increase the risk of complications during caesarean section (e.g., surgical access, difficult delivery). Antenatally, fibroids increase the risk of preterm labour and associated perinatal morbidity/mortality. 'Red degeneration', where there is haemorrhagic breakdown and necrosis of the fibroid,

is a cause of abdominal pain in pregnancy. Postnatally, fibroids may cause postpartum haemorrhage, the need for blood transfusions and prolonged hospital admission.

Subfertility and miscarriage

Up to 30% of women with fibroids will experience subfertility secondary to fibroids. Submucous and intramural fibroids are more likely to be implicated, although the precise mechanisms by which fibroids impair fertility are unknown. Theories include mechanical distortion of the endometrial cavity affecting implantation, effects on uterine blood flow and abnormal sperm migration.

There is evidence to suggest that fibroids increase the risk of first and second miscarriages. Recurrent miscarriage is more common in women with submucous fibroids, and studies have shown improved live birth rates following surgical resection.

CLINICAL NOTES

COMPLICATION OF FIBROIDS
GYNAECOLOGICAL
- Degeneration: This is when the fibroid breaks down, resulting in acute pain.
- Torsion of pedunculated fibroids.
- Malignancy (sarcomatous change): Risk of leiomyosarcoma is approximately 0.1%.

PREGNANCY RELATED
- Subfertility
- Miscarriage
- Obstruction of labour
- Preterm labour
- Postpartum haemorrhage
- 'Red degeneration': Haemorrhagic infarction and necrosis within the fibroid

SYSTEMIC
- Venous thromboembolism: Any large mass in the pelvis can cause external compression of the pelvic venous system (usually the external iliac vein), leading to venous stasis and an increased risk of deep vein thrombosis and pulmonary embolism.

ASSESSMENT OF FIBROIDS

History and examination for AUB has been described previously in Chapter 4.

INVESTIGATION

Blood tests

Perform a full blood count and haematinics to assess for anaemia. Consider renal function tests (urea and electrolytes) in women with large fibroids that have the potential to cause ureteric compression (both urea and creatinine would be raised).

Imaging

Transvaginal ultrasound is the diagnostic tool of choice for the diagnosis of fibroids. It can confirm the presence, size and location of any uterine fibroids. Visualization may be limited in women who are obese, have multiple fibroids or a very large fibroid uterus. Magnetic resonance imaging (MRI) may provide clarity in these cases and should be performed if surgical intervention is being considered.

Hysteroscopy

Submucosal fibroids are best visualized by hysteroscopy and resection can be performed concurrently if under general anaesthesia.

MANAGEMENT

Most fibroids are asymptomatic and routine intervention is not required. Management should be dictated by the patient's symptoms, preferences for uterine preservation, desire for future fertility, and the size, number and location of any fibroids.

Medical

Medical therapy in the form of nonsteroidal antiinflammatory drugs (NSAIDs), antifibrinolytics, the Combined oral contraceptive pill (COCP) and synthetic progestogens (Progesterone-only pill (POP), Levonorgestrel intrauterine system (LNG-IUS), depot injection, implant) may be useful in controlling menstrual blood loss and but do not have any impact on fibroid size.

Gonadotrophin-releasing hormone (GnRH) analogues produce a hypogonadotropic hypogonadal state leading to a temporary, reversible, chemical menopause. Since fibroid growth is hormone-dependent, GnRH analogues may be used to reduce fibroid size. Suppression of pituitary-ovarian function leads to hypo-oestrogenism, resulting in amenorrhoea and a reduction in fibroid volume by up to 40% at 6 months. Fibroids will commonly regrow to their original size within 3 months of ceasing GnRH therapy without subsequent surgical intervention. GnRH analogues are commonly used as a pretreatment adjunct to surgery and to correct anaemia,

especially when the uterus is enlarged or distorted. Shrinkage of the fibroids would hopefully enable a smaller surgical incision to be made, decrease intraoperative blood loss and reduce the risk of hysterectomy as a complication of myomectomy. GnRH analogues are usually reserved for short-term use of up to 6 months due to the risks associated with hypo-oestrogenism. These include menopausal symptoms such as hot flushes, vaginal dryness and mood changes, and loss of bone mineral density. 'Add-back' hormone replacement therapy (HRT) can be considered to alleviate symptoms and minimize adverse side effects.

Surgical

Transcervical resection of fibroids (TCRF) refers to the surgical excision of submucous fibroids using an operative hysteroscope.

Uterine artery embolization (UAE) is a minimally invasive radiological procedure involving interruption of the blood supply to the uterus and fibroids. Catheterization of the femoral artery is performed followed by embolization of the uterine arteries, resulting in thrombosis and fibroid ischaemia/infarction. This is associated with a sustained reduction in fibroid size of up to 50%. Revascularization of the myometrium occurs due to collateral circulation from the ovarian vessels. Complications of UAE include postoperative pain due to uterine ischaemia, infection secondary to fibroid degeneration, fibroid expulsion and postembolization syndrome (pain, fever, nausea, malaise, leucocytosis). UAE is a relative contraindication for women wishing to preserve fertility, due to the increased risk of subfertility, miscarriage and adverse pregnancy outcomes.

Myomectomy refers to the surgical excision of fibroids with preservation of the uterus and can be performed abdominally (open) or laparoscopically (Fig. 5.2). It involves incision of the capsule of the fibroid, enucleation of the muscle bulk and closure of the myometrial defect. Myomectomy

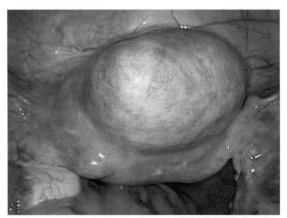

Fig. 5.2 Fibroids at laparoscopy. (Source: Kay SE, Sandhu CJ. *Crash Course Obstetrics and Gynaecology*. Elsevier; 2019:33–36.)

is associated with higher morbidity compared to hysterectomy. The commonest complication is haemorrhage due to fibroid vascularity, which may necessitate blood transfusions and potentially emergency hysterectomy in the event of life-threatening bleeding (although this is very rare). Adhesion formation is common and may lead to subfertility. Fibroid recurrence within 5 years of myomectomy occurs in up to 60% of patients, with repeat surgery required in around 20% of cases. Laparoscopic myomectomies are associated with lower morbidity compared to open procedures. Myomectomy is a surgical option for patients wishing to conceive following treatment. Chances of fertility are higher in younger women and in those with fibroids that are not distorting the endometrial cavity. Should the uterine cavity be breached during myomectomy, a caesarean section is usually advised in any subsequent pregnancy due to the increased risk of uterine rupture during labour.

For definitive removal of fibroids, the surgical procedure of choice is hysterectomy. Fibroids account for about a third of all hysterectomies in the UK. However, hysterectomy is only appropriate in women who have completed their families and have no wish for uterine preservation.

● Chapter Summary

- Fibroids are common. Their growth is hormone-dependent, hence they grow with age, during pregnancy, and shrink after the menopause.
- Around 50% of women with fibroids are asymptomatic. Others present with abnormal uterine bleeding (most common), pain, pressure symptoms, subfertility and pregnancy-related complications.
- Medical or surgical management of fibroids can be considered when they cause symptoms, factoring in preferences for uterine preservation, desire for future fertility, and the size, number and location of fibroids.

UKMLA Conditions
Anaemia
Menstrual problems
Urinary incontinence

UKMLA Presentations
Abdominal distension
Abdominal mass
Acute abdominal pain
Acute and chronic pain management
Fibroids
Pelvic mass
Pelvic pain
Urinary symptoms

Endometriosis & Adenomyosis

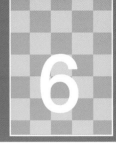

BACKGROUND

Definition

Endometriosis is the presence of endometrial-like cells (similar cells to those found in the uterine lining) outside of the uterine cavity, which induces a chronic inflammatory reaction influenced by the body's hormonal changes. Adenomyosis occurs when endometriosis-like cells are found in the myometrium (uterine muscle wall).

The most common sites for endometriosis are the ovaries, uterosacral ligaments, pelvic side wall and the pouch of Douglas. Areas of endometriosis form sticky patches and result in adhesions to nearby structures, such as the bowel, fallopian tubes and the bladder. These areas with time form plaques and tissue retraction, which can significantly distort the anatomy of the pelvis. Although endometriosis has been reported in nearly every organ, extra pelvic endometriosis is rare (Fig. 6.1).

Thoracic endometriosis is a rare form of endometriosis, which is found in the diaphragm, chest cavity and lungs. Patients may experience difficulty in breathing, cyclical haemoptysis, chest or shoulder tip pain, lung nodules or even pneumothorax. Specialist multidisciplinary team management including a cardiothoracic surgeon should be sought.

Prevalence

The true incidence of endometriosis is difficult to ascertain as not all patients are symptomatic. It is thought to affect 1 in 10 patients but has been diagnosed in up to 25% of patients at laparoscopy. It is one of the most common gynaecological conditions and therefore seen regularly in gynaecology outpatients.

Symptoms: 'The 4 Ds of pain'

- Dysmenorrhoea (painful periods)
- Dyspareunia (pain having sex – often deep)
- Dyschaezia (pain opening bowels)
- Dysuria (bladder pain/pain passing urine)
- Women can also experience chronic pelvic pain outside of their menses

Pain is thought to result from areas of endometriosis which form inflammation and adhesions in response to hormonal changes. This results in local irritation and inflammatory responses. Deep endometriosis of the rectovaginal septum is associated with symptoms such as dyschaezia and deep dyspareunia.

If endometriosis develops within an ovary, it can form a cyst called an endometrioma, otherwise known as a 'chocolate cyst' due to its characteristic liquid brown contents, which is altered blood. Like other ovarian cysts, they can rupture and release the irritant material, causing peritonism and pain. These cysts are generally less likely to result in torsion, due to neighbouring adhesions from endometriosis.

Endometriosis of the lung, bladder, bowel or umbilicus will produce cyclical inflammation and/or pain at these sites during menstruation.

DIAGNOSIS

History

Symptoms that are suggestive of endometriosis should be elicited with a focused history. This will help differentiate it from other conditions such as irritable bowel syndrome, pelvic inflammatory disease and bladder pain syndrome.

History

In addition to your standard gynaecological and obstetric history, you should ask:

- Are your periods painful? *(Dysmenorrhoea)*
- Do you have pain during sexual intercourse? Is this superficial, near the opening of the vagina, or deep within the pelvis? *(Dyspareunia)*
- Do you have pain opening your bowels? *(Dyschaezia)*
- Do you have pain passing urine? *(Dysuria)*
- Does the pain outlast the length of your period? *(More likely with adenomyosis)*
- Where do you feel the pain the most?
- Do you have pelvic pain when you're not on your period?
- What have you tried already to alleviate the pain?
- What are you using for contraception?
- What are your future fertility wishes?
- How does this impact your quality of life?

Examination

Abdominal inspection may reveal incisions from previous laparoscopic surgery. The uterus may be bulky and tender in cases of severe adenomyosis.

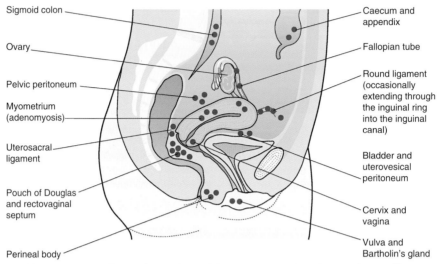

Fig. 6.1 Pelvic Pain and Endometriosis - Clinical Obstetrics and Gynaecology Potdar, Neelam; Clinical Obstetrics and Gynaecology, Chapter 8, 101-109.

A tender, retroverted, retroflexed, fixed uterus with thickening of the cardinal or uterosacral ligaments may be felt. Endometriotic nodules might be palpable in the posterior vaginal fornix and an ovarian endometrioma might be evident on bimanual palpation. The pelvic anatomy might be normal with mild disease. It is useful to assess for cervical excitation (pain on moving the cervix interiorly), as this stretches the uterosacral ligaments, which may be painful in cases of deep infiltrating endometriosis.

> **HINTS AND TIPS**
>
> A bimanual vaginal examination should be performed very gently in this cohort of patients. Awareness should be considered that for many of these women, internal examinations can be very painful.

INVESTIGATIONS

Transvaginal ultrasound

Of late, transvaginal ultrasound imaging is becoming extremely useful in the detection of endometriosis and adenomyosis; ovarian endometriomas with their typical 'ground glass' appearance can be visualized, the location and mobility of the adnexa can be assessed to look for immobile 'kissing ovaries' (Fig. 6.2), uterovesical and rectovaginal nodules can sometimes be detected, as well as the presence of pain elicited during scanning, which is a significant finding. The myometrium can also be assessed for

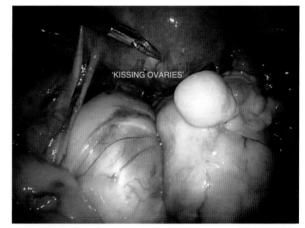

Fig. 6.2 Classic appearance of 'kissing ovaries' adherent to the posterior surface of the uterus seen at the time of laparoscopy. From Bachman EA. *Ferri's Clinical Advisor 2024*. 1st Edition. 2024: 535-537.

adenomyosis or focal adenomyomas (discrete area of adenomyosis similar to a fibroid).

Specialist tests

At present, the gold standard for diagnosis and treatment of endometriosis is with laparoscopy. The classic blue/grey 'powder-burn' lesions of endometriosis might be seen. Nonpigmented lesions can appear as opaque white areas of peritoneum, red lesions or glandular lesions. An excision biopsy should be taken to confirm diagnosis histologically. Generally, laparoscopies for endometriosis should be performed for diagnosis and treatment (if endometriosis is found). Occasionally more than one procedure is required depending on the severity of the disease. MRI may be performed prior to surgery if extensive disease is suspected, e.g., involving the bowel, which may require a colorectal surgeon to be present or the ureters, requiring a urologist.

At the time of laparoscopy, endometriosis can be classified and graded. One scoring system is the American Fertility Society Classification of endometriosis, whereby the size and location of endometriotic lesions and appearance of fallopian tubes and ovaries are assessed. More recent classification tools such as #Enzian scoring system have been devised, whereby the focus is on the main areas affected in the pelvis and whether the endometriosis is superficial (affecting the peritoneum/organ surfaces only) or deeply infiltrating (affecting the underlying structures).

Aetiology

Several theories have been suggested to explain the aetiology of endometriosis (Table 6.1). To date, the origin of this disease is still not fully understood.

TREATMENT

Treatment depends on the severity and symptoms of the disease and a holistic approach should be taken to tailor this to the patient's individual needs. The aim of treatment is to alleviate symptoms, halt progression of disease to reduce complications, optimize fertility and ensure they have adequate psychological support, if required.

Endometriosis is a chronic condition with up to 40% of women developing recurring symptoms within 1 year of stopping treatment. Maintenance therapy with medical treatments reduces the risk of symptom recurrence and significant progression. Pregnancy rates following conservative surgery are directly related to the severity of the disease and can improve within the 6 months postoperatively. Malignant change within endometriotic lesions is rare and most commonly occurs in ovarian endometriosis; this has been estimated in approximately 0.5% to 1% of endometriosis.

Psychological wellbeing may be impacted by suffering from chronic pain. This may include the impact on relationships, particularly if patients experience painful sexual intercourse, patients feeling dismissed or not listened to by clinicians and ongoing

Table 6.1 Proposed theories for the aetiology of endometriosis

Retrograde menstruation/implantation (Sampson's theory)	This is the theory that during menstruation, endometrial tissue spills into the pelvic cavity through the fallopian tubes. This ectopic endometrium then implants and becomes functional, responding to the hormones of the ovarian cycle. The implantation theory would also account for the rare cases of endometriosis found during surgical incision, for example, following open myomectomy or caesarean section. However, this theory does not account for the existence of endometriosis at the distant sites in the body (e.g., lungs).
Lymphatic and venous embolization/seeding from previous surgery	This theory hypothesizes that endometrial tissue is transported through the body by the lymphatic or venous channels and would explain the rare cases of distant sites for endometriosis. It may also explain how seeding from previous endometriosis surgery can result in port-site endometriosis. However, distant endometriotic deposits would be expected to be more common if the lymphatic and venous embolization theories were the only mechanism for the development of endometriosis.
Coelomic metaplasia	This theory relies on the principle that tissues of certain embryonic origin maintain their ability to undergo metaplasia and differentiate into other tissue types. This is certainly true of peritoneum of coelomic origin, which can undergo metaplasia and differentiate into functional endometrium. However, this does not explain the distribution of endometriosis within the peritoneal cavity itself (most common in the lower part of the peritoneal cavity) or the presence of endometriosis in sites of the body that are not of coelomic origin.
Genetic and immunological factors	The role of a genetic influence is supported by the strong family history seen in women with endometriosis, but its exact role has not yet been characterized. It is possible that women with a genetic predisposition to endometriosis have an abnormal response to the presence of ectopic endometrium, which results in endometriosis developing. There is some evidence that an altered or defective cell-mediated response is implicated. Can be seven times more likely if first-degree relative has it.
Composite theories	None of the above theories alone account for all cases of endometriosis, however, together all the theories could play a role.

fertility concerns. Subfertility may arise with endometriosis secondary to distorted adnexal anatomy inhibiting ovum capture after ovulation, impaired fertilization, inference with oocyte development of early embryogenesis and reduced endometrial receptivity.

Medical management

Endometriotic lesions regress during pregnancy and after the menopause (due to the absence of hormonal variation). Hormonal treatment for endometriosis can reduce pain but most will concurrently act as contraception (Table 6.2).

SURGICAL MANAGEMENT

Surgical options should be considered if medical management does not control symptoms, structural pain is present, or invasive fertility investigations are required.

Risks of surgery include damage to other pelvic structures, e.g., bowel, bladder and ureters. Women must also be informed about potential recurrence of endometriosis, and no change to symptoms of pelvic pain. Deep infiltrating endometriosis with bowel or ureteric involvement may require a joint procedure with colorectal or urology teams. As an adjunct to surgery for deep endometriosis, downregulation with gonadotrophin-releasing hormone agonists for 3 to 6 months prior to surgery can be considered after careful multidisciplinary team discussion.

In patients with refractory endometriosis and/or adenomyosis who have completed their family and exhausted more conservative measures, hysterectomy with bilateral salpingo-oophorectomy with excision of endometriosis can be considered. The aim of surgery is to remove all affected organs and eliminate the natural cyclical variation of oestrogen and progesterone that endometriosis responds to, as well as stop recurrence of disease in the uterus and or ovaries. As many of these women are relatively young, hormone replacement therapy is recommended afterwards. Oestrogen replacement may cause a recurrence of endometriosis in a small percentage of women. Continuous combined oestrogen and progesterone replacement might further reduce the rate of recurrence because of the protective effects of progestogens on endometriosis.

The management ladder of endometriosis is summarized in Fig. 6.3.

CLINICAL NOTES

Endometriosis is a chronic condition and can have a considerable effect on a patient's quality of life due to pelvic pain. There is a large amount of support and information available from organizations such as Endometriosis UK and clinicians should inform women about these services and support groups.

Table 6.2 Summary of medical treatment of endometriosis

Drug	Mode of action	Duration of action	Side effects
Simple analgesia; paracetamol, NSAIDs and opiates	Antiinflammatory	For as long as it is taken	Contraindicated in brittle asthmatics, gastritis, gastrointestinal bleeds
Progestogens	Pseudopregnancy – decidualizes and causes regression of endometriosis	POP – For as long as it is taken Subdermal implant – 3 years Depo injection – 3 months	Break-through bleeding, weight gain, oedema, acne, abdominal bloating, increased appetite, decreased libido
Combine oral contraceptive pill	Suppresses ovulation. Tricycling also limits the number of withdrawal bleeds.	For as long as it is taken	Least effective. Mainly acts by reducing frequency of periods
GnRH analogues/antagonists	Pseudomenopause – desensitizes pituitary gonadotrophs, leading to a temporary, reversible state of hypogonadotropic hypogonadism	1 monthly injections Maximum 6 months treatment	Hot flushes, break-through bleeding, vaginal dryness, headaches, decreased libido, bone density loss Most effective but cannot be used long term due to osteoporosis
Levonorgestrel-releasing intrauterine system (LNG-IUS)	Steady continuous delivery of progesterone causes thinning of endometrium and a degree of suppression of endometriosis lesions	Mirena – 5 years	Amenorrhoea, break-through bleeding, coil-expulsion, can take 3–6 months to take effect

GnRH, *Gonadotropin hormone-releasing hormone;* NSAIDs, *nonsteroidal anti-inflammatory drugs;* POP, *progesterone-only pill.*

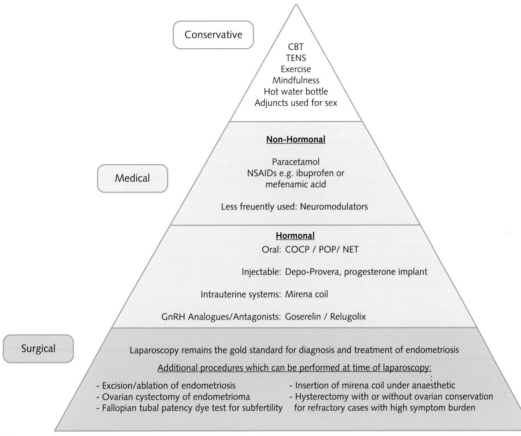

Fig. 6.3 Summary ladder of treatment and management for endometriosis and adenomyosis. *CBT,* Cognitive behavioural therapy; *COCP,* combined oral contraceptive pill; *POP,* progesterone-only pill; *GnRH,* gonadotropin-releasing hormone; *NET,* norethisterone; *NSAIDs,* nonsteroidal anti-inflammatories; *TENS,* transcutaneous electrical nerve stimulation.

● Chapter Summary

- Endometriosis is a chronic gynaecological condition characterized by cyclical pelvic pain caused by ectopic endometrial tissue.
- It is a common presentation seen in both primary and secondary care.
- A holistic approach should be taken for managing endometriosis and adenomyosis. Individualized treatment is aimed at symptom control and improving quality of life.

UKMLA Conditions
Menstrual problems

UKMLA Presentations
Acute and chronic pain management
Endometriosis
Painful sexual intercourse
Pelvic pain

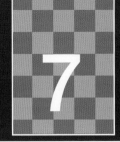

Pelvic pain and dyspareunia

BACKGROUND

Pelvic pain is a common gynaecological presentation in the emergency department, primary and secondary care. Chronic pain is thought to affect up to one in six adult women. Acute pelvic pain is sudden in onset, often secondary to new pathology, for example, an ovarian cyst torsion; whereas chronic pelvic pain is defined as intermittent or constant pelvic pain that lasts 6 months or more, not occurring exclusively with menstruation, intercourse or pregnancy. It is a symptom therefore investigations must be made to identify a possible underlying cause.

Symptoms

The type of pain experienced should be elicited through the history and examination. In terms of acute pain, it may be constant or intermittent, mild or severe, localized to the pelvis with or without radiation and exacerbated or relieved by certain factors. Chronic pain may be cyclical, related to the menses or noncyclical.

Symptoms: 'The 4 Ds of pain'

- Dysmenorrhoea (painful periods)
- Dyspareunia (pain having sex); classified as superficial or deep, depending on whether it is experienced superficially at the area of the vulva and introitus or deep within the pelvis. (Table 7.1)
- Dyschezia (pain opening bowels)
- Dysuria (bladder pain/pain passing urine)

Differential diagnosis

If a woman presents with acute pelvic pain, urgent pathologies should first be excluded:

- Ectopic pregnancy
- Ovarian cyst accidents; ruptured ovarian cyst or ovarian torsion
- Pelvic inflammatory disease (PID)

Nongynaecological causes must also be considered; for example, gastrointestinal and urinary conditions. Chronic pelvic pain may be secondary to underlying endometriosis, adenomyosis or pelvic adhesions. Again, nongynaecological causes must also be considered, such as nerve entrapment or irritable bowel syndrome (Table 7.2).

Table 7.1 Differential diagnosis of dyspareunia

Superficial	Deep
Congenital	**Congenital**
Vaginal atresia Vaginal septum	Incomplete vaginal atresia Vaginal septum
Infection	**Infection**
Vulvovaginitis (see Chapter 13)	Pelvic inflammatory disease (see Chapter 9)
Postsurgery	**Postsurgery**
Relating to childbirth, e.g., episiotomy Pelvic floor repair	Relating to childbirth Pelvic floor repair
Vulval disease	**Pelvic disease**
Bartholin cyst Vulval dystrophies Vulval cancers	Endometriosis/adenomyosis Fibroids Ovarian cysts/tumours
Psychosexual	**Psychosexual**
Vaginismus Vulvodynia	Vaginismus
Atrophic changes Postmenopausal Vulval dystrophies, e.g., lichen sclerosis (see Chapter 17) Breastfeeding (hypo-oestrogenic state)	

DIAGNOSIS

History

A detailed history of the pain is essential to distinguish between acute (Table 7.3) and chronic pain, and to differentiate between the wide range of possible differential diagnoses.

Important features in the history are:

- Last menstrual period – could she be pregnant?
- Categorizing the nature of pain
- Association with menstrual cycle
- Associated symptoms
- Gynaecological history: menstrual pattern, intermenstrual bleeding, postcoital bleeding, sexually transmitted infection (STI) and smear history
- Medical and surgical history
- Social history

Table 7.2 Differential diagnosis of pelvic pain

Acute	Chronic
PID (see Chapter 9) Tubo-ovarian abscess Post procedural: Medical termination of pregnancy, medical management of miscarriage, insertion of intrauterine contraceptive system or hysteroscopy	Endometriosis Adenomyosis (see Chapter 6) Adhesions (post surgical or post infective, e.g., PID) Subacute appendicitis
Early pregnancy complications (see Chapter 18) Miscarriage Ectopic pregnancy	
Gynaecological malignancy (see Chapter 12)	Gynaecological malignancy
Ovarian cyst (see Chapter 11) Rupture Haemorrhage Torsion	Gastrointestinal pathology Diverticulitis Irritable bowel syndrome
Fibroid necrosis (see Chapter 5)	Mass effect from large fibroid uterus
Ovulation pain (mittelschmerz)	Large ovarian cyst
Abscess Bartholin cyst Labial	
Urinary tract infection Renal calculi	Megaureter or hydronephrosis secondary to strictures from ureteric endometriosis or external compression from large fibroid uterus
Appendicitis	

PID, *Pelvic inflammatory disease.*

Targeted 'SOCRATES' pain history

S – Site of pain

O – Onset: sudden or gradual

C – Character or the pain: sharp, dull, crampy in nature

R – Radiation

A – Associated symptoms: nausea/vomiting, diarrhoea, fever, change in discharge

T – Time: how long has this pain been there?

E – Exacerbating/alleviating factors: positional, related to sexual intercourse, does analgesia help?

S – Severity: on a scale of 1 to 10, how bad is this pain?

Examination

See Chapter 1 for full gynaecological examination technique.

- Abdominal palpation

Inspect

Is the patient in pain?
Is the patient obviously pregnant?
Sick bowl / any medications around the patient?

Percuss and auscultate

Are there signs of peritonism such as guarding rebound tenderness?
Are bowel sounds present?

Palpate

Abdominal:
Using the palm of the hand, gently palpate the four quadrants of the abdomen for areas of tenderness.
Is the pain localised or generalised?
Deep or superficial?
Is the uterus palpable? (large fibroid or gravid uterus)

Bimanual:
Cervicitis? (Ectopic, PID, peritonitis)
Adnexal mass? (Ovarian cyst, ectopic, tubo-ovarian abscess)
Tender or palpable rectovaginal nodules? (Endometriosis)
Bulky tender uterus? (Adenomyosis)

Speculum examination:
Vaginal discharge? Colour / odour / amount
Cervical pathology? Cancer / ectropion

Fig. 7.1 Steps of examination for pelvic pain. PID, *Pelvic inflammatory disease.*

- Vulval/vaginal/cervical inspection
- Bimanual pelvic examination

Steps for clinical examination are shown in Fig. 7.1.

INVESTIGATIONS

Target investigations for a specific differential as highlighted by the history if possible. A summary list of the investigations used in patients who present with pelvic pain and/or dyspareunia is shown in Table 7.4.

Treatment

Management of acute or chronic pelvic pain depends on the underlying diagnoses, which are explored in other chapters. See Figs 7.2 and 7.3 for the algorithms to aid diagnosis of pelvic pain and dyspareunia.

ETHICS

As with all chronic pain it is important to consider psychological and social factors as well as physical causes of pain. Women must be supported and offered advice, for example, introduction to support groups, or referral to a pain clinic. A holistic approach should be taken to managing women with pelvic pain.

Table 7.3 Common acute presentations of pelvic pain in women

	Pathology	Typical presentation	Risk factors	Important points
Gynaecological	Ovarian torsion	Sudden onset unilateral iliac fossa pain, associated with nausea and vomiting, radiating to upper thighs.	Known ovarian cyst, previous ovarian torsion, childhood (longer infundibulo-pelvic ligaments compared with adults)	Prompt recognition and surgical management (detorsion) are necessary, to prevent irreversible ischaemia and loss of ovarian function.
	Ovarian cyst rupture	Similar presentation to torsion.	Known ovarian cyst, previous cyst rupture and ovulation.	Small self-contained cyst rupture may present with an initial severe pain followed by relief. Large cyst rupture with ongoing bleeding may present as haemodynamic instability or collapse, due to large haemoperitoneum.
	Mittelschmerz	Acute mid-cycle pain associated with ovulation.	Ovulation	Responds well to hormonal treatments which suppress ovulation, e.g., COCP
	PID	Gradually worsening diffuse lower abdominal pain, often associated with foul-smelling vaginal discharge and fever.	Multiple sexual partners, unprotected sexual intercourse, post procedure, e.g., hysteroscopy, surgical management of miscarriage/termination, intrauterine device insertion.	Management may be as an outpatient with oral antibiotics, or inpatient with intravenous antibiotics depending on the severity of infection. Large tubo-ovarian abscesses may require surgical drainage. PID can result in severe sepsis and have long-term effects on fertility, therefore prompt recognition treatment is essential.
	Bartholin/labial/vulval abscess	Bartholin abscess is an abscess of Bartholin gland (the glands are situated bilaterally towards the posterior fourchette). Labial abscesses are commonly situated on the labia majora.	Previous Bartholin cyst/abscess. Shaving of pubic hair leads to folliculitis/abscess.	Both abscesses cause acute pain, can result in systemic infection and usually require incision and drainage. Bartolin's abscess can be managed with either a Word catheter or marsupialization/enucleation, to reduce risk of recurrence. Word catheters remain in situ for a number of weeks to allow for continual drainage of abscess during this time.
	Fibroid degeneration	Severe localized abdominal pain to location of fibroids.	Fibroid uterus, pregnancy, postuterine artery embolization	Patients may have a raised C-reactive protein and fever. Treatment is usually conservative with analgesia and observation.
	Dysmenorrhoea	Cyclical pain whilst menstruating/immediately prior to menses.	Endometriosis, adenomyosis, anovulatory cycles	Important to take a thorough history to assess for acute or chronic pain with endometriosis/adenomyosis (see Chapter 7).
Gastrointestinal	Appendicitis	Initial pain in the central abdomen which radiates to McBurney's point. Rovsing's sign positive.	Appendix in situ	Acute surgical presentation with prompt diagnosis to avoid ruptured appendicitis with faecal peritonitis.
	Diverticulitis	Left iliac fossa pain, constipation, fever, age >40.	Obesity, known diverticulosis, male	Requires antibiotic treatment under surgical team to prevent bowel perforation.
Urological	Urinary tract infection (UTI)	Suprapubic pain, dysuria, hesitancy, frequency, possible haematuria, fever. Common in pregnancy.	Urological tract anatomical anomalies, previous UTIs	Treatment with oral or intravenous antibiotics depends on severity of infection. A urine dipstick to ensure clearance of the infection is good practice in high-risk patients.

COCP, *Combined oral contraceptive pill;* Hb, *haemoglobin;* MC&S *microscopy, culture and sensitivity;* PID, *pelvic inflammatory disease.*

Table 7.4 Investigations when assessing pelvic pain and dyspareunia

Investigation	Procedure
Observations: Heart rate Blood pressure Respiratory rate Oxygen saturations Temperature	Regular observations are required, particularly in acute presentations to assess for sepsis or haemodynamic instability. Pyrexia and tachycardia are associated with pelvic inflammatory disease (PID). Rupture of an ovarian cyst can cause intraperitoneal bleeding and, subsequently, hypotension with tachycardia. A ruptured ectopic pregnancy would also present with these signs. It should be noted that hypotension is a late sign in an otherwise healthy patient and its absence does not exclude these diagnoses.
Urine pregnancy test	A urine pregnancy test is mandatory in a patient of reproductive age with acute abdominal pain. It must be performed regardless of the date of the last menstrual period or if the symptoms suggest a gastrointestinal cause. It may highlight or exclude pregnancy, ectopic pregnancy or miscarriage as the cause.
Urine dipstick/midstream urine MC&S	A midstream urine sample should be sent to exclude a urinary tract infection if symptomatic or urine dipstick positive.
Blood tests	Full blood count Urea and electrolytes C-reactive protein Venous blood gas – rapid Hb assessment and lactate Group and Save
Infection screen	Midstream urine sample Vulval/high vaginal swabs Endocervical swabs to assess for STIs
Radiological investigations	Pelvic ultrasound scan (transvaginal or abdominal in children/those who are virgo intacta) to assess for ovarian, uterine or endometrial pathology or early pregnancy complications such as miscarriage/ectopic. Abdominal X-ray.
Biopsy for vulval disease	If the appearance of the vulva is abnormal, a biopsy may be indicated. This can be performed under local anaesthesia, depending on the size of the lesion.
Laparoscopy to exclude: endometriosis ovarian cyst ectopic pregnancy adhesions pelvic inflammatory disease	

Hb, *Haemoglobin;* MC&S *microscopy, culture and sensitivity;* STIs, *sexually transmitted infections.*

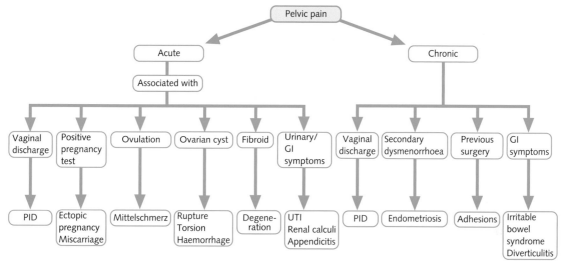

Fig. 7.2 Algorithm for pelvic pain. *GI,* Gastrointestinal; *PID,* pelvic inflammatory disease; *UTI,* urinary tract infection.

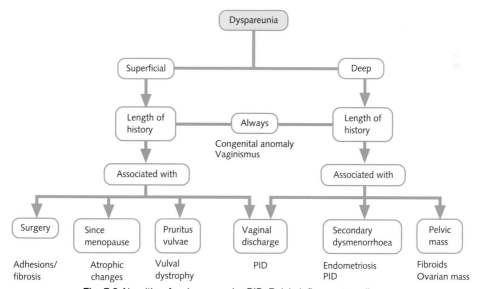

Fig. 7.3 Algorithm for dyspareunia. *PID,* Pelvic inflammatory disease.

A sexual history should be taken from the patient in a sensitive manner and in an area of privacy, with a nonjudgemental approach. Be aware of previous sexual trauma which can contribute to dyspareunia, vaginismum, vulvodynia and chronic pelvic pain.

Before palpating the abdomen, always enquire about areas of tenderness to palpate these areas last. For any intimate examination (bimanual or speculum) consent must be gained and a chaperone should be present; the examination should be performed in an area of privacy.

Chapter Summary

- Ability to identify and diagnose both acute and chronic gynaecological conditions is crucial to enable timely and appropriate management.
- In presentations of acute abdominal pain, conditions that are considered gynaecological emergencies such as an ectopic pregnancy or ovarian torsion should be considered and excluded first.
- Accurate diagnosis, effective management and communication from the first presentation may help to reduce long-term effects of acute presentations, or extensive investigations and operations in chronic conditions.
- There is a wide range of differential diagnoses for pelvic pain and dyspareunia that should be explored. It is, however, important to consider nongynaecological causes.

UKMLA Conditions
Atrophic vaginitis
Menstrual problems
Urinary tract infection

UKMLA Presentations
Abnormal urinalysis
Acute abdominal pain
Acute and chronic pain management
Ectopic pregnancy
Fibroids
Menopause
Painful sexual intercourse
Pelvic inflammatory disease
Pelvic pain
Sepsis
Urinary symptoms
Vaginal discharge

Sexually transmitted infections

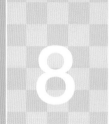

BACKGROUND

Sexually transmitted infections (STIs) are transmitted through sexual contact, including vaginal, anal and oral sex, although some can also spread via blood, or be transmitted from mother to child during pregnancy and childbirth. More than 30 different bacteria, viruses and parasites are known to be responsible. Untreated, STIs can lead to chronic pelvic pain, pelvic inflammatory disease (PID), ectopic pregnancies, gynaecological malignancies (human papillomavirus [HPV] infection and cervical cancer) and subfertility. In pregnancy, STIs can be a major cause of congenital abnormalities, miscarriage, stillbirth, prematurity and neonatal morbidity.

The World Health Organization estimates that more than 1 million STIs are acquired every day, the majority in lower- and middle-income countries. Chlamydia is the most common bacterial STI diagnosed in England (up to 46% of all STIs) and genital warts are the most common viral STI. Young adults (<25 years) are more likely to be diagnosed with an STI than older age groups. Other risk factors include earlier onset of sexual activity, previous history of STIs, frequent partner changes and non-use of barrier contraception.

History

An accurate sexual history is essential in enabling assessment of risk factors and aiding diagnosis and management. Patients may feel embarrassed, anxious or shameful, so it is important to be open and maintain a respectful and non-judgemental attitude. The interview should be conducted sensitively, using appropriate language that is understandable and avoiding euphemisms. Be aware that patients may not feel comfortable disclosing sexual history with a partner or relative present.

COMMUNICATION

A sexual risk assessment may include the following questions:

- Are you currently or have ever been sexually active?
- Have your partner(s) been men, women or both?
- Do you have regular partner(s)?
- Have you had a change in sexual partner in the last 6 months?
- When did you last have sex? What kind of sex do you engage in? Vaginal, anal, oral?
- Do you use contraception? What type of contraception do you use?
- Have you ever had unprotected sex? How regularly do you have unprotected sex?
- Have you previously been diagnosed with a sexually transmitted infection and if so was it treated?

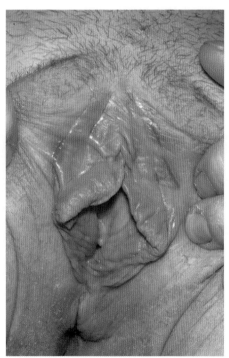

Fig. 8.1 Vaginal candidiasis. Red inflamed vulva and vagina with milky discharge is the hallmark of vaginal candidiasis. (From Dinulos JGH. *Skin Disease: Diagnosis and Treatment.* 2018: 241–281. © 2018.)

Establish the presenting symptom along with the duration and onset. This includes:

- Vaginal discharge: A description of the discharge can help identify its origin and point towards a diagnosis. Enquire about timing of onset, colour, consistency, character and smell. Some causes of vaginal discharge have a typical appearance, such as *Candida*, which appears as a thick, itchy and white discharge without an offensive smell (Fig. 8.1), whereas with bacterial vaginosis there is typically a grey, fishy-smelling discharge (Fig. 8.2).
- Unusual vaginal or rectal bleeding
- Abdominal/pelvic pain or distension
- Urinary symptoms: Dysuria, frequency
- Genital lumps, ulcers or swellings
- Dyspareunia (superficial and deep)
- Systemic symptoms: Fever, unintended weight loss, nausea and vomiting, rashes

Take a full gynaecological history. Enquire whether cervical screening is up-to-date, particularly if malignancy is suspected. A ring pessary may have been sited to relieve genital prolapse, which could be causing excess discharge. Previous history of gynaecological surgery could be linked with development of a ureterovaginal or vesicovaginal fistula. A full medical, surgical and drug history should be sought, as conditions such as diabetes or recent antibiotic use can predispose to *Candida* infection. For completion, enquire about vaginal hygiene or changes to washing powders or soaps, which can cause allergic reactions or irritation.

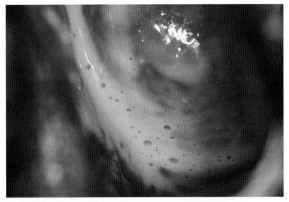

Fig. 8.2 Bacterial vaginosis. The grey, homogeneous discharge that coats the tissues is characteristic. (From Smith D, Saks E. *Ferri's Clinical Advisor 2023.* 2023: 1600–1600.e1.)

CLINICAL NOTES

VAGINAL DISCHARGE

Vaginal discharge is often a normal physiological process but can sometimes be pathological (see Table 8.1). The distinction between the two can be made by taking a history, performing an examination and conducting appropriate investigations. Treatment can then be advised based on the diagnosis.

Common *physiological* causes of vaginal discharge can be linked to fluctuating oestrogen levels during the luteal phase of the menstrual cycle and pregnancy.

Common *pathological* causes of vaginal discharge are sexually transmitted and nonsexually transmitted infections. Malignancy, especially cervical, should always be considered and excluded.

Differential	Cause of discharge
Physiological	• Cervical ectopy/ectropion
	• Vestibular gland secretions
	• Residual menstrual fluid
	• Vaginal transudate
	• Cervical mucus
Infective	• Sexually transmitted infections
	• *Chlamydia trachomatis*
	• *Trichomonas vaginalis*
	• *Neisseria gonorrhoeae*
	• Nonsexually transmitted infections
	• *Candida albicans*
	• Bacterial vaginosis
Inflammation	• Allergy to soap/contraceptives, etc.
	• Atrophic changes
	• Postoperative granulation tissue
	• Foreign body
	• Retained tampon/condom
	• Ring pessaries
	• Pregnancy related: retained products of conception (RPOC)
Malignancy	• Vulval/vaginal cancer
	• Cervical cancer
	• Endometrial cancer
Fistula	• From bowel, bladder or urethra to vagina

Management of vaginal discharge depends on its origin, and whether this is physiological or pathological. Treatment of conditions such as pelvic inflammatory disease (PID), gynaecological malignancies and vulval disease are detailed in individual chapters. Women with physiological discharge should be reassured that this is a normal process and advised on hygiene, as it can be exacerbated by practices such as excessive washing or douching.

Table 8.1 Summary of common STIs and infections of the genital tract

Organism	Clinical features	Investigations	Management
Chlamydia trachomatis (obligate intracellular bacterium)	• Asymptomatic (80%) • PCB/IMB • Lower abdominal/pelvic pain • Muco-purulent vaginal discharge (cloudy or yellow) • Cervicitis +/– contact bleeding • Dysuria, deep dyspareunia **Complications**: PID, subfertility, ectopic pregnancy, Fitz-Hugh-Curtis syndrome (liver swelling and peri-hepatic adhesions secondary to PID), neonatal conjunctivitis/pneumonitis (if acquired in pregnancy)	• **NAAT**: Urethral, endocervical and vulvovaginal swabs • First-catch urine **Note**: Contract tracing should be performed	**Nonpregnancy** - Doxycycline 100 mg BD 7/7 - Azithromycin 1 g PO + 500 mg OD 2/7 - Alt: Erythromycin 500 mg BD 10–14 days or ofloxacin 200 mg BD/400 mg OD 7/7 **Pregnancy** - Azithromycin 1 g PO + 500 mg OD for 2/7 - Erythromycin 500 mg QDS for 7/7 or 500 mg BD for 14/7 - Amoxicillin 500 mg TDS 7/7 - TOC 3/52 after completion - Avoid intercourse until completion of treatment
Neisseria gonorrhoeae (gram-negative bacterium)	• Asymptomatic (50%) • PCB/IMB • Muco-purulent vaginal discharge (yellow) • Lower abdominal/pelvic pain • Dysuria • Cervicitis +/– contact bleeding **Complications**: PID, subfertility, ectopic pregnancy, disseminated gonococcal infection/septicaemia, meningitis, endocarditis, preterm labour, neonatal conjunctivitis, neonatal infection	**Culture confirmation tests on selective media**: Monoclonal antibody test; blue agglutination is positive for gonorrhoea **Microscopy**: Gram-negative bean-shaped diplococci (stains pink) **NAAT**: Urethral, endocervical and vulvo-vaginal swabs **Note**: Contract tracing should be performed	**Nonpregnancy** - 1st: Ceftriaxone 1 g IM - 2nd: Ciprofloxacin 500 mg PO (if susceptible) - Cefixime 400 mg PO + azithromycin 2 g PO - Gentamicin 240 mg IM + azithromycin 2 g PO **Pregnancy** - 1st: Ceftriaxone 1 g IM - 2nd: Spectinomycin 2 g IM - 3rd: Azithromycin 2 g PO - TOC 3/52 after completion - Avoid intercourse until completion of treatment
Vulvovaginal candidiasis (commonly *Candida albicans*)	• Asymptomatic • Vulval/vaginal soreness • Vulval itching/excoriation • Thick, white, nonoffensive curd-like vaginal discharge (like 'cottage-cheese') • White plaques on vaginal wall • Vulval erythema/fissuring • Swelling and oedema **Associations**: Antibiotic use, immunocompromised states (diabetes, HIV, steroid use), prolonged antibiotic use	**Microscopy**: Vulval-vaginal swabs	**Nonpregnancy** - PO fluconazole 150 mg stat - PV clotrimazole 500 mg (if oral therapy contraindicated) **Pregnancy** - PV clotrimazole 500 mg nocte for up to 7 nights

Continued

Table 8.1 Summary of common STIs and infections of the genital tract—cont'd

Organism	Clinical features	Investigations	Management
Bacterial vaginosis (overgrowth of anaerobes including *Gardnerella, Mycoplasma*)	• Asymptomatic (50%) • Thin, homogeneous, greyish-white, offensive 'fishy-smelling' vaginal discharge • Vaginal pH >4.5 • Presence of 'clue cells' on wet mount microscopy **Associations**: Vaginal douching, recent change in sexual partner, multiple partners, presence of an STI, smoking **Complications**: PID, postpartum endometritis, 2nd-trimester miscarriage, preterm delivery	**Microscopy:** Vulvo-vaginal swabs	**Nonpregnancy** - Metronidazole 400 mg BD 7/7 **Pregnancy** - Asymptomatic: Not needed - Symptomatic: As above
Trichomonas vaginalis (flagellated single-cell protozoon)	• Asymptomatic (50%) • 'Frothy yellow' offensive vaginal discharge • Vulval itching/inflammation • Petechial lesions on cervix ('strawberry cervix') (Fig. 8.3) • Vulva/vaginal soreness • PCB/IMB	**NAAT**: Vulvo-vaginal swabs **Microscopy:** Detection of motile trichomonads	**Nonpregnancy** - Metronidazole 400 mg BD 7/7 **Pregnancy** - Metronidazole 400 mg BD 7/7
Genital herpes (Herpes simplex virus HSV1/HSV2)	• Asymptomatic • Vulval soreness, itching, pain • Vesicular rash, blistering or multiple painful shallow ulcers on the external genitalia or perianal region (Fig. 8.4) • Systemic infection (fever, myalgia) • Dysuria, vaginal discharge • Bilateral tender inguinal lymphadenopathy Recurrent herpes may be asymptomatic and are generally milder than in primary herpes	**NAAT**: Swabs from lesions allow direct detection of HSV **Serology**: Testing for HSV type-specific antibodies (IgG)	**Nonpregnancy** - Aciclovir 400 mg TDS 5/7 **Pregnancy** - Aciclovir 400 mg TDS 5/7 - Suppressive aciclovir 400 mg TDS OD until delivery - Advise delivery by Caesarean section if primary HSV infection is acquired in the 3rd trimester (40% risk of transmission and neonatal herpes at time of delivery)
Syphilis (*Treponema pallidum*, a spirochete bacterium)	• **Primary syphilis**: Chancre (single, painless, indurated, ulcer with rolled edges) develops around 3 weeks after exposure. Heals spontaneously. • **Secondary syphilis**: Occurs several weeks after with a generalized flu-like illness, fever, malaise, and a maculopapular rash, typically affecting the trunk, limbs and palms/soles. Wart-like papules appear in the mouth and anogenital area, known as *condylomata lata*. • **Late syphilis**: Can mimic other diseases and affect most systems in the body, especially the cardiovascular and neurological systems. **Complications in pregnancy**: Miscarriage, stillbirth, preterm delivery, congenital syphilis, neonatal death.	**Serological testing:** Treponemal enzyme immunoassay is used to detect IgG and IgM antibodies to syphilis **NAAT**: Swabs from lesions	**Early disease: Latent <2 years, primary, secondary** - IM Benzathine penicillin G 2.4 MU. 1 dose in 1st/2nd trimesters; 2 doses (1 week apart) in 3rd trimester. - Allergy: Ceftriaxone 500 mg IM OD 10 days **Late disease (latent or unknown duration)** - IM Benzathine penicillin G 2.4 MU. Weekly for 3 weeks in all trimesters **If screen positive**: Send second sample for different treponemal antibody to confirm disease. Do a rapid plasma reagin test to establish baseline titre levels before treatment. **Offer repeat testing to those at high risk**: Sex workers, multiple sexual partners, sexual contact with men who have sex with men (MSM), endemic areas

Table 8.1 Summary of common STIs and infections of the genital tract—cont'd

Organism	Clinical features	Investigations	Management
Genital warts (human papilloma virus 6 and 11)	• Asymptomatic • Flesh-coloured papules typically around the vulva, perineum and perianal area • Vulval itching and discharge	**Biopsy:** Abnormal lesions should be biopsied due to possibility of vulval/anal/vaginal intraepithelial premalignant lesions	**Medical (contraindicated in pregnancy):** Topical creams, Catephen ointment, imiquimod **Surgical (safe in pregnancy):** Ablation (electrocautery, cryotherapy, diathermy)

NAAT, *Nucleic acid amplification testing;* PCB/IMB, *postcoital bleeding;* PID, *pelvic inflammatory disease.*

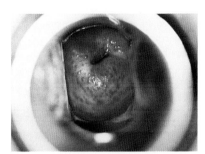

Fig. 8.3 Trichomoniasis. The vaginal mucosa is inflamed and often speckled with petechial lesions, resulting in the so-called strawberry cervix. (From Ball JW, Dains JE. *Seidel's Guide to Physical Examination.* 2023: 448–498.)

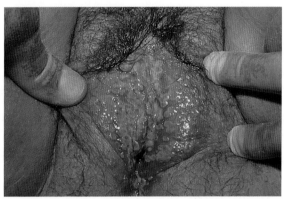

Fig. 8.4 Genital herpes caused by herpes simplex type II. (From White GM, Cox NH. Diseases of the Skin: A Color Atlas and Text. London: Mosby; 2002:282.
From Seller RH, Symons AB. *Differential Diagnosis of Common Complaints.* 2018: c1–c32.)

Examination

A full examination should be performed. This should include:

- General examination
- Abdominal examination
- Genital examination
- Bimanual pelvic examination

Does the patient appear well? General examination should be aimed at identifying signs of systemic infection, such as tachycardia, pyrexia, local lymphadenopathy or malignancy, such as cachexia or generalized lymphadenopathy. Abdominal palpation should assess for pelvic tenderness, which may be present if the patient has PID, or an abdominal mass if malignancy is suspected. If a pelvic mass is felt, it should be assessed for size, tenderness, mobility and nodularity.

Examine the pubic hair for any rash, hair loss and pubic lice. Palpate for lymphadenopathy. Can you identify any vulval or vaginal pathology? Inspect these areas carefully both externally and internally using a Cusco speculum. Look for any vaginal or cervical discharge, inflammation, erythema, excoriation, ulceration, lesions/polyps, retained foreign bodies, warts and local masses. Inspect the perineum and perianal area for the same.

Note any muco-purulent discharge coming from the cervix, contact bleeding and any ulcers. A bimanual vaginal examination should be performed, and the adnexa palpated. This may reveal adnexal tenderness or masses, cervical motion tenderness or uterine tenderness, suggesting PID. An adnexal mass may be suggestive of a pelvic tumour or tubo-ovarian abscess.

INVESTIGATIONS

Observations

Systemic illness suggests an infectious cause; pyrexia and tachycardia are associated with PID.

Urine test

A urine pregnancy test should be performed to exclude pregnancy as the cause. A midstream urine sample should be sent to exclude a urinary tract infection. Chlamydia infection can be tested using both an endocervical swab and first-void urine sample.

Microbiology swabs

Microbiology swabs and a screen for STIs, including high and low vaginal swabs, endocervical swabs and urethral swabs should be performed. Nucleic acid amplification testing (NAAT) testing is widely available for chlamydia, gonorrhoea and herpes simplex. Both chlamydia and gonorrhoea infection can be tested using vulvovaginal, endocervical and urethral swabs. If ulcers are present, swabs should be sent for NAATs for herpes and syphilis testing. Swabs of vaginal discharge for microscopy, culture and sensitivity should be sent, looking for *Candida*, *Trichomonas vaginalis* and bacterial vaginosis.

Blood tests

Raised inflammatory markers (white blood cell count, C-reactive protein level and erythrocyte sedimentation rate) may highlight an infectious cause. Blood cultures should be performed in the event of pyrexia. A blood sample should be sent for syphilis and HIV serology.

Pelvic ultrasound

Transvaginal ultrasound may identify pathology such as thickened endometrium or an adnexal mass.

Specialist tests

If abnormalities are noted on the cervix, or cervical smear is due, a cervical smear or biopsy may be taken. If malignancy is suspected, hysteroscopy with endometrial sampling can be performed as an outpatient procedure or under general anaesthetic. Laparoscopy could be performed if intraabdominal pathology is suspected or to manage PID.

MANAGEMENT

Treatment is dependent on the type of organism and should be in accordance with national guidelines. Table 8.1 summarizes

the common STIs and infections of the genital tract, along with their management. With any diagnosis of an STI it is crucial that the patient is given a detailed verbal and written explanation of the condition, including long-term implications for the health of themselves and their partner(s).

Contact tracing (or partner notification) is the process of contacting and providing healthcare to sexual contacts who may have been at risk of infection from a confirmed case, including providing treatment. The British Association for Sexual Health and HIV advises that the length of time for tracing must include typically 6 months. This process not only protects individuals, but is also important for public health to prevent onward infection and reinfection. This is most easily coordinated by a sexual health clinic and must be done sensitively and confidentially. Patients are advised to abstain from sexual intercourse until they and their partner(s) have completed treatment. A test of cure (TOC) may be performed in some conditions to ensure resolution.

CLINICAL NOTES

HIV

Human immunodeficiency virus (HIV) causes a systemic viral infection that targets the immune system by destroying and impairing the function of immune cells, resulting in immunodeficiency. It is transmitted via a variety of body fluids such as blood, breast milk, semen and vaginal secretions. It is identified by blood tests to detect the presence or absence of antibodies to HIV-1/2 and/or HIV p24 antigen. Symptoms of HIV depend on the stage of infection and individuals, but initially tend to be a generalized influenza-like illness. If the disease progresses, the state of immunodeficiency can cause opportunistic infections and malignancies affecting all body systems. Treatment is by suppression with combinations of antiretroviral therapy. This is not a cure for HIV but suppresses viral replication.

- Vaginal discharge can be a troubling symptom but does not always mean an underlying pathology.
- The most common pathological cause are infections, both sexually transmitted and nonsexually transmitted.
- Diagnosis is elicited from the history and examination, alongside screening for infection and STIs.
- STIs have a profound impact on sexual and reproductive health worldwide, with significant associated morbidity. Sexual health education regarding STIs and the use of barrier contraception is essential to reduce this impact.

UKMLA Conditions	**UKMLA Presentations**
Bacterial vaginosis	Gonorrhoea
Chlamydia	Pelvic inflammatory disease
Gonorrhoea	Urethral discharge and genital ulcers/warts
Syphilis	Vaginal discharge
Trichomonas vaginalis,	Vulval itching/lesion

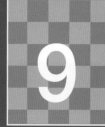
BACKGROUND

Definition

Pelvic inflammatory disease (PID) is defined as the clinical syndrome associated with ascending spread of microorganisms from the endocervix to the endometrium, fallopian tubes and related structures. It can cause endometritis, salpingitis, parametritis, oophoritis, tubo-ovarian abscess or pelvic peritonitis. Severe disease can result in adhesion formation between the liver and the peritoneum, with perihepatitis, known as Fitz–Hugh–Curtis syndrome (Fig. 9.1).

Patients can present with acute or subacute chronic infection.

Prevalence

PID can be challenging to diagnose. In some cases it can be asymptomatic and in others, it can present atypically, therefore the true incident of PID remains unknown. Studies suggest that 2% of general practitioner (GP) visits for women of reproductive age are due to PID. In most cases, PID results from sexually transmitted diseases, therefore its incidence is strongly correlated with the prevalence of sexually transmitted infections, and has increased in most countries (see Chapter 8). In the United States, the highest annual incidence is among sexually active patients in their teenage years; 75% of cases occur in patients under the age of 25. Table 9.1 outlines risk factors for the development of PID.

Aetiology

The most common causative agents for PID are *Neisseria gonorrhoeae* and *Chlamydia trachomatis*. These account for approximately a quarter of cases in the UK, with *Chlamydia* being the most common. Ten percent of women diagnosed with *Chlamydia*, develop PID within 1 year of infection. These organisms act as primary pathogens, causing damage to the protective barrier mechanisms of the endocervix and allowing endogenous bacteria from the vagina and cervix into the upper genital tract as secondary invaders. Table 9.2 lists the common organisms responsible for the development of PID.

DIAGNOSIS

History

A diagnosis of PID is made on clinical grounds, therefore a focused and sensitive history is important. The history should elicit any signs or symptoms of PID, and try to exclude possible differentials. A menstrual history and the use of contraception, in particular barrier methods, should be assessed.

> **COMMON PITFALLS**
>
> Many students can find it embarrassing to talk to patients about their sexual history both in OSCEs and in real life, but remember, if you are uncomfortable, the patient will be uncomfortable too! Always ask if it's ok to ask, and contextualize your questioning – 'Would it be ok if I ask you some personal questions about your sexual history? It is important to help me understand what might be causing your symptoms'. Always ensure you are in a private area and be mindful to sensitively screen for nonconsensual sexual acts and/or signs of sexual abuse.

Symptoms of PID to explore:

- Lower abdominal pain
- Abnormal vaginal or cervical discharge that may be purulent/malodourous
- New deep dyspareunia
- Abnormal vaginal bleeding
- Fever/general malaise/nausea/vomiting
- Asymptomatic – making its diagnosis challenging.

Risk factors to screen for:

- Number of sexual partners in the last year
- Type, if any, of contraception used
- Recent change in partner
- History of sexually transmitted infections (STI)/treatment courses
- When was the most recent STI screen

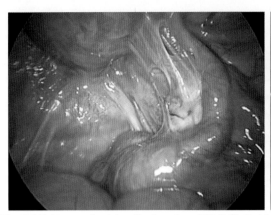 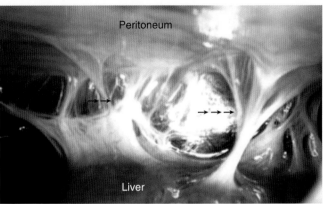

Fig. 9.1 Evidence of pelvic adhesions from PID (*left*). Peri-hepatic adhesions (*black arrows*) seen in Fitz–Hugh–Curtis syndrome (*right*). From Dassel M. *Obstetrics & Gynecology Morning Report: Beyond the Pearls*. 2018. 253-258. © 2018. (https://www.clinicalkey.com/student/search/pelvic%20inflammatory%20disease?source=home&facets=!ct~IM)

Table 9.1 Risk factors for the development of pelvic inflammatory disease

Risk factor	Description
Age	75% of patients are below 25 years
Marital status	Single
Sexual history	Young at first intercourse High frequency of sexual intercourse Multiple sexual partners
Medical history	History of sexually transmitted disease in patient or partner History of pelvic inflammatory disease in patient Recent instrumentation of uterus (e.g., termination of pregnancy)
Contraception	Use of intrauterine contraceptive device, especially insertion within 3 weeks

Table 9.2 Organisms responsible for the development of pelvic inflammatory disease (PID).

Causes	
	Chlamydia trachomatis (common)
	Neisseria gonorrhoeae (common)
	Gardnerella vaginalis (uncommon)
	Mycoplasma genitalium (rare)
	Mycobacterium tuberculosis (rare)
	Secondary to other intraperitoneal disease processes, e.g., acute appendicitis
	Secondary to instrumenting the uterus: Hysteroscopy, insertion of contraceptive intrauterine device, hysterosalpingography, laparoscopic tubal patency dye test, surgical termination of pregnancy or surgical management of miscarriage

Examination

After gaining consent for a bimanual and speculum examination, ensuring you are in a private area and have a chaperone present, gently palpate the abdomen, assessing for lower pelvic pain and/or guarding, suggestive of peritonitis. Rarely, right upper quadrant pain may be present due to Fitz–Hugh–Curtis syndrome.

Vaginal examination with a speculum may show abnormal cervical or vaginal mucopurulent discharge. This is often slight and may be transient. An endocervical, high vaginal and low vaginal swab should be taken for further analysis (see investigations).

A bimanual vaginal examination should be performed and the adnexa should be examined.

Pelvic examination may reveal adnexal tenderness (with or without a palpable mass, suggestive of a tubo-ovarian abscess), cervical motion tenderness (present in cervicitis) or uterine tenderness (suggestive of endometritis).

DIFFERENTIALS BOX

The differential diagnoses for pelvic inflammatory disease (PID) include both gynaecological and nongynaecological conditions such as an ovarian cyst accident, acute flare of endometriosis, early pregnancy complications including ectopic pregnancy, appendicitis, urinary tract infections or constipation.

INVESTIGATIONS

Initial investigations such as observations and urine pregnancy test should be performed immediately for women of reproductive age presenting with abdominal pain to the GP or accident and emergency department. Early detection and treatment of sepsis associated with PID is essential (see Table 9.3 for the full list of investigations).

TREATMENT

There should be a low threshold for empirical treatment for PID, even in the absence of definitive diagnostic criteria, as delaying treatment increases the risk of long-term sequelae, such as ectopic pregnancy resulting from damaged fallopian tubes, infertility and chronic pelvic pain from adhesions. Treatment should therefore be started prior to obtaining the results of microbiology specimens.

The principles of treatment:

- Broad-spectrum antibiotic treatment with anaerobic and aerobic cover, e.g., ceftriaxone 2 g IV once daily, plus doxycycline 100 mg oral twice daily, plus metronidazole 400 mg oral twice daily.
- Drainage of abscesses either with interventional radiology or laparoscopically/open surgery depending on case and appropriate expertise.
- Contact tracing.
- Analgesia.

Clinical suspicion of PID

Mild to moderate disease
Patient not septic, low WCC / CRP and systemically not unwell

Severe disease
Sepsis, high WCC / CRP, systemically unwell, immunocompromised state e.g. poorly controlled diabetes or pregnancy, peritonitis or tubo-ovarian abscess

Outpatient management
- Oral antibiotics as per local antimicrobial guidelines for 2 weeks
- Contact tracing of sexual partners
- 72 hour clinical review to ensure response to treatment
- Safety netting advice to seek medical attention if develops fever or worsening pain/symptoms at home

Inpatient management
- Septic screen, IV Antibiotics as per local antimicrobial guidelines, convert to oral once afebrile for 24 hours and to complete 2 week course orally
- Interventional radiological or laparoscopic/open drainage and wash out of pelvis / abscess if clinical deterioration despite 24–48 hours of IV Antibiotics
- Contact tracing of sexual partners
- Repeat ultrasound imaging 6–8 weeks to ensure resolution of tubo-ovarian abscess

LONG-TERM COMPLICATIONS OF PELVIC INFLAMMATORY DISEASE (PID)

PID and its long-term sequelae (Table 9.4) are responsible for a substantial amount of morbidity, both physical and psychological. There are also considerable financial implications, estimated at £100 million per year in the UK. Therefore, primary prevention of the disease is of great importance and needs the help of both the media and healthcare professionals. Government

Table 9.3 Investigations for patients presenting with suspected pelvic inflammatory disease (PID)

Type of investigation	
Observations	• Heart rate, blood pressure, temperature, respiratory rate and oxygen saturation should be recorded. • Pyrexia >38 °C and tachycardia (>100 bpm) should trigger a septic screen and initiation of intravenous (IV) antibiotics within 1 hour.
Urine analysis	• Urine dip to rule out UTI. • Urine MC&S to be sent if urine dip shows leucocytes or nitrites or the patient is symptomatic. • Urine pregnancy test – essential to exclude ectopic pregnancy or miscarriage as differential diagnosis.
Vaginal swabs	• A full screen for sexually transmitted infections, including high and low vaginal swabs, endocervical swabs should be performed. *Chlamydia* infection can be tested by an endocervical swab or a urine sample. The swabs are examined using nucleic acid amplification tests (NAAT) which have high detection rates. It is important to remember that negative swab results do not rule out a diagnosis of PID.
Blood tests	• Infection markers: White blood cell count, C-reactive protein level. These may be normal in mild to moderate cases of PID. • Blood cultures and serum lactate should be performed if pyrexia is present. • All patients should be offered screening for human immunodeficiency virus (HIV).
Transvaginal ultrasound scan or CT/MRI	• Transvaginal ultrasound may identify pathology such as tubo-ovarian abscess or alternative diagnoses such as an ovarian cyst accident. • Transvaginal scans should only be performed in those who have been sexually active and who give consent for this type of scan. Transabdominal is the alternative, although this type of scan can be limited in its detection as ovaries/fallopian tubes may not be so easily visualized.

CT, *Computed tomography;* MRI, *magnetic resonance imaging;* Urine MC&S, *urine microscopy, culture and sensitivity;* UTI, *urinary tract infection.*

educational programmes are currently in progress and national screening programmes are being evaluated.

COMMUNICATION

A detailed written explanation of what pelvic inflammatory disease (PID) is, its treatment and its long-term health implications for the patient and their partner should be provided. This should include an explanation of the future risk of infertility, chronic pelvic pain, possibility of repeat episodes of PID and the need to screen sexual contacts for infection to prevent reinfection. In view of increased risk of an ectopic in subsequent pregnancies, an early pregnancy scan should be sought.

Table 9.4 Complications of pelvic inflammatory disease (PID)

Potential long-term complications of PID	Infertility Ectopic pregnancy Chronic pelvic pain Dyspareunia Menstrual disturbances Psychological effects

Chapter Summary

- Pelvic inflammatory disease is an infective condition of the genital tract associated most commonly with sexually transmitted infections.
- Diagnosis of PID should be made clinically and empirical treatment should be commenced without waiting for swab results, as these may be negative.
- Early diagnosis and timely treatment reduce long-term risks.
- Primary prevention of the disease is of great importance as it is associated with high complication rates including tubal infertility, ectopic pregnancy and chronic pelvic pain.

UKMLA Conditions
Pelvic inflammatory disease
Chlamydia
Gonorrhoea

UKMLA Presentations
Acute abdominal pain
Acute and chronic pain management
Gonorrhoea
Pelvic inflammatory disease
Sepsis
Subfertility
Vaginal discharge

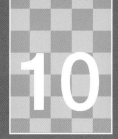

INDICATIONS

Contraception helps prevent unwanted pregnancies and provides protection against the transmission of sexually transmitted infections (STIs). Up to 65% of women of reproductive age worldwide use some form of contraception.

Contraception options vary in their method of action, mode of delivery, reversibility, pregnancy prevention, STI protection and contraindications. It is therefore crucial to have a good understanding of your patient's history, needs and priorities in order to individualize treatment. Patients should feel empowered to make an informed decision about the best type of contraception for them. To be effective, contraception must be used correctly and consistently.

When discussing contraception it is important to not only have a nonjudgemental approach but also to highlight the superior effectiveness of long-acting reversible contraception (LARC). All forms of contraception have a failure rate, based on both 'user error' and integral failure rates (Table 10.1). 'Typical use' rates are therefore lower than 'perfect use' as it includes common incorrect use such as forgotten pills and incorrectly placed condoms.

CLINICAL NOTES

Health professionals must ask women about their medication use including prescription, over-the-counter, herbal, recreational drugs and dietary supplements. Concurrent medications may increase or decrease serum levels of contraceptive hormones; similarly, hormonal contraception may increase or decrease serum levels of other medications. This can potentially cause adverse effects. Guidance regarding drug interactions and contraception is available on the Faculty of Sexual and Reproductive Healthcare website and in the British National Formulary.

HINTS AND TIPS

The UK Medical Eligibility criteria for contraceptive use guidelines in full can be easily online via https://www.fsrh.org/ukmec.

COMMUNICATION

It must be emphasized to all women that nonbarrier contraception does not protect from sexually transmitted infections and should still be used, particularly with new or occasional partners. They should be advised to attend regular sexual health checks.

POSTNATAL CONTRACEPTION

Postnatal contraception is an important part of pregnancy counselling, to prevent unplanned pregnancies following childbirth. An interval of less than 12 months can increase preterm birth, low-birthweight and small-for-gestational-age babies.

Table 10.1 Methods of contraception and their relative effectiveness

Method	Perfect use	Typical use (%)
Sterilization female	Lifetime failure rate 1 in 200–500	—
Sterilization male	Lifetime failure rate 1 in 2000	—
Combined oral contraceptive pill	>99%	91
Progesterone-only pill	>99%	91
Depot injection	>99%	94
Contraceptive implant	>99%	>99
Intrauterine contraceptive device (IUCD)	>99%	>99
Mirena intrauterine system (has the lowest failure rate in IUCD)	>99%	>99
Condom: male	98%	82
Diaphragm	95%	79
Natural fertility methods	up to 99%	76

Table 10.2 Methods of contraceptions: advantages, disadvantages and contraindications

	Type of contraception and mode of action	Advantages	Disadvantages	Contraindications
Nonhormonal	**Natural methods** Body temperature, cervical mucus and menstrual cycle length. 'Coitus interruptus' or 'withdrawal method' (withdrawal during intercourse prior to ejaculation). Basal body temperature rises 0.2°C–0.4°C when progesterone is released from the corpus luteum. Women using the 'rhythm method' will only have intercourse within their nonfertile times.	Helps avoid or plan a pregnancy. No unwanted physical side effects. Safe with any coexisting medical conditions. Acceptable to all faiths and cultures.	Relies on regular menstrual cycles, record keeping and commitment and can take three to six cycles to learn effectively. Events such as illness, stress or travel may alter the fertility indicators. At fertile times partners must avoid sex or use barrier contraception, and natural methods do not protect against STIs. The failure rate with coitus interruptus is high due to variable control of ejaculation and the presence of some sperm within pre-ejaculatory fluid.	Nil.
	Barrier contraception Condoms, femidoms, diaphragms and cervical caps. It was previously advised to use a spermicide (e.g., nonoxynol-9) to increase effectiveness of barrier contraception. However, more recent evidence, supported by the World Health Organization (WHO), shows that nonoxynol-9 offers no protection from STI, and may increase risk of human immunodeficiency virus (HIV) transmission.	Effective if used correctly. No systemic side effects. Easily available Condoms help to protect both partners against the transmission of STIs and HIV.	Must be applied prior to penetration and can reduce degree of sensation. Diaphragm and cap must be fitted and checked regularly by a trained professional. Condoms can slip or split if not used correctly or if of wrong size or shape and there can be difficulties in correct placement of a femidom. User error greatly increases barrier method failure rates.	Latex allergy, however nonlatex (polyurethane and polyisoprene) condoms are now widely available.
	Intrauterine device (IUD)* Small T-shaped plastic and copper device that works by both spermicidal action and thickening cervical mucus, and can remain in place for up to 10 years (Fig. 10.1).	No hormonal side effects. Fertility resumes almost immediately after removal.	Periods can become heavier or more painful. Complications include: expulsion, uterine perforation, 'lost threads' requiring hysteroscopic retrieval.	Cannot be inserted between 48 hours and 4 weeks postpartum. Current or recent PID. Patients who are virgo intacta (relative contraindication).
	Female sterilization Permanent method of preventing pregnancy using surgical methods – either laparoscopically outside of pregnancy or open at the time of caesarean section. The fallopian tubes are either cut, sealed or clipped, therefore preventing fertilization.	No hormonal side effects. Permanent.	Irreversible on the NHS – some women have regret. Failure rate of 1 in 200	If family is not complete or doubts about proceeding with permanent contraception.

	Male sterilization Male sterilization is known as a 'vasectomy'. Ligation of the vas deferens bilaterally via incisions in the scrotum performed under a local anaesthetic. At 3 and 4 months postoperatively, sperm samples must be tested to confirm azoospermia and barrier contraception should be used until this is confirmed.	No hormonal side effects.	Failure rate of 1:2000 after azoospermia is confirmed. Risk of chronic testicular pain.	If family is not complete or doubts about proceeding with permanent contraception.
Hormonal	**Combined hormonal contraception (CHC): e.g., combined oral contraceptive pill (COCP), patch or vaginal ring** Thickens cervical mucus preventing sperm from reaching the uterus. Thins the endometrial lining to discourage implantation. Inhibits ovulation by altering hormone levels – inhibiting follicular-stimulating hormone and preventing the follicular ripening, and preventing the luteinizing hormone surge. Effectiveness limited by some antibiotics, hepatic enzyme-inducing drugs, missed pills, vomiting and diarrhoea. The COCP is taken for 21 days of the month, followed by a 1-week pill-free period. 'Tricycling' (3 packets used consecutively) can be used in cases of menstrual disorders. The vaginal ring is worn for 3 weeks, followed by a 1-week ring-free period. The combined hormonal patch is changed once per week for 3 weeks, followed by a 1-week patch-free period.	Reliable if taken correctly, convenient and not intercourse related. Improves dysmenorrhoea, menorrhagia and premenstrual symptoms. Reduces occurrence of functional ovarian cysts and incidence of ovarian, endometrium and colon cancer. Some improve acne and menopausal symptoms.	Cardiovascular complications and thromboembolic disease, e.g., hypertension, venous thromboembolism (VTE), arterial thrombosis, heart attack or stroke. The risks increased with age, obesity, smoking, diabetes and hypertension. Small increase of cervical intraepithelial neoplasia or cervical cancer following prolonged use. There is mixed evidence regarding increased risk of breast cancer while taking COCP. Weight gain, breakthrough bleeding, headaches, nausea, breast tenderness and mood changes. Does not protect against STIs.	UK Medical Eligibility Criteria for Contraceptive Use (UKMEC) is a document produced by the Faculty of Sexual and Reproductive Healthcare that offers evidence-based guidance to providers of contraception regarding who can use contraceptive methods safely, particularly contraindications linked to particular medical conditions. It categorizes contraceptive options with various medical conditions from 'no restriction' to 'unacceptable health risk' (Table 10.3). Examples of absolute contraindications to CHC include atrial fibrillation and previous personal history of VTE (see Table 10.4).

(continued)

Table 10.2 Methods of contraceptions: advantages, disadvantages and contraindications—Cont'd

Type of contraception and mode of action	Advantages	Disadvantages	Contraindications
Progesterone-only pill (POP) Thickens cervical mucus. Thins endometrium. Ovulation is only suppressed in 50%–60% of cycles. It is very important to take the POP at the same time every day; late pills, vomiting and severe diarrhoea can make it less effective.	Good contraceptive choice for women with contraindications for COCP, such as age over 35, smokers or breastfeeding. Can improve dysmenorrhoea and menorrhagia.	Irregular breakthrough bleeding tends to settle within 6 months. Acne, breast tenderness, weight gain and headaches.	As per UKMEC, there are few contraindications to progesterone-only methods. One absolute contraindication is a current diagnosis of breast cancer.
Intrauterine system (IUS)* **e.g., Mirena/Jaydess** Small T-shaped plastic device that releases progesterone locally into the uterus for up to 5 years. Two fine threads are left through the cervical os which can be examined to ensure the coil is still in place/be used for removal.	Periods usually become shorter, lighter and can even stop, although this may take up to 6 months. Highly effective at preventing unwanted pregnancies. Fertility resumes almost immediately once removed.	Insertion of the IUS can cause discomfort particularly if the patient is nulliparous and often a local anaesthetic is injected into the cervix. Complications include: expulsion, uterine perforation, 'lost threads' requiring hysteroscopic retrieval. If a pregnancy does occur, it is more likely to be ectopic.	Cannot be inserted between 48 hours and 4 weeks postpartum. Current or recent PID Patient who are virgo intacta (relative contraindication).
Contraceptive subdermal implant* **e.g., Nexplanon/Implanon** The contraceptive implant is a small, flexible rod put under the skin of the upper arm which releases progestogen. It requires a small procedure under local anaesthesia for implantation and removal. Last for up to 3 years. Thickens cervical mucus. Thins endometrium.	Periods usually become shorter, lighter and can even stop (20% of patients), although this may take up to 6 months. Highly effective at preventing unwanted pregnancies.	Breakthrough bleeding common. Uncommonly, there can be challenges with removal.	As per UKMEC.
Depot progesterone injections* Thickens cervical mucus. Thins endometrium. Lasts for 3 months.	Periods usually become shorter, lighter, less painful and can even stop (50% amenorrhea).	Can delay fertility for up to 1 year after stopping. Acne, breast tenderness, breakthrough bleeding, weight gain and headaches.	Osteoporosis. Under 20 years of age or over 45. Previous VTE (UKMEC 2).

*Long-acting reversible contraceptive (LARC).

Table 10.3 Definition of UK Medical Eligibility Criteria for Contraceptive Use (UKMEC) categories

UKMEC category	Definition
1	A condition for which there is no restriction for the use of the method.
2	A condition where the advantages of using the method generally outweigh the theoretical or proven risks.
3	A condition where the theoretical or proven risks usually outweigh the advantages of using the method. The provision of a method requires expert clinical judgement and/or referral to a specialist contraceptive provider, because use of the method is not usually recommended unless other more appropriate methods are not available or not acceptable.
4	A condition that represents an unacceptable health risk if the method is used.

This is relevant for both breastfeeding and nonbreastfeeding women as soon as possible, as ovulation can resume as early as 3 weeks postpartum.

Most methods of contraception including progesterone-only pill (POP) and progesterone implants can be initiated safely immediately, with the exception of combined hormonal contraception (CHC). Women can initiate the combined oral contraceptive pill (COCP) from 21 days after childbirth if they are not breastfeeding and have no additional venous thromboembolism (VTE) or hormonal contraception risk factors. If breastfeeding or any additional VTE risk factors are present, COCP can only be started from 6 weeks postnatally. Intrauterine devices/systems can be inserted immediately after birth, even at the time of caesarean section, up to 48 hours after delivery. If 48 hours have passed, insertion should be after 28 days.

POSTTERMINATION OF PREGNANCY/MISCARRIAGE

Termination services should offer methods of contraception, particularly LARC to women prior to their discharge. In the event of miscarriage or ectopic pregnancy we should allow women to discuss their conception plans and offer contraception if requested. Any method of contraception can be initiated after an uncomplicated abortion or miscarriage, as long as there is no presence of sepsis.

BREASTFEEDING

Breastfeeding can be an effective form of contraception if less than 6 months postpartum, amenorrhoeic and fully breastfeeding. However, if breastfeeding decreases, menstruation returns or if it is over 6 months postpartum, risk of pregnancy increases.

Progesterone-based contraception methods have no adverse effects on lactation, infant growth or development. The COCP should not be started until 6 weeks postpartum if breastfeeding; due to minimal evidence of effect of COCP in breastmilk on child development.

EMERGENCY CONTRACEPTION

Emergency contraception is aimed to prevent unplanned pregnancy in the event of contraceptive failure or unprotected sexual intercourse (UPSI). Patients must be counselled about the risks of failure, and therefore pregnancy even after taking emergency contraception. Pregnancy must be excluded prior to providing the medication. There are three methods currently available over the counter in the UK; levonorgestrel (Levonelle), ulipristal acetate (EllaOne) and the copper IUD (Cu-IUD) (Table 10.5).

Levonorgestrel is a synthetic progestogen taken in a single 1.5-mg tablet that must be used within 72 hours (3 days) of the episode of UPSI. If taken before the preovulation oestrogen surge, ovulation can be inhibited for 5 to 7 days and fertilization prevented. Side effects include dizziness, nausea, headaches, breast tenderness or abdominal pain. Vomiting occurs in approximately 1% of patients, and the treatment should be repeated if vomiting occurs within 3 hours of ingestion.

Ulipristal acetate is a selective progesterone receptor modulator taken in a single-dose 30-mg tablet that must be used within 120 hours (5 days) of UPSI. It inhibits ovulation and alters endometrial lining to prevent implantation. It has a similar side-effect profile to levonorgestrel.

Cu-IUD can be inserted up to 120 hours (5 days) following UPSI or more, if not more than 5 days after the earliest predicted date of ovulation. Copper has a toxic effect on the sperm and ovum, which prevents fertilization. It has the advantage of providing ongoing contraception.

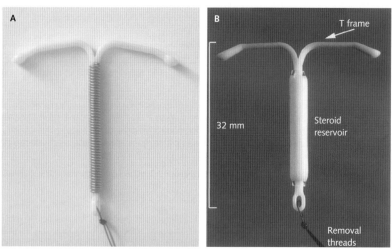

Fig. 10.1 (A) Copper IUD. (B) Intrauterine hormonal device. (https://www.clinicalkey.com/student/search/contraception?source=search-results&facets=!ct~IM&page=2)

Table 10.4 Contraindications to combine hormonal contraception

Degree of contraindication	Description
Absolute	Heavy smoker
	Vascular disease/ischaemic heart disease/stroke
	History of/current venous thromboembolism
	Thrombogenic mutations
	Atrial fibrillation
	Migraine with aura
	Current breast cancer
	Liver disease
	Systemic lupus erythematosus with antibodies
	Pregnancy
	Oestrogen-dependent tumour
Relative	Age >35
	Family history of thrombosis
	Diabetes with nephropathic complications
	Hypertension
	Body mass index >35 kg/m²

It is important to offer a regular method of contraception and risk assessment for STIs following use of emergency contraception.

TERMINATION OF PREGNANCY

The Abortion Act 1967, amended by the Human Fertilisation and Embryology Act 1990, instructs abortion care in England, Scotland and Wales. Two registered medical practitioners must agree that an abortion is justified within the terms of the Act, agreeing on one of five circumstances. Over 98% of abortions are undertaken due to risk to mental or physical health of the woman or her children. Nonconsensual sexual intercourse should be carefully screened for in all patients and subsequent support should be provided if required.

Medical termination

Medical abortions can be performed at any gestation using regimes of mifepristone, an antiprogesterone, and

Table 10.5 Emergency contraception

	Levenelle 1.5 mg (levonorgestrel)	EllaOne (ulipristal acetate 30 mg)	IUCD
Mode of action	Prevents ovulation and fertilization	Delays ovulation	Spermicidal
Licence use	72 hours (3 days) from UPSI	120 hours (5 days) from UPSI	Up to 5 days from UPSI or up to 5 days after ovulation
Contraindications	• Interacts with warfarin. Recheck INR within 48 hours post pill	• Severe asthma on steroids • Antiepileptic drugs (AEDs) • Proton pump inhibitors (PPIs)/antacids	• Increased risk of perforation if breastfeeding
Failure rate	Failure rate: 1%–2%	Failure rate: 1%–2%	
Comments	• Good for patients using progesterone-based contraceptives • Give same pill if second one is needed in the same cycle. Do not repeat dose within 5 days • Repeat dose if patient vomits within 3 hours • Does not affect breastfeeding Indications for use of high dose (3 mg): • If patient is taking AEDs • If >70 kg or BMI >26	• Affects efficacy of returning back to contraceptive pill • Give same pill if second one is needed in the same cycle. Do not repeat dose within 5 days • Effectiveness reduced if pill taken 7 days prior or 5 days after • Repeat dose if vomit within 3 hours • Discard breastmilk for 7 days if breastfeeding	• Highest efficacy for patients with a high BMI • Highest efficacy for patient taking AEDs
Restarting contraceptives	• Resume pill as usual	• COCP: Advise to use barrier protection for 12 days • POP: Advise to use barrier protection for 7 days • Qlara: Advise to use barrier protection for 14 days • Contraceptive implant: advise to use barrier protection for 7 days	

misoprostol, a prostaglandin analogue. In early pregnancy (<63 days) mifepristone (200 mg) is taken orally followed by misoprostol (800 mcg) after 24 to 48 hours orally or vaginally. At later gestations the misoprostol can be read-ministered every 3 hours up to four further doses. Feto-cide should be performed before medical abortion after 21 weeks and 6 days of gestation to ensure there is no risk of a live birth. Complete abortion occurs in 95% of patients. If there is clinical evidence that the abortion is incomplete or heavy bleeding occurs, then surgical evacuation may be required.

Surgical termination

Vacuum aspiration is an appropriate method of surgical abortion up to 14 weeks of gestation and is the most commonly used method up to 12 weeks. During vacuum aspiration, the uterus is emptied using a suction cannula. After 14 weeks surgical abortion by dilatation and evacuation can be performed; this may require uterine contents to be removed with forceps, a 'destructive termination'. Cervical preparation should be considered in all cases, particularly in nulliparous women, with either prostaglandin priming (misoprostol) or osmotic dilators at later gestation.

Complications

Abortion is a safe procedure with major complications being uncommon. Complications are more common with surgical methods. These include pain, infection, bleeding and trauma to the cervix and uterus including perforation. Prior to an abortion it is advised to screen for STIs and give prophylactic antibiotics. Retained products of conception following the procedure may result in heavier bleeding, and a second evacuation may be required. It is crucial to determine rhesus status, as if rhesus negative, anti-D is required.

ETHICS

It is crucial to appreciate the physical symptoms and psychological sequelae experienced after a termination of pregnancy. It is important to provide patients with information regarding counselling, support and contraceptive advice.

● Chapter Summary

- There is a huge variety of contraceptive methods available to help prevent unwanted pregnancies and provide protection against sexually transmitted infections.
- Clinicians should educate patients about these options, so they are able to make the most appropriate choice for them.
- It is important to identify risk factors and contraindications for various methods and encourage the use of long-acting reversible contraception methods when appropriate.

UKMLA Conditions
Contraception request/advice
Termination of pregnancy

UKMLA Presentations
Unwanted pregnancy and termination

Benign gynaecological tumours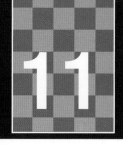

BACKGROUND

A neoplasm or tumour refers to an abnormal mass of a tissue characterized by excessive growth. They may be benign or malignant.

Ovarian tumours are common in both pre- and postmenopausal women – 1 in 10 women will have surgery during their lifetime for this indication. The exact prevalence is unknown due to the lack of consistent reporting and the fact that most ovarian tumours are asymptomatic with a high likelihood of spontaneous resolution. In premenopausal women, the vast majority of ovarian tumours are benign, with an incidence of malignancy of 1 in 1000. In postmenopausal women, this incidence increases to 3 in 1000 women.

Apart from physiological cysts, germ cell tumours are the most common type of ovarian tumours seen in premenopausal women. In postmenopausal women, epithelial ovarian tumours are the most common.

This chapter will focus primarily on benign ovarian tumours. Uterine leiomyomas (fibroids) are discussed in Chapter 5, endometriotic cysts (endometriomas) in Chapter 6 and gynaecological malignancies in Chapter 12.

PRESENTATION

Benign ovarian tumours are usually asymptomatic and therefore discovered incidentally, for example, at the time of a routine antenatal scan. Nevertheless, ovarian tumour pathology is one of the most common causes for gynaecological hospital admissions. Common presenting symptoms include:

- **Acute abdominal/pelvic pain:** Usually secondary to an ovarian cyst accident. This includes ovarian torsion (twisting of a large tumour on the ovarian pedicle resulting in ischaemia and necrosis), cyst rupture or haemorrhage within the cyst. Pain may be severe and associated with vomiting in the case of ovarian torsion. Patients can also present with an acute abdomen and haemorrhagic shock if intraabdominal blood loss is severe.
- **Abdominal swelling:** Due to tumour enlargement or malignant ascites.
- **Symptoms from pressure effects on the bowel or bladder:** Increased urinary frequency or urgency, constipation, change in bowel habit.

- **Symptoms of hormonal disturbance:** Androgen-secreting tumours may present with symptoms of virilization such as hirsutism, clitoromegaly and deepening of the voice. Oestrogen-secreting tumours may present with abnormal uterine bleeding such as heavy menstrual bleeding (HMB), post-menopausal bleeding (PMB) and irregular bleeding.

ASSESSMENT

The diagnosis of an ovarian mass is aided by thorough history-taking and examination (see Chapters 1 and 2). Important features of the history include:

- Characteristics of any pain (SOCRATES)
- Menstrual and gynaecological history
- Associated symptoms

It is important to consider possible differential diagnoses as approximately 10% of suspected ovarian masses are ultimately found to be nonovarian in origin (Table 11.1).

TYPES OF TUMOURS

Ovarian tumours can be physiological (functional cysts which are benign) or pathological (benign, borderline and malignant). They are classified based on the tumour's tissue of origin, and principally arise from three types of cell lines in the ovary:

- **Epithelial cells:** Cells from the surface epithelium of the ovary.
- **Sex cord stromal cells:** Hormone-producing and connective/fibrous tissue cells that hold the ovary together.
- **Germ cells:** Cells destined to become eggs.

These can be further divided into different histological subtypes (Table 11.1).

Physiological cysts

These are usually asymptomatic and tend to occur in younger women. As the name suggests, these cysts occur due to normal physiological processes that take place in the ovary and the majority resolve spontaneously.

Follicular cysts

Follicular cysts are simple cysts that occur due to nonrupture of the dominant follicle during the normal ovarian cycle, or failure

Table 11.1 Classification of ovarian tumours

Category	Type of tumour	Subtype
Physiological (functional)		Follicular cysts Luteal cysts
Benign ovarian tumours	Epithelial	Serous cystadenomas Mucinous cystadenomas Brenner tumours
	Sex cord stromal	Fibromas Thecomas
	Germ cell	Mature cystic teratomas (dermoid cysts) Mature solid teratomas
Benign nonovarian tumours		Paratubal cyst Hydrosalpinges Tubo-ovarian abscess Appendiceal abscess Diverticular abscess Pelvic kidney Fibroids (leiomyomas)
Malignant ovarian tumours (primary)	Epithelial	Serous cystadenocarcinoma Mucinous cystadenocarcinoma Endometroid cystadenocarcinoma Clear cell cystadenocarcinoma Transitional cell carcinoma of the ovary, malignant Brenner
	Sex cord stromal	Granulosa cell tumours Sertoli-Leydig cell tumours
	Germ cell	Dysgerminomas Endodermal sinus (yolk sac) tumours Embryonal carcinomas Immature teratomas Choriocarcinomas
Malignant ovarian tumours (secondary)	Krukenberg	Gastrointestinal cancers: classically gastric cancer Breast cancer Lung cancer
Borderline ovarian tumours	Epithelial	Serous borderline tumours Mucinous borderline tumours
Other benign ovarian tumours		Endometriomas (endometriotic cysts)

of atresia of the nondominant follicles. They are usually small, asymptomatic and resolve spontaneously within a few months. They may occur as a result of ovarian stimulation with clomiphene during fertility treatment.

Luteal cysts

Luteal cysts originate from the corpus luteum following ovulation and are of two types:

- **Granulosa luteal cysts**
  - Arise during the second half of the menstrual cycle and typically rupture on days 20 to 26, causing pain.

- May cause delayed menstruation due to persistent progesterone production.
- **Theca luteal cysts**
  - Arise due to excessive physiological stimulation from high levels of beta human chorionic gonadotrophin (β-HCG), for example, during pregnancy or in gestational trophoblastic disease.

Luteal cysts are typically haemorrhagic and can rupture and cause intrabdominal bleeding. Surgical intervention may be required if there is significant haemoperitoneum or signs of haemorrhagic shock. Otherwise, spontaneous resolution is the usual outcome.

Endometriotic cysts (endometriomas)

Women with endometriosis may develop cysts known as 'endometriomas'. They are often called 'chocolate cysts' due to the accumulation of altered menstrual blood and can enlarge over time. They have a typical 'ground glass' appearance on ultrasound as a result of haemorrhagic debris (Fig. 11.1). Treatment is usually with ovarian cystectomy, ablation or sclerotherapy if symptomatic, as these cysts typically do not resolve spontaneously.

Benign epithelial tumours

The majority (70%) of all ovarian tumours arise from the surface epithelium of the ovary, making epithelial tumours the commonest type of ovarian neoplasm. They develop from coelomic epithelium over the gonadal ridge of the embryo and can therefore be derived from the epithelium of any of the pelvic organs or renal tract, sharing histological similarities. Epithelial tumours can be benign, borderline or malignant.

Serous cystadenomas

Serous cystadenomas are the commonest benign epithelial tumours, occurring primarily in women of reproductive age. They are usually unilocular, cystic (containing serous fluid) with no solid areas or papillary projections, and unilateral in 90% of cases. Histologically, the epithelial lining of a serous cystadenoma is similar to that found in the fallopian tube (simple ciliated columnar epithelium).

Mucinous cystadenomas

Mucinous cystadenomas are typically unilateral, multilocular and cystic, containing thick mucinous fluid. They can grow to very large sizes occupying the peritoneal cavity. Histologically, mucinous cystadenomas are lined by simple columnar (glandular) epithelium. Mucin-secreting cells are likely to indicate an endocervical or gastrointestinal derivation.

Borderline ovarian tumours

Borderline tumours are a distinct subgroup comprising 10% to 15% of all epithelial ovarian tumours. Histologically, cells exhibit moderate dysplastic changes when compared to benign tumours, including cellular atypia, high cytoplasmic-to-nuclear ratio and increased mitotic activity. However, there is no breach of the basement membrane or stromal invasion to make them malignant. They are therefore also known as 'tumours of malignant potential'. Borderline tumours tend to occur in younger women aged 25 to 40. The most common histological subtypes are serous and mucinous tumours.

The majority of borderline tumours are asymptomatic and discovered incidentally. Up to 20% are indistinguishable from benign simple cysts on ultrasound and they can be difficult to distinguish from early ovarian epithelial tumours. Most tumours will have suspicious ultrasound features although

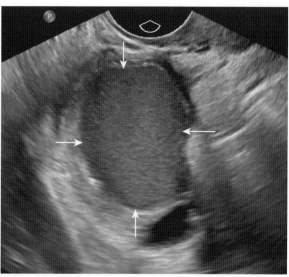

Fig. 11.1 Endometrioma on ultrasound with typical 'ground glass' appearance. (From: Wang PS. *Learning Radiology*. 2024: 201–222. 2024.)

the diagnosis is usually only confirmed following ovarian cystectomy and histological analysis. Prognosis is generally good compared to other ovarian malignancies, although long-term follow-up is required due to the risk of late recurrences.

CLINICAL NOTES

Both serous and mucinous cystadenomas tend to occur in women of reproductive age and are usually removed by ovarian cystectomy. If surgery is indicated, a laparoscopic approach is preferred for the management of benign ovarian tumours. Laparoscopy may be contraindicated in certain cases, for example, in very large cysts or if malignancy is suspected.

It is important to always consider borderline or malignant ovarian tumours as a possible diagnosis when undertaking any surgery for an ovarian mass. As much as possible, rupturing of a cyst should be avoided to avoid seeding of tumour cells into the peritoneal cavity. This may have implications should histology results come back as borderline or malignant. In the case of dermoid cysts, spillage of cyst contents intraoperatively may cause chemical peritonitis. Rupturing of a mucinous tumour may lead to pseudomyxoma peritonei, a condition where seeding of mucinous cells within the peritoneal cavity results in the formation of a gelatinous tumour.

Brenner tumours

Brenner tumours are usually benign although they may rarely undergo malignant transformation. Histologically, the epithelium of Brenner tumours resembles transitional cell/uroepithelium. They are solid, sharply circumscribed and pale yellow–tan in colour with 90% being unilateral.

Benign sex cord stromal tumours

These tumours are uncommon (5%–10% of all ovarian neoplasms) and arise from hormone-producing and connective/fibrous tissue cells within the ovary. They can be benign or malignant, and may present with hormonally mediated symptoms.

Thecomas

These cysts are nearly always benign, unilateral, solid tumours, occurring mostly in postmenopausal women. Those which produce oestrogen can cause endometrial hyperplasia and abnormal uterine bleeding, especially PMB. Those that secrete androgens may present with symptoms of virilization, such as hirsutism, clitoromegaly and deepening of the voice.

Fibromas

Fibromas are benign, unilateral, solid tumours, mostly derived from stromal cells with intersecting bundles of spindle cells producing collagen. They do not produce hormones. Meigs syndrome is seen in 1% of cases. This is the classic triad of ascites (nonmalignant), pleural effusion (usually right sided) and an ovarian fibroma.

Benign germ cell tumours

Germ cell tumours are a heterogeneous group of tumours that can be benign (95%) or malignant (5%). They comprise 20% to 25% of all ovarian neoplasms, and are the commonest type of ovarian tumours in premenopausal women.

Teratomas

Teratomas arise from pluripotent germ cells and contain elements of all three embryonic germ cell layers. This includes gastrointestinal tissue from the endoderm, bone and cartilage from the mesoderm, and ectodermal derivatives such as teeth and hair (Fig. 11.2).

Mature cystic teratomas are commonly known as 'dermoid cysts'. They are the most common type of germ cell tumours, and the commonest ovarian tumours in children and young women. The median age of presentation is 30 years. Dermoid cysts are almost always benign although they may rarely undergo malignant transformation in <1% of cases (usually

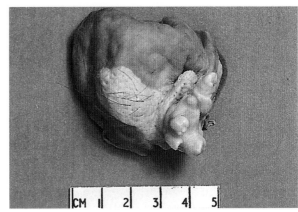

Fig. 11.2 Dermoid cyst (mature cystic teratoma) containing teeth and hair. (From: Ngan HYS, Chan KKL. *Essential Obstetrics and Gynaecology*. 2020: 328–351. 2020.)

squamous cell carcinoma). The majority are asymptomatic, but they can present with abdominal pain and torsion (10%–15% of cases), or rarely, rupture. Dermoid cysts are usually removed by laparoscopic ovarian cystectomy. Care should be taken to avoid rupturing the cyst intraoperatively as spillage of cyst contents into the peritoneal cavity may lead to chemical peritonitis.

Mature solid teratomas are solid tumours commonly with neural elements. They are less common compared to dermoid cysts, and must be histologically distinguished from immature solid teratomas, which are malignant.

INVESTIGATIONS

Reviewing the observations is crucial to assess whether the patient is haemodynamically stable. A patient unwell with an ovarian torsion or ruptured haemorrhage cyst may present with tachycardia and hypotension.

Pregnancy test

A urinary pregnancy test or serum β-HCG should be performed to exclude pregnancy.

RED FLAGS

In any woman presenting with abdominal/pelvic pain it is crucial to first exclude an ectopic pregnancy by performing a urinary pregnancy test. It is also important to consider differential diagnoses that require urgent management, such as appendicitis (see Table 11.2).

Blood tests

A full blood count or venous blood gas should be performed to assess current haemoglobin (Hb) levels. Serial Hbs trending downwards may indicate a ruptured haemorrhagic cyst and ongoing intra-abdominal haemorrhage. White blood cell count and C-reactive protein may be elevated in the case of appendicitis or a tubo-ovarian abscess.

Tumour markers are often used in the investigation of ovarian cancer. Cancer antigen-125 (CA-125) is a glycoprotein widely distributed in adult tissues. Its use as a tumour marker is well established and allows for the calculation of the Risk of Malignancy Index (RMI; see Chapter 12). A CA-125 cut-off level of <35 IU/mL is widely used. It is important to note that CA-125 should not be used in isolation to determine malignancy due to its nonspecific nature. CA-125 levels may be elevated in benign gynaecological conditions such as endometriosis, pelvic inflammatory disease and ovarian torsion. It can also be elevated in heart failure, hepatic failure and other nongynaecological conditions causing peritoneal irritation such as appendicitis, hepatitis and pancreatitis. Other cancers that metastasize to the peritoneum including breast, colon and lung cancer can also cause an elevated CA-125.

Other tumour markers that can be performed include cancer antigen 19-9 (CA 19-9), inhibin B, lactate dehydrogenase (LDH), alpha-fetoprotein (α-FP) and human chorionic gonadotrophin (HCG).

Sexually transmitted infection screen

Microbiology swabs and a screen for STIs, including high and low vaginal swabs, endocervical swabs and urethral swabs, should be performed if there is suspicion of pelvic inflammatory disease or a tubo-ovarian abscess.

Imaging

Transvaginal pelvic ultrasound is the diagnostic tool of choice for evaluating ovarian pathology. Because different types of ovarian tumours have typical ultrasound appearances, both the presence and type of tumour can usually be identified. Pelvic ultrasound can also help to detect the presence of ascites, evaluate blood flow on Doppler studies, and exclude other nonovarian masses such as fibroids. Transabdominal ultrasound should be performed if the transvaginal route is not appropriate.

A 'simple cyst' is associated with five ultrasound features and is usually benign:

- A round or oval shape
- Thin or imperceptible wall
- Posterior acoustic enhancement
- Anechoic fluid
- Unilocular: Absence of septations or nodules

A 'complex ovarian cyst' is associated with a higher risk of malignancy, with the following features:

- Multilocular: Presence of septations
- Solid nodules
- Papillary projections

The International Ovarian Tumour Analysis (IOTA) group has also developed an ultrasound classification system to help distinguish between benign and malignant ovarian masses (Table 11.3). Simple ultrasound rules based on five ultrasonic features typical for benign and malignant tumours are used to classify masses as benign (B features) or malignant (M features). Patients with an ovarian mass classified as malignant should be referred urgently to a gynaecological oncology service.

Table 11.2 Differential diagnoses for adnexal masses

Symptom	Differential diagnosis
Abdominal/pelvic pain	Ectopic pregnancy Spontaneous miscarriage Pelvic inflammatory disease Appendicitis Diverticulitis
Abdominal swelling	Pregnancy Fibroid uterus Full bladder
Pressure effects on bowel or bladder	Stress/urge urinary incontinence Vaginal prolapse
Hormonal disturbance	Menstrual irregularity Postmenopausal bleeding Precocious puberty

Table 11.3 IOTA group ultrasound rules and classification of benign and malignant ovarian masses

Benign 'B' features	Malignant 'M' features	Classification
• Unilocular cyst • Presence of solid components where the largest is <7 mm in diameter • Acoustic shadowing • Smooth multilocular tumour • No detectable blood flow on Doppler examination	• Irregular solid tumour • Presence of ascites • At least four papillary structures • Irregular multilocular solid tumour with largest diameter ≥100 mm • Strong blood flow on Doppler examination	• Benign: Only B features present • Malignant: Only M features present • Inconclusive: Both B and M features present, or no features apply

If malignancy is suspected, further imaging with computed tomography (CT) or magnetic resonance imaging (MRI) may be required.

MANAGEMENT

Conservative

Ovarian tumours can generally be managed conservatively if they are asymptomatic, depending on the woman's age and size of the mass.

Simple ovarian cysts measuring <5 cm are associated with a low risk of malignancy. These are likely to be physiological/functional, and usually resolve over 2 to 3 menstrual cycles without the need for intervention. Simple cysts between 5 and 7 cm in diameter can be managed with yearly ultrasound follow-up. Larger cysts should be considered for further evaluation with MRI and/or surgical intervention (Fig. 11.3). Simple cysts that persist or increase in size are unlikely to be physiological and may require surgery.

Conservative management is preferred in premenopausal women who wish to retain fertility, as along with common surgical risks, cystectomy carries the risk of oophorectomy should the ovary be too damaged from the cyst or if there is severe haemorrhage.

Surgical

Surgical management of an ovarian tumour may be indicated in the following scenarios:

- Suspicion of borderline or malignant tumour
- Complex ovarian cysts
- Failure of conservative management with nonresolution of a cyst or an increase in size
- Cysts >5 cm in diameter, due to the risk of ovarian torsion
- Symptomatic cysts
- Acute ovarian cyst accidents: Torsion, cyst rupture or haemorrhage

Women who present with acute abdominal/pelvic pain and a suspected ovarian cyst accident may require emergency laparoscopy or laparotomy depending on the clinical situation. Ovarian torsion should be treated as an emergency as any delay results in prolonged ischaemia and unrecoverable necrosis of the ovary requiring oophorectomy.

If surgery is indicated, a laparoscopic approach is preferred for the management of benign ovarian tumours. This is associated with decreased intraoperative blood loss, shorter recovery periods, lower postoperative morbidity and shorter inpatient admissions. Cystectomy is the procedure of choice over cyst aspiration as the latter is less effective and associated

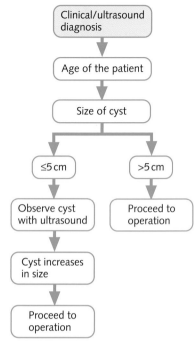

Fig. 11.3 Management of an asymptomatic benign ovarian tumour in a premenopausal woman. (From: Kay SE, Sandhu CJ. *Crash Course Obstetrics and Gynaecology*. 2019: 65–69. 2019.)

with a high rate of recurrence. Women should always be counselled preoperatively about the possibility of oophorectomy. Postmenopausal women should undergo a bilateral salpingo-oophorectomy rather than cystectomy. Care should be taken to avoid rupture and spillage of cyst contents as there is always a possibility of the tumour being borderline or malignant. Spillage of a dermoid cyst may also lead to chemical peritonitis. If inadvertent spillage occurs, extensive peritoneal washings should be performed.

Laparotomy may be more appropriate in certain cases, for example, suspected malignancy, borderline tumours and very large cysts. Women with suspected ovarian malignancy as indicated by suspicious features on imaging, raised serum tumour markers or an RMI ≥200, require a full laparotomy and staging procedure consisting of total hysterectomy with bilateral salpingo-oophorectomy, omentectomy, peritoneal washings, assessment/dissection of pelvic and para-aortic lymph nodes and biopsy of any suspicious areas including the peritoneal surfaces. Fertility-sparing surgery may be considered following careful counselling regarding the risks and benefits.

If a borderline tumour or ovarian malignancy is diagnosed during surgery or from subsequent histology (including frozen section), women should be referred to a gynaecological oncology service for further management.

Chapter Summary

- Ovarian cyst accidents are a common acute gynaecological presentation to hospital.
- Any woman presenting with abdominal/pelvic pain must be investigated for possible differential diagnosis such as ectopic pregnancy and appendicitis.
- Ovarian torsion should be treated as an emergency as the ovary twisting can cause decreased perfusion, and therefore unrecoverable necrosis of the ovary requiring oophorectomy.
- Transvaginal ultrasound is the optimum investigation to highlight an ovarian cyst and identify its probable aetiology.
- Management should be tailored to the particular patient considering their age, cyst size and risk of malignancy as calculated using the Risk of Malignancy Index.

UKMLA Presentations
Abdominal mass
Acute abdominal pain
Acute and chronic pain management
Pelvic mass
Pelvic pain

Globally, cancer remains a major health burden, and its incidence and mortality are predicted to rise significantly worldwide, a reflection of population growth and ageing, and the prevalence of cancer risk factors, many of which are associated with socioeconomic development. Gynaecological malignancies include cancers affecting the ovary, uterus, cervix, vagina and vulva. In the UK, ovarian and endometrial cancers are the most common, together accounting for 10% of all new cancer cases in women. Cervical cancer is the commonest gynaecological cancer in women worldwide, with >80% of cases occurring in developing countries.

GENETIC MUTATIONS

It is estimated that up to 10% of all cancers worldwide are inherited. While representing only a small fraction of the overall cancer burden, hereditary cancers tend to be of earlier onset with poor prognosis and have a devastating impact on young women and their families. Two of the most common hereditary cancer syndromes related to women's cancers include hereditary breast and ovarian cancer syndrome (HBOC) and Lynch syndrome (LS), predominantly caused by mutations in *BRCA* and DNA mismatch repair genes (*MLH1*, *MSH2*, *MSH6* and *PMS2*), respectively.

The best-known cancer susceptibility genes are the breast cancer associated (*BRCA*) 1 and 2 genes, located on chromosomes 17 and 13. These are tumour suppressor genes that play a role in the DNA repair pathway and regulating cell growth. Mutations in these genes result in an inability to repair DNA damage or undergo apoptosis (programmed cell death), leading to the uncontrolled cell growth and proliferation seen in cancer. Individuals who carry mutations in cancer susceptibility genes such as *BRCA* have a substantially higher risk of developing certain cancers compared to noncarriers. For example, *BRCA1/BRCA2* mutation carriers are at higher risk of developing breast and/or ovarian cancer, and carriers of mutations in Lynch syndrome genes (*MLH1*, *MSH2*, *MSH6* and *PMS2*) are predisposed to the development of endometrial, colorectal and ovarian cancers. Recently, other genes have also been found to confer an increased risk of ovarian cancer, including *RAD51C*, *RAD51D*, *BRIP* and *PALB2*.

Overall, an estimated 15% to 20% of ovarian cancers, 4% of breast cancers, 3% of endometrial cancers and 4% of colorectal cancers are attributable to inherited genetic mutations in cancer susceptibility genes. These are inherited in an autosomal dominant manner denoting a 50% risk of carriage in first-degree relatives, and are potentially preventable. The lifetime risks for the development of *BRCA* and Lynch syndrome-associated cancers are shown in Table 12.1.

The importance of thorough family history-taking in gynaecological oncology followed by referral to genetic clinics should not be underestimated. The identification of at-risk mutation carriers before they develop cancer would enable these individuals to access effective cancer risk management and preventive interventions to reduce their risk, including screening, chemoprevention (e.g., aspirin for bowel protection) and risk-reducing surgery. It can also enable personalized treatments for cancer patients that improve cancer survival, such as using poly-ADP-ribose-polymerase (PARP) inhibitors in BRCA mutation carriers with ovarian cancer. Additionally, knowledge of carrier status will enable women to make better-informed lifestyle, contraceptive and reproductive choices, and allow access to risk-reduction strategies for all carriers and affected family members through cascade testing.

OVARIAN CANCER

Background

Ovarian cancer is the sixth most common cancer in women in the UK with approximately 7,500 new cases diagnosed each year. It is the second most common gynaecological malignancy after endometrial cancer, with a lifetime risk of around 2% (1 in 50 women). Incidence increases with age – over 80% of all new ovarian cancer cases in the UK are diagnosed in women over the age of 50, with a peak incidence between the ages of 75 and 79. Ovarian cancer has been labelled the 'silent killer' due to its lack of (and often vague) symptoms. Consequently, around 60% of women present late in advanced stages of the disease (stages III and IV). Despite advances in cancer therapies, the overall 5-year survival remains at 43%, making ovarian cancer the leading cause of death in women with gynaecological malignancies.

Risk factors

The risk of developing ovarian cancer correlates with the amount of 'work' an ovary has undergone, i.e., the higher the number of ovulation cycles, the greater the risk. Conversely, factors that suppress ovulation will confer some degree of protection against ovarian cancer (Box 12.1).

Table 12.1 Hereditary cancer syndromes, cancer susceptibility genes and cancer risks

| Syndrome | Cancer susceptibility gene | Lifetime cancer risks (%) | | | |
		Breast	Ovarian	Colorectal	Endometrial
HBOC	*BRCA1*	72	44		
	BRCA2	69	17		
LS	*MLH1, MSH2, MSH6, PMS2*		3–17	10–50	40–60
Background population risk (no mutation)		12–15	2	5.6	2.7

BRCA 1,2, *Breast cancer associated 1 and 2 genes;* HBOC, *hereditary breast and/or ovarian cancer syndrome;* LS, *Lynch syndrome.*

BOX 12.1 RISK FACTORS FOR OVARIAN CANCER

Factors increasing risk	Factors decreasing risk
Increasing age	Pregnancy
Nulliparity	Multiparity
Late motherhood (>35 years)	Breastfeeding
Early menarche	Use of the COCP
Late menopause	Tubal ligation or hysterectomy (interruption of blood flow to the ovaries)
Obesity	
Family history of ovarian cancer	
Known carrier of a cancer gene mutation: *BRCA1, BRCA2,* Lynch syndrome genes	Risk-reducing surgery: bilateral salpingo-oophorectomy (RRSO), bilateral salpingectomy with delayed oophorectomy (RRESDO; research context only)
Use of HRT after the menopause	

BRCA 1,2, *Breast cancer associated 1 and 2 genes;* COCP, *combined oral contraceptive pill;* HRT *hormone replacement therapy.*

Pathogenesis

Primary ovarian cancers

As discussed in Chapter 11, ovarian neoplasms are classified based on the type of ovarian tissue from which they arise: epithelial cells, sex cord stromal cells and germ cells. These can be further divided into different histological subtypes (Table 12.2).

Epithelial ovarian cancers account for 90% of all ovarian malignancies. The commonest and most lethal subtype is high-grade serous ovarian carcinoma (HGSOC). In recent years, there has been increasing evidence that the majority of HGSOCs do not originate from the ovary but from precursor lesions in the fallopian tube, known as serous tubal intraepithelial carcinoma (STIC). Histologically, STIC lesions have been found to be on a continuum with early tubal and ovarian cancers, with the potential to seed onto the ovary and progress to HGSOC. Cancer of the peritoneum (primary peritoneal cancer) and fallopian tube are histologically similar to epithelial ovarian cancer and are treated the same way.

Secondary ovarian cancers (metastatic spread)

The ovary is a common site for secondary spread, and the most common metastases is from endometrial cancer. A Krukenberg tumour refers to a secondary deposit in the ovary that has metastasized from a primary malignancy elsewhere in the body. Cancers of the gastrointestinal tract, classically the stomach, are the most common primary tumours to metastasize to the ovaries, followed by breast and lung cancer. Histologically, Krukenberg tumours are characterized by mucin-secreting cells with a 'signet ring' appearance.

Staging and prognosis

The mode of spread is primarily trans-coelomic (direct seeding of tumour cells onto surfaces and organs within the peritoneal cavity). Lymphatic and haematogenous spread may also occur. Staging helps to determine prognosis and management. Ovarian cancer is staged according to the FIGO (International Federation of Gynecology and Obstetrics) classification system (Table 12.3).

Presentation

Ovarian cancer often presents with diverse and nonspecific symptoms widely experienced by the general population, requiring a high index of suspicion, especially in those with risk factors. Patients presenting with persistent vague or nonspecific symptoms require careful clinical assessment and diagnostic evaluation to exclude ovarian cancer. Symptoms associated with ovarian cancer include:

Table 12.2 Classification of malignant ovarian tumours

Type	Subtype	Description
Epithelial (90% of ovarian cancers)	Serous	• May be benign (see Chapter 11), borderline or malignant • Malignant tumours may be high grade or low grade • High-grade serous carcinomas: aggressive tumours; commonest and most lethal histological subtype • Generally unilocular, bilateral (50% of cases), cystic (containing serous fluid) and may have both solid and cystic components • Lined by simple ciliated columnar epithelium similar to the fallopian tube
	Mucinous	• May be benign (see Chapter 11), borderline or malignant • Tumours can grow to large sizes • Generally multilocular, cystic (containing mucinous fluid) and lined by simple columnar glandular epithelium • Histologically similar to gastrointestinal and endocervical cells • May coexist with pseudomyxoma peritonei • May be associated with appendiceal cancer
	Endometroid	• Second most common histological subtype; aggressive tumours • Associated with endometriosis: histologically similar to endometrial glands/stroma; resemble endometrial carcinomas • May coexist with endometrial carcinoma in 20% of cases
	Clear cell	• Histological variant of endometroid tumours • Commonest ovarian cancer associated with endometriosis • Cells have a typical hobnail appearance with clear cytoplasm
	Transitional cell/ urothelial-like	• Usually benign (Brenner tumour; Chapter 11) but rarely can undergo malignant transformation (malignant Brenner tumour) • Histologically similar to uroepithelium • Transitional cell carcinoma (TCC) of the ovary (non-Brenner type) is an aggressive tumour resembling TCC of the bladder
Sex cord stromal (5% of ovarian cancers)	Granulosa cell	• Commonest sex cord stromal and oestrogen-secreting tumours • Arise from granulosa cells: secrete inhibition B and oestradiol • Characterized by cells with 'coffee bean' nuclei and 'Call–Exner bodies' which are pathognomonic of the disease • Presentation depends on age of onset: precocious puberty, endometrial hyperplasia, abnormal uterine bleeding (prolonged/irregular/heavy menstrual bleeding, postmenopausal bleeding (PMB))
	Sertoli–Leydig	• Arise from Sertoli–Leydig cells: androgen-secreting tumours • Present with symptoms of virilization: hirsutism, clitoromegaly, deepening of the voice
	Fibromas/thecomas	• Usually benign (see Chapter 11)
Germ cell (5% of ovarian cancers)	Dysgerminomas	• Commonest malignant germ cell tumour • Tumour marker: lactate dehydrogenase (LDH) and human chorionic gonadotrophin (HCG)
	Endodermal sinus (yolk sac)	• Second most common malignant germ cell tumour • Tumour marker: alpha-fetoprotein (α-FP)
	Embryonal Carcinomas	• Usually coexists with an endodermal sinus tumour • Tumour marker: α-FP and HCG
	Teratomas	• Derived from all 3 embryonic germ cell layers • Mature cystic teratomas (dermoid cyst): majority benign but may undergo malignant transformation – see Chapter 11 • Immature teratomas (1% of all teratomas): malignant, secrete α-FP and LDH, tend to occur in children
	Choriocarcinomas	• Nongestational type (different from gestational trophoblastic disease; see Chapter 18) • Originate from trophoblastic tissue • Tumour marker: HCG • Present with precocious puberty

Table 12.3 FIGO staging classification for cancer of the ovary, fallopian tube and peritoneum

Stage	Description	5-year survival (%)
I	Confined to the ovaries or tubes	93%
A	One ovary (capsule intact) or tube, no ascites	
B	Both ovaries (capsules intact) or tubes, no ascites	
C	One or both ovaries/tubes: breached capsule(s) or ascites	
II	Spread within pelvis (below pelvic brim) or primary peritoneal cancer	68%
A	To uterus and/or tubes and/or ovaries	
B	To other pelvic organs	
III	Spread outside pelvis and/or metastasis to retroperitoneal lymph nodes	27%
A	Microscopic peritoneal metastasis and/or retroperitoneal lymph nodes	
B	Macroscopic peritoneal metastasis ≤2 cm +/– retroperitoneal lymph nodes	
C	Macroscopic peritoneal metastasis >2 cm +/– retroperitoneal lymph nodes	
IV	Distant metastases	13%
A	Pleural effusion with positive cytology	
B	To liver, spleen or other extraabdominal organs/lymph nodes	
Overall		43%

- Abdominal/pelvic pain or discomfort
- Abdominal bloating, distension or swelling
- Early satiety and/or loss of appetite
- Unexplained weight loss
- Increased urinary frequency or urgency
- Postmenopausal bleeding (PMB)
- Change in bowel habit
- Fatigue/general malaise
- Night sweats

Investigations

Transvaginal pelvic ultrasound is usually the first-line investigation for the evaluation of ovarian pathology. The International Ovarian Tumor Analysis (IOTA) ultrasound classification system is used to help distinguish between benign and malignant ovarian masses (see Chapter 11). Patients with an ovarian mass classified as malignant should be referred urgently to a gynaecological oncology service.

Serum CA-125 levels should be measured to allow calculation of the risk of malignancy index (RMI). CA-125 is shed by around 75% of epithelial ovarian cancers and 30% of mucinous tumours. Conversely, a normal CA-125 level (<35 IU/mL) does not exclude ovarian cancer as it is only raised in 50% of early-stage disease (stages I and II). CA 19-9 levels are raised in mucinous tumours. Serum LDH, α-FP and HCG should be measured in all women under the age of 40 with a complex ovarian mass due to the possibility of germ cell tumours. Inhibition B should be measured in the case of suspected granulosa cell tumours.

CLINICAL NOTES

RISK OF MALIGNANCY INDEX

Estimating the risk of malignancy is essential in the assessment of women with an ovarian mass. The risk of malignancy index (RMI) is the most utilized, widely available and validated model, and should be calculated to help guide further management.

$$RMI = \text{Ultrasound score (U)} \times \text{Menopausal status (M)} \times CA\text{-}125\ (IU/mL)$$

Calculation of the RMI requires the following:
- Serum CA-125 level (IU/mL)
- Menopausal status
  - M = 1 (Premenopausal)
  - M = 3 (Postmenopausal – defined as women who have had no period for >1 year or women over the age of 50 who have had a hysterectomy)
- Ultrasound score
  - 1 point for each of the following characteristics: multilocular cysts, solid areas, metastases, ascites and bilateral lesions
  - U = 0 (No characteristics present)
  - U = 1 (1 characteristic present)
  - U = 3 (2 or more characteristics present)

An RMI ≥200 is associated with a higher risk of malignancy and women should be referred to a gynaecological oncology service for further workup and management.

Further imaging and assessment should be performed in patients with suspicious features on ultrasound, raised serum tumour markers or an RMI ≥200. Magnetic resonance imaging (MRI) should be used as the second-line imaging modality for the characterization of indeterminate ovarian masses when ultrasound is inconclusive or limited due to body habitus.

Computed tomography (CT) of the chest, abdomen and pelvis can be undertaken to assess for metastases, pleural effusions, peritoneal implants, lymphadenopathy and to stage the disease.

CLINICAL NOTES

Patients with suspected or confirmed ovarian malignancy should be referred urgently to a gynaecological oncology service for further workup and management, and are best cared for within a multidisciplinary team consisting of gynaecological oncologists, medical oncologists, radiologists, specialist nurses, menopause specialists, pathologists and psychologists. Women cared for in dedicated cancer units/centres have higher satisfaction rates and improved prognosis.

Management

Chemotherapy

Chemotherapy may be required depending on the stage, grade and type of tumour. It is usually indicated in patients with high-grade disease (even at early stages), stage 1C or above, aggressive histological subtypes or cancer recurrence.

Chemotherapy can be administered on its own or in combination with surgery:

- **Adjuvant chemotherapy**: Chemotherapy given after primary debulking surgery to destroy any remaining cancer cells.
- **Neoadjuvant chemotherapy**: Chemotherapy given before surgery to shrink the tumour and decrease the amount of disease so that there is a higher chance of achieving complete resection at the time of cytoreductive surgery (interval debulking). This is then followed by further chemotherapy.

For epithelial ovarian cancer, conventional treatment involves the use of carboplatin (a platinum-based chemotherapy agent) along with paclitaxel for six cycles at 3-week intervals. Germ cell tumours are usually highly chemosensitive. The most common chemotherapy regimen is a combination of bleomycin, etoposide and cisplatin (BEP). Common side effects of chemotherapy agents include nausea, nephrotoxicity, neurotoxicity, bone marrow suppression and alopecia.

Surgery

Surgery is the mainstay of treatment for ovarian cancer. In early cancers, the aim is to resect all macroscopic disease (complete cytoreductive/debulking surgery) and establish stage. This staging procedure involves a midline laparotomy, total hysterectomy with bilateral salpingo-oophorectomy, omentectomy, peritoneal washings, assessment/dissection of pelvic and para-aortic lymph nodes, and biopsy of any suspicious areas including the peritoneal surfaces. An appendicectomy is performed in the case of mucinous cancers. Young women keen on fertility-sparing surgery (unilateral salpingo-oophorectomy with preservation of the uterus and contralateral ovary) should be counselled carefully regarding the risks and benefits so as to make an informed decision.

In patients with advanced disease, the aim is to achieve complete resection of all macroscopic disease. Prognosis is dependent on the amount of disease remaining following primary surgery, and complete resection is associated with improved overall survival. Primary debulking surgery followed by six cycles of adjuvant chemotherapy is the standard treatment, especially when complete resection is possible. Interval debulking (neoadjuvant chemotherapy for three cycles followed by cytoreductive surgery and then further chemotherapy) may be more appropriate in some advanced cases. Surgery in advanced disease may involve bowel resections with the formation of a colostomy/ileostomy, splenectomy and diaphragmatic stripping.

Targeted therapies

The use of bevacizumab, a monoclonal antibody and anti-angiogenic agent, has been shown to improve progression-free (but not overall) survival. For *BRCA* mutation carriers, maintenance therapy with PARP inhibitors such as olaparib prolongs progression-free survival in ovarian cancer. Many other agents are undergoing development.

CLINICAL NOTES

The rationale for screening for any condition is to enable early detection of disease and allow earlier clinical intervention in order to improve overall survival. Unfortunately, screening for ovarian cancer is difficult, partly because there is no premalignant stage, but also because there is no single test to diagnose ovarian cancer. Currently, there is no evidence to support screening for ovarian cancer in the general population or in women at increased risk. Studies have so far failed to demonstrate any significant reduction in mortality with ovarian cancer screening, despite detecting a higher proportion of women with earlier-stage disease.

Risk-reducing surgery

Given the absence of a national screening programme, the most effective way of preventing ovarian cancer is risk-reducing salpingo-oophorectomy (RRSO). Surgery is usually offered upon completion of childbearing, and involves the removal of both fallopian tubes and ovaries, usually through a laparoscopic procedure. RRSO is associated with an 80% to 96% reduction in ovarian cancer risk although a small residual risk (2%–4%) of primary peritoneal carcinoma remains. In the UK, current guidelines recommend offering prophylactic RRSO to women with a >4%–5% lifetime risk of ovarian cancer. This includes *BRCA1/BRCA2* mutation carriers, women with Lynch syndrome and women with a strong family history of ovarian cancer. RRSO is typically offered from 35 to 40 years for *BRCA1* carriers and 40 to 45 years for *BRCA2* carriers. Concomitant hysterectomy can be considered for women with Lynch syndrome due to the 40% to 60% lifetime risk of endometrial cancer, usually after completion of childbearing and not before 35 to 40 years.

The average age of natural menopause in most industrialized countries is 51 years. RRSO in premenopausal women leads to premature iatrogenic menopause, with detrimental short- and long-term health sequelae. Examples of short-term effects include vasomotor symptoms (hot flushes, night sweats), mood changes, sexual dysfunction (dyspareunia, reduced libido, vaginal dryness) and sleep disturbance. Oestrogen also has a protective effect on bone strength, cardiovascular health and neurocognitive function. Long-term effects include an increased risk of stroke, osteopenia and osteoporosis, neurocognitive decline, dementia and coronary heart disease. Current clinical practice recommends the use of hormone replacement therapy (HRT) up to the age of natural menopause for symptomatic relief and to mitigate the adverse long-term health consequences of premature menopause. This does not increase breast cancer risk and is safe in the absence of any contraindication. HRT is usually contraindicated in women with a personal history of breast cancer, especially if hormone sensitive. Nevertheless, in women with triple-negative breast cancer, short-term HRT may be considered on an individual basis following multidisciplinary team discussion and informed counselling. Alternative pharmacological, nonpharmacological and complementary therapies may be considered for women unable to take HRT, although the evidence for these is limited.

The tubal hypothesis for the origin of ovarian cancer, coupled with the detrimental effects of premature menopause, has led to the proposal of a novel two-step alternative surgical approach for women at high risk but who wish to delay or decline RRSO. Risk-reducing early salpingectomy followed by delayed oophorectomy (RRESDO) involves removal of the tubes followed by the ovaries at a later date or at the time of menopause. This has the benefit of providing some degree of risk reduction, while conserving ovarian function and avoiding the negative health sequelae associated with premature menopause. Nevertheless, there is paucity of evidence on the extent of ovarian cancer risk reduction afforded by only removing the tubes, the effectiveness of the approach, and long-term outcomes. RRESDO is currently being offered solely within the context of several ongoing clinical trials.

ENDOMETRIAL CANCER

Background

Endometrial cancer is the fourth most common cancer in women in the UK after breast, bowel and lung cancer, with almost 10,000 new cases diagnosed each year. It is the commonest gynaecological malignancy in developed countries, with a lifetime risk of around 3% (1 in 36 women). Over 90% of endometrial cancer cases occur in postmenopausal women, although younger women (aged <40 years) with Lynch syndrome are also at increased risk.

Risk factors

The risk of developing endometrial cancer correlates with prolonged high levels of oestrogen, i.e., hyperoestrogenic states are associated with increased risk. Prolonged stimulation of the endometrium with unopposed oestrogen (i.e., oestrogen only without the use of progestogens) may lead to the development of endometrial hyperplasia and malignancy. Oestrogens may be exogenous or endogenous. Factors that oppose the proliferative effects of oestrogen help to protect the endometrium and reduce the risk of endometrial cancer (Box 12.2).

Endometrial hyperplasia

Endometrial hyperplasia is the precursor lesion of endometrial cancer. It is a premalignant condition characterized by precancerous changes in the endometrium that if left untreated can progress to cancer. Endometrial hyperplasia develops when persistent and prolonged high levels of oestrogen, unopposed by progesterone, stimulates endometrial cell growth by binding to oestrogen receptors in endometrial cells, resulting in a thickened endometrium. The most common presentation of endometrial hyperplasia is abnormal uterine bleeding (AUB), including heavy menstrual bleeding (HMB), intermenstrual bleeding (IMB), PMB and irregular bleeding. Diagnosis requires an endometrial biopsy followed by histological examination of the endometrial tissue. There are two types of endometrial hyperplasia:

- **Endometrial hyperplasia without atypia**
  - Risk of progression to endometrial cancer is 5% over 20 years if left untreated.
  - Majority of cases (95%) regress spontaneously during follow-up.
  - Progestogen treatment encourages regression (95%–99% regression rate). The levonorgestrel intrauterine system (LNG-IUS) is first-line and is more effective compared to oral progestogens.

- Endometrial surveillance incorporating biopsies should be carried out at 6-month intervals to detect disease progression or regression.
- Modifiable risk factors should be addressed: Encouraging weight loss, stopping systemic oestrogen-only HRT, switching tamoxifen to letrozole.
- **Endometrial hyperplasia with atypia (atypical hyperplasia)**
  - Risk of progression to endometrial cancer is 25% (1 in 4 women) if left untreated.
  - 40% of women are found to have coexisting endometrial carcinoma.

RED FLAGS

Atypical endometrial hyperplasia has a high likelihood of progression to endometrial cancer if left untreated, and in many cases might indicate that a carcinoma is already present in another part of the uterus. Total hysterectomy is the recommended treatment due to the risk of underlying malignancy or progression to cancer. Peri- and postmenopausal women should be offered bilateral salpingo-oophorectomy together with total hysterectomy. For premenopausal women, the decision for oophorectomy should be individualized and requires careful counselling on the short- and long-term consequences of premature menopause, its impact on quality of life, as well as the risks, benefits and limitations of hormone replacement therapy (HRT). Bilateral salpingectomy should be considered as this may reduce the risk of future ovarian malignancy.

Women wishing to retain their fertility should be carefully counselled about the risks of underlying malignancy and subsequent progression to endometrial cancer. First-line treatment with the levonorgestrel intrauterine system (LNG-IUS) is recommended, with oral progestogens as a second-best alternative. Endometrial surveillance incorporating endometrial biopsies should be performed at 3-month intervals. Hysterectomy should be performed once fertility is no longer required or if there is evidence of disease progression.

Pathogenesis

Endometrial cancer is an adenocarcinoma and can be classified into two types (Table 12.4). The vast majority are sporadic type I (endometroid) endometrial carcinomas which develop on a background of endometrial hyperplasia. The most common histological subtype is endometrioid adenocarcinoma. Type II (nonendometroid) carcinomas refer to other histological subtypes including serous and clear cell carcinomas and are unrelated to excess oestrogen.

BOX 12.2 RISK FACTORS FOR ENDOMETRIAL CANCER

Factors increasing risk	Factors decreasing risk
Obesity	Use of the
Increasing age	combined oral
Nulliparity	contraceptive
Early menarche	pill (COCP)
Late menopause	Progestogen
Use of tamoxifen in breast cancer	treatment
Lynch syndrome (previously known as hereditary nonpolyposis colorectal cancer; HNPCC)	
Polycystic ovarian syndrome (PCOS)	
Systemic oestrogen-only hormone replacement therapy (HRT)	
Oestrogen-secreting tumours: granulosa cell tumours	
Type II diabetes mellitus	
Endometrial hyperplasia	

Table 12.4 Type I and II endometrial carcinomas

Type I endometrial carcinomas	Type II endometrial carcinomas
• Commonest type of endometrial cancer • Usually refers to endometroid adenocarcinomas (commonest histological subtype) • Oestrogen dependent • Have a precursor lesion: develop on a background of endometrial hyperplasia • Generally diagnosed at earlier stages, are slow-growing, less likely to spread, and have better prognosis	• Less common than type I • Histological subtypes: serous, clear cell • Not related to hyper-oestrogenism • No premalignant phase • Tend to be fast-growing aggressive tumours with high likelihood of metastases and poor prognosis

Staging and prognosis

Endometrial cancer spreads by direct local invasion into the myometrium followed by surrounding organs. Lymphatic and haematogenous spread may also occur. Endometrial cancer is staged according to the FIGO classification system (Table 12.5). Prognosis is largely dependent on tumour stage, grade and histological subtype. The overall 5-year survival for endometrial cancer is around 75%.

Table 12.5 FIGO staging classification for endometrial carcinoma

Stage	Description	5-year survival (%)
I	Confined to the body of the uterus	90%
	A <50% myometrial invasion	
	B ≥50% myometrial invasion	
II	Spread to the cervix	75%
III	Spread outside the uterus but within the pelvis	50%
	A Adnexae or serosa of the uterus	
	B Vagina or parametrium (local supporting tissues)	
	C Pelvic or para-aortic lymph nodes	
IV	Regional/distant metastases	15%
	A Bladder or bowel mucosa	
	B Abdominal metastases or inguinal lymph nodes	
Overall		75%

Presentation

Abnormal uterine bleeding, most commonly PMB, is the cardinal symptom of endometrial carcinoma and should be appropriately investigated. The probability of endometrial cancer in women presenting with PMB is 5% to 10%. Other symptoms include:

- IMB
- Watery, blood-stained or purulent vaginal discharge
- Unscheduled bleeding on HRT
- Change in menstrual bleeding pattern: e.g., new-onset HMB or irregular bleeding
- Back pain, fatigue/general malaise, weight loss or night sweats (late stages)

RED FLAGS

Postmenopausal women presenting with PMB should be referred urgently for assessment and investigation. They should be treated as having endometrial cancer until proven otherwise.

Premenopausal women over the age of 40 presenting with abnormal uterine bleeding should also be investigated, especially in the presence of risk factors for endometrial cancer.

Investigation

Imaging

Transvaginal ultrasound is often the first-line investigation used to assess the appearance of the endometrium and measure endometrial thickness (ET). In postmenopausal women, an ET of ≤4 mm is associated with a low risk of endometrial cancer. An ET >4 mm, irregularity of the endometrium, or the presence of intrauterine structural lesions such as polyps should warrant further investigation with hysteroscopy and endometrial biopsy.

Once a tissue diagnosis is obtained, an MRI can be performed to assess the extent of myometrial invasion, involvement of surrounding tissues/organs and lymph node involvement. This allows staging of the disease, and helps to determine prognosis and management.

Endometrial biopsy

Diagnosis of endometrial hyperplasia or cancer requires histological examination of endometrial tissue. Sampling of the endometrium can be performed in the outpatient setting, as a stand-alone procedure (pipelle biopsy) or in conjunction with hysteroscopy. A pipelle biopsy involves the passage of a thin plastic tube through the cervix and into the uterine cavity, using aspiration to obtain an endometrial sample. This technique, however, only samples <5% of the endometrial surface area and may miss the cancer if present.

Hysteroscopy and endometrial biopsy are considered the gold standard investigation as they allow direct visualization and biopsy of the uterine cavity. It can be performed under general anaesthesia or in the outpatient setting (with the option of local anaesthetic). Hysteroscopy can be used to facilitate an endometrial biopsy when sampling fails or is nondiagnostic, and if intrauterine structural abnormalities such as polyps are suspected on pelvic ultrasound.

Management

Surgery is the mainstay of treatment for patients with endometrial cancer. This involves a total hysterectomy with bilateral salpingo-oophorectomy and peritoneal washings. Adjuvant radiotherapy may be required depending on the stage and grade of disease, and is given to reduce the risk of recurrence. Vaginal brachytherapy refers to radiotherapy directed to the vaginal vault, while external beam radiotherapy is directed to the whole pelvis. In advanced disease, the use of chemotherapy in addition to radiotherapy has been associated with improved survival.

Risk-reducing surgery

Women with Lynch syndrome have an up to 17% lifetime risk of ovarian cancer and a 40% to 60% lifetime risk of endometrial cancer (Table 12.1). Risk-reducing total hysterectomy and bilateral salpingo-oophorectomy is the most effective way of preventing endometrial and ovarian cancer in these individuals. Manchester Consensus guidelines recommend offering risk-reducing surgery from the age of 35 to 40, following completion of childbearing. Women who have not completed their family or decline surgery may opt to undergo endometrial surveillance with transvaginal ultrasound, hysteroscopy and endometrial biopsies. While this provides regular review and reassurance, there is no evidence that this leads to earlier diagnosis or improved survival in Lynch syndrome-associated endometrial cancer.

UTERINE SARCOMAS

Background

Uterine sarcomas are rare, accounting for only 2% of all uterine malignancies, typically with an aggressive nature and poor prognosis. As discussed earlier, the majority of cancers arising from the uterus are endometrial adenocarcinomas arising from the endometrial glands. Uterine sarcomas may arise from the myometrium (leiomyosarcomas), stroma of the endometrium (endometrial stromal sarcomas) or a mixture of both endometrial stroma and epithelium (carcinosarcomas).

Leiomyosarcomas

Leiomyosarcomas are a type of soft-tissue sarcoma that can be described as a 'malignant fibroid', although only 5% to 10% of them arise from an existing fibroid. They are smooth muscle tumours that arise from the myometrium, and account for 1% of all uterine malignancies and 35% to 40% of all uterine sarcomas, making them the most common gynaecological sarcoma. An index of suspicion should be raised in women who present with a rapidly growing abdominal mass, which on imaging appears to be consistent with a fibroid. Treatment is with total hysterectomy. Leiomyosarcomas have a poor prognosis with recurrence rates of up to 70% and an overall 5-year survival of around 40%.

Endometrial stromal sarcomas

Endometrial stromal sarcomas arise from the stroma of the endometrium and can be classified into the following categories:

- Endometrial stromal nodule – benign
- Low-grade endometrial stromal sarcoma (LGESS) – malignant
- High-grade endometrial stromal sarcoma (HGESS) – malignant
- Undifferentiated uterine sarcoma (UUS) – malignant

Endometrial stroma sarcomas are more common in younger women aged 45 to 50 years. They may be associated with endometriosis. Treatment is with total hysterectomy and bilateral salpingo-oophorectomy. HGESS and UUS are aggressive tumours with high recurrence rates despite surgical management. The overall 5-year survival is around 40%.

Carcinosarcomas

Carcinosarcomas consist of a mixture of both endometrial stromal and epithelial elements, and therefore have features of both endometrial carcinoma and uterine sarcoma. They are aggressive tumours that metastasize early – over 75% of patients present with disease that has spread beyond the endometrium. Carcinosarcomas are managed similarly to type II endometrial carcinomas as they have similar risk factors and behaviours.

CERVICAL CANCER

Background

Cervical cancer is the fourth most common cancer in women and the most common gynaecological malignancy worldwide. Nearly all cervical cancer cases are preventable, due to the presence of a precursor/premalignant lesion known as cervical intraepithelial neoplasia (CIN), detectable through screening. The introduction of cervical screening programmes in many countries worldwide has led to a significant decline in cervical cancer incidence and mortality. More recently, the introduction of the human papillomavirus (HPV) vaccine into national vaccination programmes is aimed at preventing HPV infection as a primary preventive measure. Nevertheless, cervical cancer remains the commonest cancer and leading cause of death in women in developing countries without established cervical screening programmes. In the UK, cervical cancer is the 14th most common cancer in women, with a lifetime risk of <1% (1 in 142 women). The overall 5-year survival for cervical cancer is 60%.

Risk factors

HPV is a DNA virus belonging to the *Papillomaviridae* family. Over 100 different types of HPV have been described, around 40 of which affect the genital area. HPV is mainly transmitted by sustained direct skin-to-skin contact, especially during sexual intercourse which includes vaginal, anal and oral sex. It is the most common sexually transmitted infection worldwide, and the majority of sexually active individuals would have been infected by HPV at some point during their lifetime. Most HPV infections are asymptomatic and transient – 90% are cleared by the body's immune system. Some HPV types are termed 'high risk' as they are oncogenic. Persistent infection with high-risk HPV is linked to the development of premalignant lesions and cancers of the cervix, vulva, vagina, penis, anus and oropharynx (head and neck).

Over 99% of cervical cancers are caused by persistent infection with high-risk HPV. There are at least 12 high-risk types of HPV, 2 of which cause the majority of HPV-related cancers – HPV 16 and 18. Between them, these two types are responsible for over 80% of cervical cancer cases. High-risk HPV types can also cause genital, and head and neck cancers as mentioned earlier. HPV 6 and 11 are low-risk HPV types that are responsible for causing 90% of genital warts.

Factors leading to persistent and/or increased risk of HPV infection are risk factors for cervical cancer. These include:

- Early age of first intercourse
- Multiple sexual partners
- Low socioeconomic status
- Immunosuppression
- Cigarette smoking
- Use of the combined oral contraceptive pill (COCP)

Premalignant lesions of the cervix

There are two main types of carcinomas of the cervix, each with its own precursor lesion:

- **Squamous cell carcinomas (70%–80% of cases)**
  - Arise from squamous epithelium of the ectocervix
  - Precursor lesion is CIN
- **Adenocarcinomas (20%–30% of cases)**
  - Arise from glandular epithelium of the endocervix
  - Precursor lesion is cervical glandular intraepithelial neoplasia (cGIN)

Both CIN and cGIN arise due to persistent HPV infection of the cervical epithelium, causing premalignant changes that if left untreated can progress to cancer. CIN is graded according to the degree of dysplasia (histological term referring to cellular abnormalities) and the extent to which normal squamous epithelium has been placed by abnormal dysplastic cells (Fig. 12.1). There are three stages, thought to represent a continuum from low-grade (CIN I) to high-grade dysplasia (CIN II and III). CIN grade is determined histologically following a biopsy.

Not every woman with CIN or cGIN will develop cervical cancer. As most HPV infections are transient, dysplastic changes typically resolve on their own once the virus clears. Around 40% of low-grade CIN (CIN I) will resolve spontaneously without the need for intervention. In persistent HPV infection, CIN has the potential, if left untreated, to progress to high-grade disease and eventually cervical cancer over time, usually over a period of 10 to 20 years. Given that premalignant lesions tend to be asymptomatic, this provides a window of opportunity to screen and treat patients before they develop cancer.

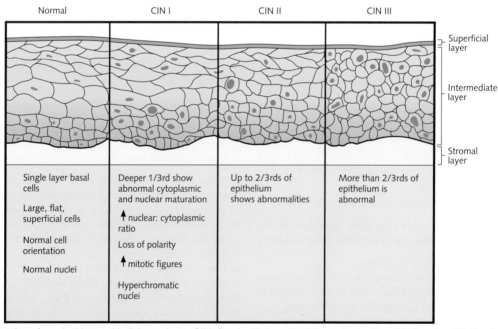

Fig. 12.1 Grades of cervical intraepithelial neoplasia. *CIN,* Cervical intraepithelial neoplasia. (Kay SE, Sandhu CJ. *Crash Course Obstetrics and Gynaecology.* 4th ed. 2019: 71–80. © 2019.)

Cervical screening

Screening intervals

The UK has an established cervical screening programme that invites women and anyone with a cervix (including trans men and nonbinary individuals assigned female at birth) aged 25 to 64 to undergo cervical screening. In England and Northern Ireland, patients are invited for screening every 3 years between the ages of 25 and 49, and then every 5 years until the age of 64. In Wales and Scotland, the recall interval is every 5 years between the ages of 25 and 64. This may vary in other countries and healthcare settings.

Procedure and process

Cervical screening involves sampling cells from the transformation zone of the cervix, an area where columnar cells are continuously undergoing squamous metaplasia, and is the commonest place for precancerous changes to develop (see Chapter 1). Cells are then examined under a microscope for the presence of cellular abnormalities (dyskaryosis). Conventionally, cells are taken and smeared onto a glass slide for analysis, hence the term 'cervical smear' or 'Pap smear' after the inventor of the test, Georgios Papanicolaou. In the UK, liquid-based cytology (LBC) has now replaced conventional smear tests. Instead of glass slides, cells are sampled and placed into a container of fluid medium.

Currently, the NHS cervical screening programme utilizes high-risk HPV testing as its primary cervical screening method, with secondary triage by cytology if found to be positive. This has been shown to be more sensitive compared to cytology in the detection of precursor lesions. Cervical screening samples are tested for high-risk HPV types:

- **High-risk HPV negative**: Women are returned to routine recall and will be invited for screening again in 3 or 5 years' time depending on age.
- **High-risk HPV positive**: Cytology triage will be carried out on the same sample. Cells are assessed to see whether HPV infection has caused cervical cellular abnormalities. Patients who are high-risk HPV positive with abnormal cytology results will be referred for colposcopy and may require more frequent screening depending upon findings and treatment.
    - **Cytology negative**: Women are invited for repeat screening in 12 months' time.
    - **Cytology positive**: Women are referred for colposcopy.

Classification of cervical cytology

Dyskaryosis is a cytological term describing cells with abnormal nuclear changes. Cells will usually exhibit varying degrees of cellular abnormalities and lie on a continuum from normal to malignant. The degree of dyskaryosis seen on cytology tends to correlate with the degree of dysplasia and CIN confirmed on histology (i.e., low-grade, moderate and severe dyskaryosis = CIN 1, II and III, respectively) (Table 12.6).

Table 12.6 Classification of cervical cytology results

Negative
Borderline change in squamous cells
Borderline change in endocervical cells
Low-grade dyskaryosis
High-grade dyskaryosis (moderate)
High-grade dyskaryosis (severe)
High-grade dyskaryosis/? invasive squamous cell carcinoma
? Glandular neoplasia of endocervical type
? Glandular neoplasia of noncervical type

Colposcopy

It is important to remember that HPV testing and cervical cytology are screening and not diagnostic tests. A diagnosis of CIN, cGIN or malignancy can only be made histologically and requires a biopsy. Colposcopy, or examination of the cervix, is usually performed as an outpatient. A colposcope is a binocular microscope used to visualize and assess the surface of the cervix under magnification. The patient is positioned in a modified lithotomy position and the cervix is visualized following insertion of a Cusco's (bivalve) speculum. The cervix is then viewed through the colposcope.

Two types of solutions can be applied to the cervix to aid in the identification of any abnormal areas or lesions. This is because dyskaryotic cells contain a higher amount of nuclear protein and lower amount of glycogen compared to normal cervical epithelium.

- **5% acetic acid**: Abnormal cells give an intense 'acetowhite' appearance, due to the coagulation of nuclear proteins by the acetic acid. Areas of CIN appear as distinct 'acetowhite' lesions with demarcated edges.
- **Lugol's iodine**: Abnormal cells contain lower amounts of glycogen and take up less iodine, giving a pale appearance. Normal cells will stain dark brown with the uptake of iodine.

The extent of any lesions should be noted along with any extension into the endocervical canal. All abnormal or suspicious looking areas should be biopsied in order to make a histological diagnosis.

CLINICAL NOTES

Suspicious features at colposcopy:
- Intense acetowhite appearance with 5% acetic acid solution
- Pale appearance with Lugol's iodine staining
- Mosaicism and punctation due to increased capillary vasculature with atypical patterns and bizarre branching
- Friable tissue with contact bleeding
- Raised or ulcerated areas with abnormal vessel formation

Management of premalignant lesions of the cervix

Low-grade CIN (CIN I) can be managed conservatively with regular cytological surveillance, as many of these lesions will resolve spontaneously. High-grade CIN (CIN II and III) and cGIN generally require treatment, either by excising or destroying/ablating the affected area.

Excision techniques include large loop excision of transformation zone (LLETZ) and cone biopsy. LLETZ can be performed in the outpatient setting under local anaesthetic and involves excision with a diathermy wire loop. A deeper cone biopsy can be performed in the case of cGIN or if the lesion affects the endocervical canal. Excisional methods allow abnormal tissue to be removed and sent for histology to confirm the diagnosis and check tissue margins, ensuring complete excision. Removal of cervical tissue inevitably results in shortening of the cervix with a small risk of cervical stenosis, insufficiency and preterm labour.

Ablative techniques include cold coagulation (coagulation diathermy), cryocautery and laser vaporization. Disadvantages include the lack of tissue available for histological assessment and the fact that the depth of tissue destruction is often unknown.

Initial treatment is associated with a 95% success rate. Following treatment, patients should be followed up with repeat screening, usually after 6 months.

Human papillomavirus (HPV) vaccination

The introduction of the HPV vaccine into national vaccination programmes is aimed at preventing HPV infection as a primary preventive measure. These vaccines have been developed to protect against the most common oncogenic HPV types, and are most effective when administered prior to any exposure to the virus (i.e., before children become sexually active). Cervarix and Gardasil are widely used in many countries. Studies have demonstrated long-term protection against HPV infection for at least 10 years, although vaccination is predicted to confer lifelong immunity.

In the UK, HPV vaccination was added to the NHS vaccination programme for girls in 2008 and extended to boys in 2019. Currently, girls and boys aged 12 to 13 years are routinely offered HPV vaccination with the nanovalent vaccine Gardasil 9, which protects against nine types of HPV – HPV 6, 11, 16, 18, 31, 33, 45, 52 and 58. HPV 6 and 11 cause around 90% of genital warts while the rest are high-risk oncogenic HPV types which together account for over 95% of cervical cancers. Use of the vaccine should help to reduce the incidence of HPV-related cancers (cervical, vulval, vaginal, anal, penile, head and neck), as well as genital warts.

It must be emphasized that HPV vaccination does not replace cervical screening. The HPV vaccine does not protect against all types of HPV and therefore not every case of cervical cancer can be prevented. All women who receive the HPV vaccine should also undergo regular cervical screening once they reach the age of 25.

Presentation

Cervical cancer may be completely asymptomatic in the early stages and only diagnosed as an incidental finding on cervical cytology. Symptoms of invasive disease include:

- Abnormal uterine bleeding: PCB, IMB and PMB
- Offensive vaginal discharge which may be blood stained
- Bladder symptoms: increased urinary frequency, urgency, dysuria, haematuria
- Bowel symptoms: change in bowel habit, tenesmus, diarrhoea, constipation, rectal bleeding
- Abdominal, pelvic or back pain
- Systemic symptoms: unexplained weight loss, fatigue/general malaise, night sweats

A thorough history should be taken, including a history of cervical screening and any previously abnormal results. All patients should have a speculum examination to identify any abnormality on the cervix, and any features of concern should prompt urgent referral for colposcopy. Examination may reveal the presence of an irregular, friable, warty-looking mass arising from the ectocervix, which exhibits contact bleeding. Tumours that arise from within the endocervical canal may not be visible externally but cause the cervix to become cylindrical and 'barrel-shaped'. Ulcerative tumours are associated with seropurulent discharge and erosion of parts of the cervix.

Staging and prognosis

Cervical cancer spreads by direct local invasion into adjacent surrounding structures such as the parametrium, upper and lower vagina and pelvic wall. Lymphatic and haematogenous spread may also occur. Involvement of the pelvic side wall may lead to ureteric obstruction, hydronephrosis and renal failure. Lymphatic spread is usually to the pelvic (common iliac, external/internal iliac) and para-aortic nodes. Cervical cancer is staged according to the FIGO classification system (Table 12.7).

In countries with effective cervical screening programmes, cervical cancer tends to be diagnosed at earlier stages, with associated improved survival rates (95% for stage I disease). Unfortunately, worldwide, the majority of women present in advanced stages. Overall 5-year survival is 60% but is as low as 15% for stage IV disease. In the coming years, data on the effectiveness of the HPV vaccine and predicted reduction in cervical cancer diagnoses should become available.

Table 12.7 FIGO staging classification for cervical cancer

Stage			Description	5-year survival (%)
I	Confined to the cervix			95%
	A	Microscopic invasion only (max depth <5 mm)		
		IA1	Stromal invasion <3 mm	
		IA2	Stromal invasion ≥3 mm and <5 mm	
	B	Invasion with depth ≥5 mm		
		1B1	≥5 mm depth and <2 cm greatest dimension	
		1B2	≥2 cm and <4 cm greatest dimension	
		1B3	≥4 cm greatest dimension	
II	Invasion to upper 2/3 of vagina +/– parametrium			70%
	A	Upper 2/3 vagina (without parametrium)		
		IIA1	<4 cm greatest dimension	
		IIA2	≥4 cm greatest dimension	
	B	Upper 2/3 vagina (with parametrium)		
III	Invasion to lower 1/3 of vagina/pelvic wall/lymph nodes/affects kidney			40%
	A	Lower 1/3 of vagina		
	B	Pelvic wall or hydronephrosis/nonfunctioning kidney		
	C	Pelvic or para-aortic lymph nodes (r = imaging, p = pathology)		
IV	Regional or distant metastases			15%
	A	Bladder or rectal mucosa		
	B	Distant organs		
Overall				60%

Management

Treatment of cervical cancer is with surgery, radiotherapy and chemotherapy. Factors to take into consideration when planning management include patient age, disease stage, comorbidities and fertility concerns. Treatment options and decisions are usually made within a multidisciplinary team.

Stage IA (microinvasive) disease may be treated by local excision, either by LLETZ or cone biopsy, in patients keen to preserve fertility. With clear tissue margins, no further treatment is necessary. Simple hysterectomy may be performed in those who have completed their family.

Stages IB to IIA may be treated with surgery or chemoradiotherapy with equivalent results, although there are significant differences in morbidity with radiotherapy due to fistula formation, vaginal stenosis and sexual dysfunction. Radical hysterectomy with pelvic lymphadenectomy involves a total hysterectomy, excision of the parametrium and upper vagina and excision of the pelvic lymph nodes. The ovaries may be conserved in young women. Radiotherapy usually consists of external beam radiation to the pelvis and vaginal brachytherapy. Chemotherapy in conjunction with radiotherapy has been shown to improve survival. Surgery is generally preferred over chemoradiation for tumours <4 cm, while for tumours ≥4 cm, chemoradiation is preferred. In patients keen for fertility preservation, a radical trachelectomy (removal of the cervix, upper vagina and parametria only) with pelvic lymphadenectomy and prophylactic cervical cerclage (to reduce the risk of preterm delivery) can be considered.

Stages IIB and above are generally treated with chemoradiotherapy.

VULVAL CANCER

Background

Vulval cancer is rare, with an incidence of around 3 in 100,000 women per year. Almost half of all new cases are diagnosed in females aged 75 and over. The lifetime risk is <0.5% (1 in 232 women). Around 90% of vulval cancers are squamous cell carcinomas (SCC). The rest are malignant melanomas, basal cell carcinomas, adenocarcinomas, Bartholin gland tumours and sarcomas. Risk factors for vulval cancer are similar to those of cervical cancer, with high-risk HPV infection playing a central role. Risk factors include:

- Persistent infection with high-risk HPV
- Low socioeconomic status
- Immunosuppression
- Cigarette smoking
- Lichen sclerosis
- Vulval dermatoses
  - Lichen sclerosus: 5% lifetime risk of progression to vulval cancer
  - Lichen planus: 3% lifetime risk of progression to vulval cancer
- Precursor lesions: vulval intraepithelial neoplasia (VIN), Paget disease of the vulva

Presentation

The most common presenting symptoms are:

- Pruritus (itching)
- Irritation or discomfort
- Pain (often described as a burning sensation)
- A lump or ulcer
- Bleeding
- Discharge
- Dysuria
- Dyspareunia

Vulval cancer commonly develops over the labia majora (50% of cases). Other sites include the labia minora, clitoris, Bartholin glands, perineum and posterior fourchette (Fig. 12.2).

RED FLAGS

Consider a suspected cancer pathway referral (for an appointment within 2 weeks) for vulval cancer in women with an unexplained vulval lump, pruritus, ulceration or bleeding.

Premalignant lesions of the vulva

Vulval intraepithelial neoplasia

VIN is the precursor lesion of vulval SCC. It is a premalignant condition characterized by the presence of abnormal dysplastic cells that can progress to cancer if left untreated. Most cases of VIN are asymptomatic, although patients may present with pruritus, pain, ulcers or lesions. Lesions may be raised, erythematous, ulcerated, pigmented, wart-like or keratotic. They may be multifocal or unifocal, and can take the form of macules, papules or plaques. VIN is most commonly seen over the labia and posterior fourchette. There are two main types of VIN, each with distinct features (see Table 12.8).

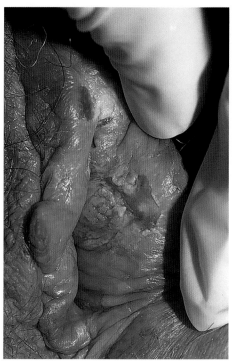

Fig. 12.2 Squamous cell carcinoma of the vulva. (Toma H, Chatterjee-Paer S. *Ferri's Clinical Advisor 2023*. 1st ed. 2023: 1619.e2–1619.e5. © 2023.)

Table 12.8 Types of vulval intraepithelial neoplasia

'Usual-type' or 'classic' VIN	Differentiated VIN
Multifocal and multicentric (multiple lesions)	Unifocal and unicentric (single ulcer/lesion)
Same grading as CIN – VIN I, II, III	Usually high grade
Low risk of progressing to SCC	High risk of progressing to SCC
More common in premenopausal women	More common in postmenopausal women
Associated with HPV infection, cigarette smoking and immunosuppression	Associated with lichen sclerosis/planus
May coexist with intraepithelial neoplasia of the cervix (CIN), vagina (VAIN) and peri-anal region (AIN)	Not classically associated with intraepithelial neoplasia

CIN, *Cervical intraepithelial neoplasia*; HPV, *human papillomavirus*; SCC, *squamous cell carcinomas*; VIN, *vulval intraepithelial neoplasia*.

Diagnosis of VIN is made by histological examination of a biopsy, usually obtained at the time of vulvoscopy. Opportunistic examination of the cervix, vaginal and peri-anal region should be performed due to the risk of intraepithelial neoplasia at these sites.

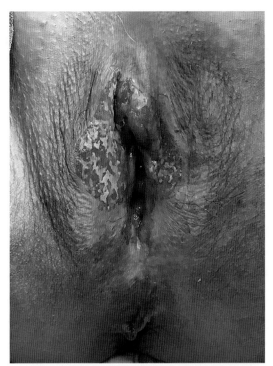

Fig. 12.3 Paget disease of the vulva. (Ngan HYS, Chan KKL. *Essential Obstetrics and Gynaecology.* 2020: 328–351. 2020.)

VIN may be treated by surgical excision, imiquimod (an immune modulator) or laser ablation. Surgical excision with clear margins reduces the risk of progression to SCC and is associated with higher cure rates compared to laser ablation or medical treatment. Reconstruction may be necessary in the case of multiple or extensive excisions. Around 15% of patients undergoing local excision are found to have coexisting SCC. The risk of progression to SCC is 4%, increasing to 40% to 60% in patients who have not undergone surgical excision. Regular follow-up in these patients with vulvoscopy is essential due to the risk of malignant progression. Long-term follow-up for all patients is also important due to the high risk of recurrence.

Paget disease of the vulva (extra-mammary Paget disease)

Paget disease of the vulva is the precursor lesion of vulval adenocarcinomas and arises from glandular epithelium. It has a characteristic appearance of a scaly, erythematous, poorly demarcated lesion resembling eczema, with scattered white islands of hyperkeratosis, progressing to plaque-like, multifocal lesions (Fig. 12.3). The presence of Paget disease of the vulva is associated with a coexisting adenocarcinoma elsewhere in the body in 20% of cases, with the most common sites being the breast, bowel, urinary tract and genital tract (vulva).

Staging and prognosis

Vulval cancer spreads locally to the vagina, perineum, urethra and anus. Lymphatic spread is to the inguinofemoral nodes and then pelvic (common iliac, external/internal iliac) lymph nodes. Cancers originating from the midline (from the urethra, clitoris, introitus or anus) will spread to lymph nodes on both sides. In lateral lesions (i.e., ≥1 cm from the midline), only the nodes on the affected side will be involved.

Vulval cancer is staged according to the FIGO classification system (see Table 12.9). Prognosis is determined primarily by the extent of lymph node involvement. Five-year survival in stage I disease is 80%, halving to 40% in stage III disease. Bilateral lymph node metastases are associated with a 5-year survival of 30%, falling to 10% to 15% if pelvic lymph nodes are involved.

Management

As vulval cancers are rare, it is best practice for them to be managed in dedicated gynaecological cancer centres by a multidisciplinary team. The aim is to achieve complete surgical resection and minimize the risk of recurrence while preserving as much function as possible. Treatment is dependent on disease stage.

Stage 1A disease is treated by wide local excision of the primary tumour with a disease-free tissue margin of at least 15 mm. This is usually sufficient as the risk of lymph node involvement is low. Stage 1B disease requires wide local excision and groin lymphadenectomy. Unilateral groin node dissection may be performed for lateral lesions (≥1 cm from the midline). In all other cases, bilateral groin lymphadenectomy is required. Stages II to IV disease should be treated by radical vulvectomy and bilateral groin lymphadenectomy. In some centres, sentinel lymph node biopsy can be performed to determine the presence of lymph node involvement. If malignant cells are not present in the sentinel node, lymphadenectomy may not be required. This helps to reduce morbidity associated with groin lymphadenectomy.

Patients unsuitable for radical vulvectomy can be offered radiotherapy in conjunction with chemotherapy. Neoadjuvant chemoradiation can help to reduce tumour volume prior to primary surgery. Adjuvant chemoradiotherapy can also be given to patients with lymph node involvement, if the lesion extends close to the excision margin, or in extensive disease. Primary and recurrent vulval cancer does respond to chemotherapy, but responses are variable, and toxicity may be a problem in elderly patients.

Complications of treatment are shown in Table 12.10. Because of the large area involved, wound breakdown is, sadly, relatively common. Some surgeons advocate performing skin grafts at the time of initial surgery. Plastic surgery reconstruction may be required for large defects and when radiotherapy has been used. The vulva is a challenging area for wound healing and faecal and urinary diversion is often required.

Table 12.9 FIGO staging classification for vulval cancer

Stage		Description	5-year survival (%)
I		Confined to the vulva	80%
	A	Stromal invasion ≤1 mm and tumour ≤2 cm in size	
	B	Stromal invasion >1 mm or tumour >2 cm in size	
II		Spread to adjacent perineal structures	50%
		Tumour of any size with invasion into the lower 1/3 of urethra, lower 1/3 of vagina or anus	
III		Spread to inguinofemoral lymph nodes	40%
	A	1 lymph node metastasis (≥5 mm) or 1–2 lymph node metastasis (<5 mm)	
	B	≥2 lymph node metastasis (≥5 mm) or ≥3 lymph node metastasis (<5 mm)	
	C	Positive nodes with extracapsular spread	
IV		Regional/distant metastases	15%
	A	Invasion into the upper 2/3 urethra, upper 2/3 vagina, bladder mucosa, rectal mucosa, fixed to the pelvic bone or fixed/ulcerated inguinofemoral lymph nodes	
	B	Distant metastasis including pelvic lymph nodes	
Overall			67%

Table 12.10 Complications of treatment for vulval cancer

Treatment	Complication
Radical vulvectomy + groin lymphadenectomy	• Wound breakdown • Lymphocyst formation and lymphoedema • Venous thromboembolism • Haemorrhage • Infection – wound, urinary tract • Vulval mutilation, deformity and scarring • Sexual dysfunction • Psychological morbidity
Radiotherapy	• Erythema • Necrosis of the femoral head or pubic symphysis • Fistula formation – urethrovaginal, vesicovaginal, rectovaginal

VAGINAL CANCER

Background

Vaginal cancer is rare and the majority of cases (75%) are preventable. It is usually either a primary SCC or secondary cervical, vulval or endometrial carcinoma that has spread to the vagina. Almost half of vaginal cancer cases in the UK are diagnosed in females aged 70 years and over. Risk factors for vaginal cancer are similar to that of cervical and vulval cancer, with high-risk HPV infection playing a central role. Risk factors include:

• Persistent infection with high-risk HPV
• Coexisting CIN
• Current or previous history of another gynaecological malignancy
• Precursor lesions: vaginal intraepithelial neoplasia (VAIN).
• In utero exposure to diethylstilboestrol: Associated with vaginal adenocarcinoma, typically clear cell adenocarcinoma, although the incidence of this has declined sharply since the drug was banned from use in pregnancy.

Premalignant lesions of the vagina

VAIN is the precursor lesion of vaginal SCC. It is a premalignant condition characterized by the presence of abnormal dysplastic cells that can progress to cancer if left untreated. Most cases of VAIN are asymptomatic and discovered incidentally at the time of cervical screening or during colposcopy. Lesions are usually multifocal and associated with CIN. Treatment is by surgical excision, laser ablation or cryosurgery.

Presentation

The upper third of the vagina is the most common site. Common presenting symptoms include:

• Abnormal vaginal bleeding
• Offensive vaginal discharge
• The presence of a mass which may be ulcerated or necrotic

Table 12.11 FIGO staging classification for vaginal cancer

Stage	Description	5-year survival (%)
I	Confined to the vagina	
II	Spread to the paravaginal tissues	
III	Spread to the pelvic side wall	
IV	Regional/distant metastases	
A	Bladder or rectal involvement	
B	Distant metastasis	
Overall		60%

Staging and prognosis

A diagnosis of vaginal carcinoma is made by histological examination of a biopsy. Vaginal cancer spreads by direct local invasion and through the lymphatic system. Invasion into the bladder or rectum may result in fistula formation. Vaginal cancer is staged according to the FIGO classification system (see Table 12.11). About 70% of women who present have stage I or II disease, with 5-year survival rates of around 60%.

Management

Radiotherapy is the mainstay of treatment and is usually a combination of external beam radiation and brachytherapy. Complications include fistulae formation (as with vulval radiotherapy) and stenosis of the vagina and rectum. Surgical excision may be appropriate in selected patients. This may involve radical hysterectomy, vaginectomy, pelvic lymphadenectomy and pelvic exenteration, depending on the stage of disease and its location. Stage 1 disease in the lower vagina can usually be removed by wide local excision while a radical hysterectomy (including vaginectomy) may be considered in patients with lesions in the upper vagina.

Chapter Summary

- Early diagnosis of all gynaecological cancers will result in improved prognosis. However, it is well-known that some of these cancers, such as ovarian cancer, typically present late.
- Screening programmes, such as the National Cervical Cytology Programme, have already improved early diagnostic rates and outcomes of cervical cancer. It is hoped that these rates will continue to improve since the introduction of the human papillomavirus (HPV) vaccination programme.
- Red flag symptoms, particularly in the postmenopausal population, such as postmenopausal bleeding, abdominal distention or masses, should prompt urgent 2-week wait referrals to a gynaecology department.

UKMLA Conditions
Cervical cancer
Cervical screening (HPV)

UKMLA Presentations
Abdominal distension
Abdominal mass
Abdominal cervical smear result
Endometrial cancer
Ovarian cancer
Pelvic mass
Pruritus
Urethral discharge and genital ulcers/warts
Vulval itching/lesion
Vulval/vaginal lump

Disorders of the vulva are common, and symptoms can cause considerable discomfort to patients. Many of them are chronic conditions that have a negative impact on quality of life and may cause anatomical disfiguration, with associated functional problems and psychosexual issues. When considering the aetiology, while infection and vulval dermatoses are common, malignancy should always be considered and excluded.

The term 'vulva' is used to describe all of the external female genitalia (Fig. 13.1) – the mons pubis, labia majora and minora, clitoris, external urinary meatus, vaginal vestibule, vaginal orifice (introitus) and hymen. The surface of the vulva up to the inner aspect of the labia minora is covered by keratinized stratified squamous epithelium, with a superficial cornified layer. The vaginal mucosa is made up of nonkeratinizing squamous epithelium. The labia majora contains hair follicles, sebaceous glands and sweat glands. As the vulva is essentially skin, dermatological conditions such as psoriasis, eczema and dermatitis can also affect the vulva. Vulval skin care is therefore the cornerstone of treatment in the management of vulval conditions (see clinical notes).

PRESENTATION

Common presenting symptoms of benign vulval disease include:

- Pruritus vulvae (vulval itching)
- Irritation or discomfort
- Pain (often described as a burning sensation)
- A lump or ulcer
- Bleeding
- Discharge
- Dysuria
- Dyspareunia

ASSESSMENT

History taking

The diagnosis of benign vulval disease is strongly reliant on a thorough history due to the varied possible underlying aetiology.

A full medical and gynaecological history should be taken, including age and menopausal status. Postmenopausal women presenting with PMB should be referred urgently for assessment and investigation due to the possibility of malignancy. Establish the presence of a personal or family history of dermatological conditions (e.g., psoriasis, eczema, dermatitis), autoimmune disease (e.g., Crohn, thyroid disease), immunosuppression and chronic conditions (e.g., type I diabetes mellitus) as these can all affect the vulva. Over 90% of individuals presenting with vulval dermatitis will have a history of atopy including hay fever, eczema and asthma.

Enquire about the onset of symptoms, possible triggers, the length of time symptoms have been present and exacerbating/relieving factors. An acute onset of symptoms in conjunction

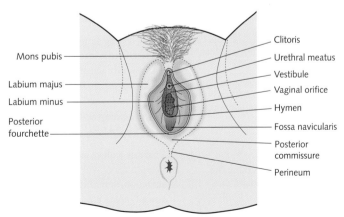

Fig. 13.1 The anatomy of the vulva. (From Kay SE, Sandhu CJ. *Crash Course Obstetrics and Gynaecology.* 2019: 81–85. © 2019.)

with abnormal vaginal discharge is suggestive of infection, and a detailed sexual history should be taken. The colour and odour of discharge may suggest the underlying cause. Take note of any new exposure to or changes to skincare products such as soaps, perfumed hygiene products and washing detergents, as these may irritate vulval skin and cause contact dermatitis. Ask about drug history, including over-the-counter medications, and known allergies. Self-treatment with topical emollients and antifungals is common and any response to this may be relevant.

Examination

A general dermatological examination should be performed as this may give useful information. Psoriasis is typically seen over the scalp, extensor surfaces of the elbows and knees, umbilicus, natal cleft and nail beds (pitting). Lichen planus can affect oro-genital mucous membranes, with the presence of Wickham striae on buccal mucosa. Vulval eczema or dermatitis is often seen over flexor surfaces and in skin folds (intertrigo).

Examine for palpable lymph nodes. Inguinal lymphadenopathy can occur secondary to infection or malignancy. The vulva should be inspected externally for visible lesions, lumps or swellings, plaques, ulcers, erythema and obvious excoriation marks. A speculum examination should be performed to assess the vagina and cervix. Any bleeding or vaginal discharge should be noted. Generalized vaginitis, ulcers and vaginal discharge suggest an infective cause, but ulcers should also raise the suspicion of malignancy (Table 13.1).

Table 13.1 Differential diagnoses of ulcers

Condition	Description of ulcer
Vulval malignancy	A raised lesion which may ulcerate and bleed, focal necrosis may produce purulent/offensive vaginal discharge
Herpes	Usually multiple and painful ulcers
Syphilis	Usually a solitary, indurated, painless ulcer (chancre)
Lichen planus	Superficial erosions or ulcers may be seen on vaginal mucosa +/− Wickham striae, these are more painful than itchy
Behcet disease	Multiple aphthous (yellow-based) painful ulcers found in oral and vaginal mucosa
Vulval Crohn	Granulomatous lesion affecting the perineum and perianal region, can ulcerate and bleed, leading to abscess and fistula formation

INVESTIGATIONS

Microbiology swabs/sexually transmitted infection (STI) screen

Microbiology swabs and a screen for STIs (if applicable), including high and low vaginal swabs, endocervical swabs and urethral swabs, should be performed.

Biopsy

A histological diagnosis is often required to confirm the diagnosis, due to close similarities between the presentation and appearances of various vulval dermatoses. Punch biopsies can be performed under local anaesthetic in a vulval clinic or under general anaesthesia if more extensive samples are required. The threshold for biopsy should be low especially if the diagnosis is uncertain, there are atypical features, symptoms are refractory to treatment or if there are any changes in appearance of chronic disease.

Pelvic ultrasound

This should be performed in any postmenopausal woman presenting with PMB to assess endometrial thickness and ensure a potentially malignant cause is not being missed. A postmenopausal endometrial thickness of >4 mm is considered abnormal and warrants further investigation with hysteroscopy and endometrial biopsy.

Blood tests

Where systemic disease is suspected, investigations such as thyroid, liver and renal function should be performed. Women presenting with lichen sclerosus or planus should be investigated for autoimmune disease due to its associations with these conditions.

Skin patch testing

Patch testing is indicated if allergy or hypersensitivity is suspected in the case of vulval dermatitis. This should be performed with dermatological input.

AETIOLOGY

Pruritus vulvae and pain are the most common presenting symptoms of vulval disease with varied aetiology including infection, systemic illness, neoplastic disease and vulval dermatoses (Table 13.2). Common dermatological conditions involving the vulva include lichen sclerosus, lichen planus, dermatitis, psoriasis and eczema. Infective causes include candidiasis, STIs and scabies. Vulval candidiasis will be covered here while other STIs including syphilis and herpes will be discussed in Chapter 8. Systemic causes of pruritus vulvae include diabetes mellitus, renal failure and Crohn disease. An algorithm for the management of pruritus vulvae can be found in Fig. 13.2.

Vulval candidiasis

Around 75% of women will experience at least 1 episode of symptomatic *Candida* infection in their lifetime. Most

Table 13.2 Aetiology of vulval disease

Classification	Condition
Infection	• Fungal: *Candida,* tinea • Parasitic: *Trichomonas vaginalis,* scabies • Bacterial: bacterial vaginosis, syphilis, *Neisseria gonorrhoeae* • Viral: herpes, vulval warts, human papilloma virus (HPV)
Systemic	• Autoimmune disease: thyroid disease, diabetes mellitus, Crohn • Immunosuppression: steroid use • Renal failure
Neoplastic	• Vulval intraepithelial neoplasia • Paget disease of the vulva • Vulval malignancy
Vulval dermatoses	• Lichen sclerosus • Lichen planus • Vulval dermatitis • Vulval psoriasis • Vulval eczema • Atrophic vulvovaginitis

infections are caused by *Candida albicans* (80%–90%) although other species have been reported. Risk factors for vulval candidiasis include:

- Pregnancy
- Poorly controlled diabetes mellitus
- Iron deficiency anaemia
- Immunosuppression such as prolonged steroid use
- Antimicrobial therapy such as antibiotics causing disturbances in vaginal flora

Vulval candidiasis presents with vulval itching and pain, often described as a soreness or burning sensation. Vaginal discharge is often thick, nonoffensive and curdy, with a typical cottage cheese-like appearance. There may be white plaques over the vaginal walls. Vulval erythema, fissuring and excoriation marks are often seen. *Candida* infection can spread beyond the vulva, giving rise to satellite lesions which appear as a papular eruption. The genitocrural skin folds are commonly affected due to the moist and warm environment (intertrigo).

Treatment is with azole antifungal agents, most commonly oral fluconazole 150 mg as a single dose. Oral therapy is contraindicated in pregnancy and breastfeeding. Topical azoles are safe and equally effective. Clotrimazole 500 mg vaginal pessaries for up to seven consecutive nights has a cure rate of over 90%.

Atrophic vulvovaginitis

This condition affects postmenopausal women due to the fall in oestrogen levels following the menopause. Anatomically there is thinning of the vulval skin and fusion of the labia minora across the midline resulting in burying of the clitoris and narrowing of the introitus. Women may present with pain, vaginal dryness, dysuria and dyspareunia. Management is with topical

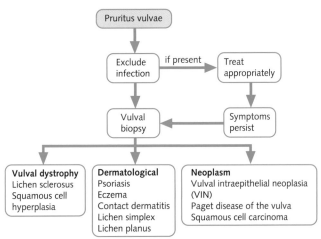

Fig. 13.2 Algorithm for the management of pruritus vulvae. (From Kay SE, Sandhu CJ. *Crash Course Obstetrics and Gynaecology.* 2019: 81–85. © 2019.)

oestrogen therapy (oestriol) for 6 weeks. This is safe and associated with minimal systemic absorption.

Lichen sclerosus

Lichen sclerosus is the most common of the vulval dermatoses. It is a chronic, relapsing autoimmune skin condition that can develop at any age but is more common in postmenopausal women. The exact aetiology is unknown, although autoimmune factors are thought to be involved in its pathogenesis. Lichen sclerosus is associated with other autoimmune diseases including pernicious anaemia, thyroid disease (Hashimoto thyroiditis), vitiligo and type 1 diabetes mellitus. It is unrelated to hormones, menopause, combined oral contraception or hormone replacement therapy use.

Vulval itching is the hallmark of lichen sclerosus. This is classically worse at night and can lead to skin splitting and bleeding (itch-scratch cycle). Other symptoms include vulval pain (often described as a soreness, irritation or burning), dyspareunia (secondary to introital narrowing) and difficulty passing urine (due to midline fusion of the labia).

Diagnosis is usually made on the characteristic clinical appearance of lichen sclerosus and histological findings of a thinned epidermis with hyalinization and deep inflammation on biopsy. Lichen sclerosus affects the whole vulval and perianal region with pale/whitened atrophic plaques ('leucoplakia') in a characteristic 'hourglass' or 'figure-of-8' distribution. Subepidermal atrophy and hyalinization cause thinning and crinkling of the skin, giving a 'cigarette' or 'parchment paper' appearance. Fibrosis and adhesions cause scarring and loss of normal vulval anatomical architecture such as absorption of the labia minora, recession of the clitoral hood and midline fusion of the labia leading to narrowing of the vaginal introitus and burying of the clitoris (Fig. 13.3). Subepithelial haemorrhages (ecchymosis) are commonly seen underneath the skin. The vaginal mucosa is not involved.

Biopsy is mandatory if the diagnosis is uncertain or if there is no response to treatment. Treatment is aimed at managing symptoms and preventing further vulval anatomical disfiguration. High-potency topical corticosteroids (e.g., clobetasol propionate or 'Dermovate') are the first-line treatment and should be used daily before being reduced gradually to a maintenance dose once symptoms are under control. Topical tacrolimus is a second-line option. Laser ablation or surgery is usually avoided and should only be used to restore anatomy and function and not to treat symptoms. Patients with lichen sclerosus should be reviewed yearly with vulvoscopy due to a 5% risk of developing vulval squamous cell carcinoma. Lichen sclerosus is responsible for 30% of all vulval cancers.

CLINICAL NOTES

General vulval skin care advice should be given to all women with vulval conditions:

- Avoid irritants: Examples include panty liners, soaps, bubble baths, fabric softeners, bleaches, shampoos, bath additives, perfumed hygiene products, powders, baby wipes, deodorants, washing detergents (especially fragranced), flavoured lubricants, douches.
- Apply an unscented emollient (moisturizer) cream/lotion/ointment regularly. These soothe, protect and act as a barrier. The aim is to promote healing and ensure that the skin is not exposed to repeated insults. Emollients should also be used as a soap substitute. Examples include Diprobase and Dermol 500.
- Advise 100% cotton underwear and loose clothing, avoiding tight-fitting clothes such as tights and nylon pants.
- Emphasize local hygiene and weight loss (where appropriate).
- Keep the area dry and well-ventilated.
- Avoid spermicide-lubricated condoms.
- Be aware that oil-based products may damage/degrade condoms, leading to possible breaks and risk of pregnancy. They also pose a fire risk and should not be handled near cigarettes or an open flame.

Lichen planus

Lichen planus is another chronic autoimmune skin condition that affects women from all age groups. It may occur anywhere on the body, but predominantly over the vulval and flexor surfaces. Unlike lichen sclerosus, lichen planus can affect oro-genital mucous membranes.

The main presenting symptoms are vulval pain and itching although the condition may be asymptomatic. Pain is usually more significant than itching due to the presence of ulcers. Dyspareunia and difficulty passing urine are also features. Lesions are commonly polygonal, planar (flat-topped), purpuric papules and plaques with fine white lines forming a reticular pattern on their surface (Wickham striae). Wickham striae are more easily visible on buccal mucosa. Superficial erosions or ulcers may be

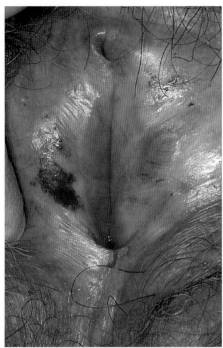

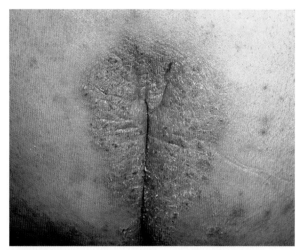

Fig. 13.4 Lichen simplex chronicus. Patient with atopic dermatitis and secondary lichenification manifesting as thickened skin with accentuation of skin markings. Secondary excoriations are also present. (From Swanson E. *Dermatology Secrets*. 2021: 10–20. © 2021.)

Fig. 13.3 Lichen sclerosus. (From Carseldine W, Symonds I. *Talley & O'Connor's Clinical Examination.* Elsevier; 2022: 778–796. © 2022.)

seen on vaginal mucosa along with a well-demarcated glazed erythema around the introitus. Like lichen sclerosus, there is fibrosis and scarring with loss of normal vulval anatomical architecture.

Treatment options include high-potency topical corticosteroids followed by maintenance treatment of a weaker steroid preparation. In cases of complex disease, ciclosporin, topical tacrolimus, retinoids or oral steroids may be required. Surgical excision should be avoided. Patients with lichen planus have a 3% risk of developing vulval squamous cell carcinoma and should be reviewed annually with vulvoscopy.

Vulval dermatitis

Vulval dermatitis is an overarching term used to describe hypersensitivity and inflammation of the vulval skin, usually secondary to allergic or irritant contacts (contact dermatitis). The main symptoms are vulval itching and pain. Allergens/irritants include washing detergents and soaps (see clinical notes). Vulva eczema is a form of dermatitis that occurs more commonly due to an allergen or irritant rather than existing atopy. It is associated with the risk of secondary bacterial or fungal infection.

Vulval intertrigo is a moist, inflammatory dermatitis that occurs in skin folds, especially genitocrural skin, due to apposition and chafing of the skin surfaces. Obesity and tight clothing are common triggers. The skin is often inflamed, erythematous and macerated. *Candidiasis* infection may coexist with intertrigo.

Lichen simplex chronicus

Lichen simplex is a chronic condition characterized by vulval itching and pain. Aetiology can be due to vulval dermatitis, eczema, systemic illness causing pruritis such as iron deficiency, environmental factors, exogenous irritants such as washing detergents and soaps (see clinical notes), and psychiatric disorders such as schizophrenia and depression.

On examination, there is poorly demarcated erythema and inflammation extending beyond the vulval skin. Chronic irritation and scratching results in skin thickening and hypertrophy. There is lichenification and evidence of excoriation along with thickened, scaly skin (Fig. 13.4). Erosions and macerations are present due to excoriation (itch-scratch cycle), often with fissuring and loss of pubic hair. The vaginal mucosa is not involved.

The cornerstone of treatment is general vulval skin care (see clinical notes), avoidance of precipitating factors and the use of emollient soap substitutes. Patch testing can be offered to help identify allergens/irritants. Topical corticosteroids titrated depending on severity may be necessary to help break the itch-scratch cycle and reduce local inflammation caused by scratching. These can be combined with an antifungal or antibiotic in cases of secondary infection. Symptomatic relief may be obtained from antihistamines, moisturizers and emollients. A biopsy should be performed if there is no response to treatment to confirm the diagnosis and exclude malignancy.

Vulval psoriasis

Psoriasis is a chronic autoimmune inflammatory skin disease presenting with typically well-circumscribed, symmetrically distributed, erythematous plaques with 'silver scaling'. The most common sites are the scalp, elbows, nails, natal cleft and knees although any part of the body may be affected. Over the vulva, psoriatic erythematous plaques are typically uniform, symmetrical and smooth, but without 'silver scaling'. Patients typically complain of vulval itching and pain. The presence of coexisting extra-genital psoriasis and nail involvement is suggestive as the vulva is rarely the only area affected. Treatment is as for psoriasis in general, including topical corticosteroids, coal-tar preparations and vitamin D analogues.

FEMALE GENITAL MUTILATION

Definition

The World Health Organization (WHO) defines female genital mutilation (FGM) as any procedure that involves partial or total removal of the external female genitalia, or other injury to the female genital organs for nonmedical reasons.

Prevalence

Worldwide, over 200 million women and girls have been subjected to FGM in at least 30 countries in Africa, the Middle East and Asia, with around 3 million girls estimated to be at risk annually. It also takes place within parts of Europe and other developed countries, primarily among immigrant and refugee communities. FGM is almost exclusively performed on young girls between the ages of infancy and adolescence. It is a traditional cultural practice and multiple socio-cultural factors exist within families and communities for perpetuating FGM.

ETHICS

Female genital mutilation (FGM) is illegal in the UK, as per the Female Genital Mutilation Act 2003 in England, Wales and Northern Ireland and the Prohibition of Female Genital Mutilation (Scotland) Act 2005. It is an offence for any person (regardless of nationality or residence status) to:

- Perform FGM within the UK.
- Aid/abet a girl to undergo FGM within the UK.
- Arrange or assist in arranging (from within the UK) for a UK national/resident to be taken overseas for the purpose of FGM.
- Aid/abet (from within the UK) a non-UK person to perform FGM overseas on a UK national/resident.

For UK nationals/residents (even in countries where FGM is not illegal), it is an offence to:

- Perform FGM outside of the UK.
- Aid/abet a girl to undergo FGM outside the UK.
- Arrange or assist in arranging (from outside the UK) for a UK national/resident to be taken overseas for the purposes of FGM.
- Aid/abet (from outside the UK) a non-UK person to perform FGM overseas on a UK national/resident.

Additionally, it is an offence for those with parental/guardian responsibility to fail to protect a girl under the age of 16 from the risk of FGM. Health and social care professionals have a mandatory duty to notify the police if they discover that FGM has been carried out on a girl under 18 years of age during the course of their work.

Reinfibulation (resuturing of FGM) such as after childbirth or on patient request is illegal. Female genital cosmetic surgery such as labiaplasty can be performed only if necessary for the patient's physical or mental health. All surgeons who undertake female genital cosmetic surgery must be sufficiently trained, and ensure any surgery complies with FGM laws.

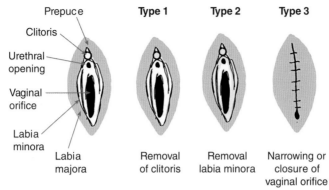

Fig. 13.5 Classification of areas removed by female genital mutilation are highlighted in yellow. Illustrated by Hollie Blaber. (From Punter H, Magnus D. *Medicine in a Day*. 2023: 390–424. © 2023.)

Types

FGM varies in extent and severity, and can be classified into four main types (Fig. 13.5):

Type 1 (clitoridectomy): Partial or total removal of the clitoris and/or the prepuce/clitoral hood.

Type 2 (excision): Partial or total removal of the clitoris and labia minora, with or without removal of the labia majora.

Type 3 (infibulation): Narrowing of the vaginal introitus through the creation of a covering seal by cutting and appositioning the labia minora and/or the labia majora, sometimes through stitching, with or without removal of the clitoris and prepuce/clitoral hood.

Type 4: Encompasses all other harmful procedures to the female genitalia for nonmedical purposes, e.g., pricking, piercing, incising, scraping and cauterizing the genital area.

Complications

There are no health benefits associated with FGM. The procedure involves the removal of healthy and anatomically normal female genital tissue, and interferes with normal sexual function. Short- and long-term complications of FGM are shown in the table below.

Short-term complications	Long-term sequelae
• Severe pain and swelling • Haemorrhage • Infection • Urinary retention • Poor wound healing • Shock • Death	• Wound healing: keloid formation, genital scarring • Urinary dysfunction: dysuria, recurrent urinary tract infections, retention, scarring, difficulty urinating • Sexual dysfunction: chronic pain, dyspareunia • Psychological trauma: depression, anxiety, posttraumatic stress disorder (PTSD) • Genital infection, discharge, itching • Obstetric complications: obstructed labour, difficult vaginal delivery, haemorrhage, caesarean section • Need for deinfibulation to allow sexual intercourse and childbirth (vaginal delivery)

Management

Women with FGM should be managed by a multidisciplinary team of gynaecologists, obstetricians and midwives trained to identify and manage the condition. Consultations should be appropriately sensitive and nonjudgemental, taking into consideration the psychological impact of FGM on patients. There should be an awareness of the techniques for management of FGM which adhere to the FGM Act 2003, particularly if clinical signs and symptoms suggest recent FGM or if the patient presents with pain, haemorrhage, infection and urinary retention.

Deinfibulation refers to the division of scar tissue in order to reopen the vaginal introitus. This may be required for women who have undergone type 3 FGM to enable sexual intercourse, normal passage of urine and menstrual blood, cervical screening, vaginal delivery and other gynaecological procedures. Deinfibulation can be performed under local or regional anaesthesia. For expectant women, it can be carried out antenatally or during labour. Women should be advised on the legal position of FGM both within the UK and abroad. This is especially important if the foetus/baby is female or there are other young girls in the household.

● Chapter Summary

- Vulval disease is a common presentation, particularly in the postmenopausal population. It is associated with severe discomfort, itching, dyspareunia and anatomical changes with secondary complications including infection and risk of developing squamous cell carcinoma.
- Aetiology of vulval disease is varied and systemic conditions, infectious cause and malignancy (see Chapter 12) must be considered as differentials.
- Female genital mutilation is an illegal practice with complex short- and long-term complications. All healthcare professionals should be trained to identify and sensitively manage this presentation.

UKMLA Conditions
Atrophic vaginitis

UKMLA Presentations
Painful sexual intercourse
Pruritus
Vulval itching/lesion

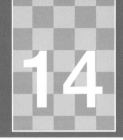
Background

Definition

A prolapse is the protrusion of an organ or structure beyond its normal anatomical site. Pelvic floor organ prolapse results from weakness of the supporting structures (pelvic floor muscles, fascia and ligaments) of the pelvic organs leading to descent from their normal positions. In the female genital tract the type of prolapse depends on the organ involved and its position in relation to the anterior or posterior vaginal wall. Table 14.1 defines and names the different types of prolapse. Prolapse can occur to different degrees, ranging from first (uterine descent only within the vagina) to complete descent outside of the body (procidentia; Fig. 14.1).

Prevalence

Pelvic floor prolapse is common, particularly in older women. It is thought that 50% of women over 50 years of age have some symptoms of pelvic organ prolapse and by the age of 80 years more than 10% would have had surgery for prolapse.

Symptoms

The most common symptom that patients complain of is the sensation of a lump 'coming down', which may have an associated dragging discomfort or heaviness in the vagina. This tends to increase after periods of standing and is relieved when in a supine position. A cystocoele (bladder prolapse) may cause increased urinary frequency, incomplete bladder emptying or recurrent urinary tract infections (UTIs). A rectocoele (bowel prolapse) can cause lower back pain, constipation or incomplete bowel emptying. Prolapses may also cause discomfort during intercourse.

Anatomy

The pelvic floor consists of a series of forward-sloping muscles that form a hammock consisting of the levator ani muscles, coccygeus, piriformis and obturator internus. The levator ani consists of a pubococcygeal part anteriorly and the iliococcygeal part posteriorly and is covered by pelvic fascia. The vagina and urethra pass through the urogenital aperture formed by the medial border of the levator ani. The rectum passes posteriorly with muscle fibres from the pubic bone uniting at the anorectal junction. Thus the muscles provide an indirect support for these structures.

The pelvic fascia condenses to form strong ligaments which support the upper portion of the vagina, cervix and uterus. The transverse cervical (cardinal) ligaments support the cervix to the pelvic side wall and the uterosacral supports the cervix to the sacrum. The round ligament passes from the cornu of the uterus through the inguinal canal to the labia majora, and has a minimal role in support.

Aetiology

Causes of pelvic organ prolapse:

- Obstetrics factors (most common cause): Vaginal delivery with a prolonged second stage, assisted operative vaginal delivery, macrosomia and multiparity are common risk factors.

Table 14.1 Diagnosing and defining type of prolapse

Organ that has prolapsed	Name of prolapse
Bladder	**Cystocoele:** Prolapse of the upper anterior wall of the vagina, attached to bladder by fascia.
Bladder and urethra	**Cystourethrocoele:** A cystocoele extending into the lower anterior vaginal wall, displacing urethra downwards.
Rectum	**Rectocoele:** Weakness in the levator ani muscles causes a bulge in the midposterior vaginal wall which incorporates the rectum.
Small bowel	**Enterocoele:** True hernia of the pouch of Douglas. Prolapse of the upper third of the posterior vaginal wall and contains loops of small bowel.
Uterus and cervix	**Uterine descent:** Uterus descends within the vagina and may even lie outside it (called 'procidentia'). May be associated with a cystocoele and/or rectocoele. Graded according to the position of the cervix on vaginal examination: *First degree:* Cervical descent within the vagina. *Second degree:* Cervical descent to the introitus. *Third degree:* Cervical descent outside the introitus (procidentia).
Vaginal vault	**Vault descent:** After hysterectomy, the proximal end of the vaginal vault can prolapse within or outside the vagina.

- Postmenopausal atrophy: The hypo-oestrogenic state of menopause leads to atrophy of connective tissues.
- Raised intraabdominal pressure: Obesity, weight-lifting and chronic cough, e.g., in chronic obstructive pulmonary disease (COPD) or in smokers with recurrent bronchitis.
- Genetic predisposition: Connective tissue disorders and abnormal collagen production.
- Posthysterectomy vault prolapse: Hysterectomy predisposes to future prolapse of the vagina by surgical division of the transverse cervical and uterosacral ligaments which support the upper vagina.

Diagnosis

History

The diagnosis of pelvic floor prolapse can often be made from its typical presenting symptoms alone. However, it is important to not miss alternative diagnoses. A full medical and gynaecological and obstetric history should be taken, including menopausal status.

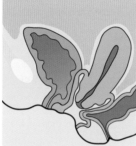

1st degree
descent within the vagina

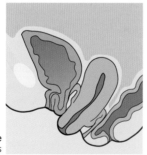

2nd degree
descent to the vaginal introitus

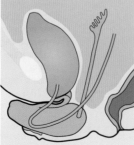

3rd degree/procidentia
descent outside the vagina

Fig. 14.1 Degree of uterine prolapse.

HINTS AND TIPS

Key questions to ask when taking a urogynaecology history:

- Have you noticed a lump from the vagina or a dragging sensation? Does this worsen with prolonged episodes of standing/walking? *(Prolapse symptoms)*
- How many times do you need to pass urine during the daytime?
- Do you wake at night to pass urine? If so, how many times? *(Nocturia)*
- Do you have pain/burning when passing urine? *(Dysuria)*
- Have you seen any blood in your urine? *(Red flag for bladder cancer)*
- Do you suffer from abnormal vaginal discharge? Have you noticed any blood in the discharge? (May result from ulcerated vaginal prolapse or can be a red flag symptom for endometrial cancer in postmenopausal patients)
- Do you have pain when having sex?
- When you need to pass urine, are there times when you struggle to initiate the stream? *(Hesitancy)*
- Do you have to run to the toilet very quickly to pass urine? *(Urgency)*
- Do you have any leaking of urine? *(Urinary incontinence)*
- Is this caused by coughing, sneezing, laughing or running? *(Stress incontinence)*
- Do you have continual leaking throughout the day and night? *(Fistula)*
- How many caffeinated/carbonated drinks do you have per day?
- How much fluid in total do you drink per day?
- Do you smoke? *(Risk factor for chronic cough)*
- Do you struggle to open your bowels? *(Constipation causes straining, which increases intraabdominal pressure)*
- How is this affecting the quality of your life? *(Important when considering management options)*
- Do you take any regular medications? *(Some may cause urinary retention, e.g., anticholinergics, or increased urinary production, e.g., diuretics)*

Examination

General observations are important in the assessment – for example, what is the patient's body mass index and general mobility?

On abdominal examination are there any scars from previous surgery? Are there any palpable abdominal masses?

A Cusco's speculum can be used to examine the patient vaginally with the patient's consent and a chaperone present. Alternatively, the patient can be examined with a Sims speculum in the left lateral position. With the posterior vaginal wall retracted, an anterior prolapse can be easily seen; conversely if the anterior wall is retracted, a posterior prolapse can be assessed. Does the cervix appear normal? Does the vaginal tissue appear healthy?

A bimanual pelvic examination should be performed both with the patient at rest and when performing a Valsalva manoeuvre as prolapses may otherwise be missed in a lying down position. Is there uterine descent? Is there urinary leakage on straining or coughing? A vaginal examination can be performed with the patient standing for a thorough assessment of descent.

The degree and location of pelvic organ prolapse can be assessed using universally recognized grading and staging systems. The Baden–Walker halfway system allows for descriptive grading, while the pelvic organ prolapse quantification (POP-Q) allows for more quantitative grading (see Fig. 14.2).

Investigations

Few investigations tend to be required as prolapse is a clinical diagnosis. However, if the patient has urinary symptoms it is important to investigate these appropriately.

- **Urine test**: Perform a midstream urinary test to exclude UTI as a cause or contributing factor for the symptoms.
- **Urodynamics**: Urodynamics are a series of specialist tests that looks at how well the bladder, sphincters and urethra are storing and releasing urine by showing what happens to the bladder on filling, under stress (e.g., with coughing) and emptying. This is performed in cases where the patient has a history suggesting stress or urge incontinence.

Management

Prevention

As pelvic organ prolapse is such a common phenomenon, it is crucial that we emphasize to patients the importance of preventative measures to strengthen the pelvic floor such as pelvic floor exercises.

It is important to limit the length of the first and second stages of labour and to provide written information on the importance of postnatal pelvic floor exercises.

Baden–Walker halfway system	
Grade 0	Normal position for each respective site
Grade 1	Descent halfway to the hymen
Grade 2	Descent to the hymen
Grade 3	Descent halfway past the hymen
Grade 4	Maximum possible descent for each site

POP-Q Examination and staging	
Stage 0	No prolapse
Stage I	Leading edge ≥1 cm above hymenal ring
Stage II	Leading edge ≤1 cm above hymenal ring but ≤1 cm below hymenal ring
Stage III	Most distal point is >1 cm but < (TVL-2) cm below the hymenal ring
Stage IV	Leading edge ≥ (TVL-2) cm below hymenal ring

Fig. 14.2 Baden–Walker halfway system and the pelvic organ prolapse quantification (POP-Q) for staging and grading pelvic floor prolapse. https://www.clinicalkey.com/student/content/book/3-s2.0-B978032375573300696X. Pelvic Organ Prolapse - Ferri's Clinical Advisor 2023; Hodges, Ashley, MD; Fagan, Matthew J., MD, FACOG; Ferri's Clinical Advisor 2023, 1165-1167.e1.

Conservative

- Weight loss: if BMI is >30.
- Smoking cessation: Reduces chronic cough.
- Managing other causes of chronic cough: Optimizing asthma/chronic obstructive pulmonary disease (COPD) control.
- Avoiding constipation: Dietary changes and/or use of laxatives.
- Avoiding heavy lifting.
- Referral for guided pelvic floor physiotherapy: Apps have also be developed to help guide and remind patients to perform pelvic floor exercises.
- Treating atrophy: In women who are postmenopausal, the presence of atrophic pelvic tissues may be contributing. Hormone replacement therapy, particularly topical vaginal oestrogen treatment, can help increase collagen content and reduce friability of atrophic tissue.
- Pessaries: A pessary is a removable plastic or silicone device placed into the vagina that is designed to support areas of

pelvic organ prolapse. There are various types and sizes that are chosen as per patient suitability, but the most commonly used type is a ring pessary. After a vaginal examination is performed and appropriate size is chosen, the pessary is passed into the vagina so that it sits behind the pubic bone anteriorly and in the posterior fornix of the vagina posteriorly, thereby enclosing the cervix. Fitting the correct size of pessary is important and may take more than one attempt. You do not want the pessary to be too small and risk falling out, but if it is too large it can cause discomfort or urinary difficulty. On occasions pessaries can cause local inflammation or bleeding and granulation tissues can develop. Pessaries should be changed or removed, cleaned and reinserted regularly to reduce this risk, ideally every 6 months. Oestrogen cream is used when changing the pessary, to minimize soreness. It is possible to have intercourse when a ring pessary is in situ. A pessary insertion is a very good alternative to surgical options in situations where the patient is not medically fit for surgery, would prefer conservative management or if their family is not yet complete.

Surgical

Surgery should be considered for those who have trialled conservative management and have ongoing severe symptoms. Surgery aims to relieve symptoms while optimizing bladder and bowel function. It is not recommended if a patient's family is not yet complete. It is important to counsel about the risks and benefits of the procedure including dyspareunia which may result from narrowing and shortening of the vagina. No operation guarantees a permanent solution for prolapse, but it often has a good chance of improving symptoms. Up to 30% of women having surgery for prolapse however will develop another prolapse in the future.

- A **pelvic floor repair** can be performed if there is prolapse of the anterior or posterior wall of the vagina. An anterior repair (**anterior colporrhaphy**) is indicated for the repair of a cystocoele. A portion of redundant anterior vaginal wall tissue mucosa is excised and the exposed fascia is plicated to support the bladder. This operation is done via the vagina without abdominal incisions. Postoperatively there is a risk of worsening urinary symptoms. A posterior repair (**posterior colporrhaphy**) is indicated for the repair of a rectocoele using a technique similar to an anterior colporrhaphy on the posterior vaginal wall. It is possible to perform anterior and posterior repairs simultaneously.
- A **vaginal hysterectomy** (removal of the uterus) can be performed for uterine prolapse and can reduce the risk of recurrence of cystocoele or rectocoele. Anterior or posterior repair can also be performed at the same time. At the time of hysterectomy, a **McCall culdoplasty** can be performed, which opposes the uterosacral ligaments to support the remaining vaginal vault.

Operations can also be performed to lift and support the vaginal vault.

- **Sacrospinous fixation** fixes the apex of the vault to the sacrospinous ligament via a transvaginal approach.
- **Sacral colpopexy** is an abdominal procedure that suspends the vaginal vault from the sacral promontory using strips of fascia or a synthetic mesh or suture. Complications can include nerve damage, bleeding and infection.

See Fig. 14.3 for management summary.

> **HINTS AND TIPS**
>
> There has been much controversy in recent years regarding the use of mesh for pelvic floor surgeries, resulting in a 'Mesh ban' across many countries. Patients are presenting with late complications of mesh erosion including chronic pelvic pain, dyspareunia and persistent vaginal discharge/chronic infections. Patients with complications from mesh require referral to a specialist unit for consideration of mesh removal.

URINARY INCONTINENCE

Background

Definition

Urinary incontinence (UI) is the complaint of any involuntary leakage of urine. It is a common symptom that can affect women of all ages. The bladder has two major roles: the retention of urine and the expulsion of urine. Failure to retain urine or loss of normal voiding control are the two aetiologies of incontinence.

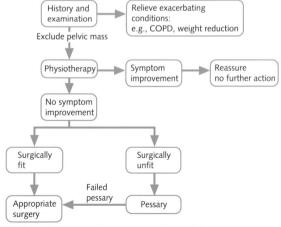

Fig. 14.3 Summary of management for pelvic organ prolapse.

- Stress urinary incontinence (SUI) is involuntary urine leakage on effort or exertion such as with sneezing, coughing or laughing and accounts for 50% of incontinence.
- Urge incontinency, or detrusor overactivity (DO), is involuntary urine leakage proceeded by a sudden compelling urge to urinate when the bladder is either unstable or overactive and accounts for 40% of incontinence.
- Mixed urinary incontinence (MUI) is a combination of SUI and DO. Overactive bladder is urgency that occurs with or without incontinence and commonly with frequency and nocturia. It is suggestive of DO (Table 14.2).

Prevalence

The prevalence of UI increases with increasing age with 8.5% of women aged under 65 years, 11.6% over 65 years and 43.2% over 85 years affected.

Table 14.2 The causes of female urinary incontinence in order of frequency of occurrence

1.	Stress urinary incontinence (SUI)	50%
2.	Detrusor overactivity (DO)	40%
3.	Mixed SUI and DO	5%
4.	Sensory urgency	4%
5.	Chronic voiding problems (chronic retention)	<1%
6.	Fistula	<1%

Diagnosis

Stress incontinence

The bladder acts as a low-pressure reservoir. As the volume of urine increases, the bladder pressure rises slightly. Urethral closure pressure, produced by the passive effect of elastic and collagen fibres and active striated and smooth muscle, causes the urethra to remain closed at rest. In the resting state the urethral closure pressure is higher than the relatively low bladder pressure, and continence is maintained (Fig. 14.4).

Raised intraabdominal pressure, such as when coughing or sneezing, increases the bladder pressure and bladder neck pressure. If the bladder neck and proximal urethra are above the pelvic floor, the positive pressure gradient and continence are maintained. However, if the bladder neck and proximal urethra are below the pelvic floor, then the positive pressure gradient is lost and incontinence occurs. Therefore SUI has an association with pelvic floor prolapse.

SUI increases with increasing age due to parity, postmenopausal status and as maximal urethral closing pressure decreases. Vaginal tissue atrophy and pelvic floor surgery are also associated.

Urge incontinence/detrusor overactivity

In women with DO the urethra functions normally, but if the uninhibited detrusor activity increases bladder pressure above maximal urethral closure pressure, urinary leakage can occur.

The majority of women with DO have idiopathic aetiology with no demonstrable abnormality, but it increases with age. However, causes can include surgery to the bladder neck and proximal urethra, such as surgery for SUI. Neurological

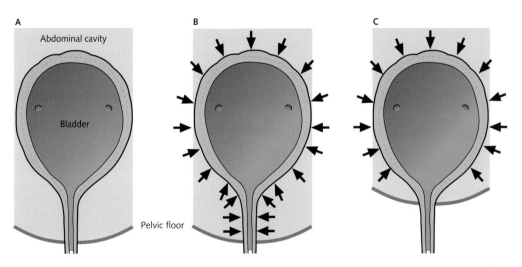

Fig. 14.4 Mechanism of stress urinary incontinence (SUI). (A) Bladder at rest; (B) intraabdominal pressure transmitted to the bladder and urethra (normal); and (C) intraabdominal pressure not transmitted to the bladder/urethra (SUI).

Table 14.3 Neurological causes of voiding difficulties (acute and chronic retention)

Type of lesion	Neurological cause of voiding difficulty
Central (suprapontine)	Cerebrovascular accident Parkinson disease
Spinal	Spinal cord injury Multiple sclerosis
Peripheral	Prolapsed intervertebral disc Peripheral autonomic neuropathies (e.g., diabetic)

conditions such as multiple sclerosis, autonomic neuropathy and spinal lesions lead to uninhibited detrusor contractions, causing detrusor hyperreflexia (Table 14.3).

Sensory urgency

Irritation of the bladder mucosa, due to acute infection, chronic infection, bladder stones or tumours can cause sensory urgency. The aetiology of primary vesicle sensory urgency is not well understood but accounts for almost 4% of incontinent women.

Voiding disorders

Voiding difficulties can present as acute or chronic urinary retention with overflow incontinence. Chronic overdistension of the bladder is then likely to be exacerbated, worsening symptoms with additional detrusor ischaemia and denervation.

Voiding difficulties can occur secondary to mechanical obstruction, medication or neurological conditions. Impaction of a pelvic mass, for instance, a fibroid uterus, bladder polyps or malignancy might obstruct the urethra. It is also common to have a temporary blockade caused by swelling following bladder neck surgery. Postoperative pain can cause reflex inhibition of micturition, as can severe inflammation of the bladder, urethra and vulva.

Central, spinal and peripheral neurological lesions can produce voiding difficulties. Approximately 25% of women with multiple sclerosis will present with acute urinary retention.

Medications can cause voiding difficulties, the most common example being epidural or spinal anaesthesia during labour. Tricyclic antidepressants, anticholinergic agents, α-adrenergic agonists and ganglion blockers can all impact voiding.

Fistulae

The most common cause of urogenital fistulae worldwide is obstructed labour, which is almost eradicated in the UK due to our care of prolonged labour. Fistulae can also occur secondarily to urogynaecological surgery, malignancy or pelvic radiotherapy. These may occur from the rectum, ureter, bladder or urethra to the vagina.

History

A detailed history is important as patients can present with multiple symptoms of varying degrees (Table 14.4). It is important to correlate the history with a bladder diary. A specific urogynaecology history should be taken as per pelvic floor dysfunction described earlier in this chapter.

COMMUNICATION

It is important to acknowledge the considerable psychosocial impact of urinary incontinence symptoms. Some hospitals have the benefit of a continence specialist nurse to provide additional support. Support groups are available, such as ERIC (https://www.eric.org.uk/) for children, and Bladder Health UK (bladderhealthuk.org) for adults. Histories should be taken in a sensitive manner and should always be in a confidential environment to ensure the patient feels as comfortable as possible discussing this.

Examination

Examination focusses on the same features as pelvic floor prolapse (see earlier discussion).

Examine the external genitalia – are there signs of excoriation or chronic inflammation of the bladder? Are the vaginal tissues healthy or are there signs of tissue atrophy?

While performing a pelvic examination assess for uterine descent – is there descent on straining or coughing? Is there urinary leakage on straining or coughing? A vaginal examination can be performed with the patient standing and often stress incontinence can be demonstrated by coughing with a moderately full bladder.

If there is suspicion from the history of neurological cause of incontinence, a full neurological examination should be performed including a digital rectal examination.

Investigations

- **Urine test:** Perform a urinary dipstick to exclude UTI as the cause.
- **Bladder diary:** This is a recording of times and volumes of urine passed, leakage and pad usage along with type and amount of fluid intake, degree of urgency and degree of incontinence. It is recommended that this is kept for a minimum of 3 days on both working and leisure days. It will highlight triggers for incontinence episodes related to lifestyle that may be adjustable, such as high caffeine intake.

Table 14.4 Commonly used urogynaecological terms

Term	Definition
Cystometry	The measurement of bladder pressure and volume
Detrusor overactivity	An overactive bladder is one that is shown objectively to contract spontaneously or on provocation during the filling phase while the patient is attempting to inhibit micturition
High frequency of micturition	Voiding more than seven times per day
Stress urinary incontinence	The involuntary loss of urine when the intravesical pressure exceeds the maximum urethral pressure in the absence of detrusor activity
Nocturia	Voiding more than twice per night
Nocturnal enuresis	The involuntary passage of urine at night
Stress incontinence	Involuntary loss of urine associated with raised intraabdominal pressure
Urge incontinence	Urinary leakage associated with a strong and sudden desire to void
Urgency of micturition	A strong and sudden desire to void
Urinary incontinence	Involuntary loss of urine that is a social or hygienic problem and is objectively demonstrable
Uroflowmetry	The measurement of urine flow rate
Videocystourethrography	Combines radiological with pressure and flow studies

- **Urodynamic studies:** This term encompasses tests that assess the function of the lower urinary tract, and therefore the ability to void. Flow studies, using a flowmeter, assess the rate of flow of urine that normally should be above 15 mL/s. A low flow rate suggests poor action of the detrusor muscle, or an outflow obstruction.

  Cystometry measures bladder pressure during filling and voiding using pressure catheters inserted in the bladder (intravesical pressure) and the rectum (intraabdominal pressure). The bladder pressure can be subtracted from the intraabdominal pressure to give the detrusor pressure. This can detect detrusor instability, contractility and outflow resistance (Fig. 14.5).

Video cystourethrography involves real-time radiological monitoring of the bladder during cystometry using contrast material in the bladder. This can concurrently help to identify anatomical anomalies – such as diverticula and fistula, stress incontinence or bladder neck descent – seen on coughing or outflow pathology visualized on voiding.

- **Cystoscopy:** This is an investigation involving a narrow camera being introduced in the bladder via the urethra, which allows inspection of the bladder neck and internal bladder anatomy. It will enable identification of polyps, calculi, chronic inflammation and malignancies. However, it elicits no information regarding bladder function, so it has no role in the initial assessment of women with UI alone. Fig. 14.6 summarizes the investigation and diagnosis pathways.

Management

Conservative

As per pelvic organ prolapse, conservative measures include weight loss, fluid management and caffeine reduction. Stopping smoking and treating constipation and chronic cough can improve urinary symptoms.

Physiotherapy and pelvic floor exercises can improve urinary control and symptoms in up to 60% of women with SUI. Techniques can range from simple muscular exercises to more complex therapy involving vaginal cones. However, symptoms can return if exercises are stopped.

Bladder retraining aims to improve bladder control in women with DO. Patients are taught how to 'reset' bladder function by micturating by the clock rather than by felling of need, gradually increasing voiding intervals. Offer a trial of supervised pelvic floor muscle training of at least 3 months duration as first-line treatment to women with SUI or mixed incontinence. This may be successful in up to 80% of patients. Hypnotherapy and acupuncture have also been shown to be beneficial.

Medical

There is a strong placebo effect in the drug treatment of DO.

- **Antimuscarinic medications** act to increase bladder capacity by delaying initial desire to void, decreasing the strength of detrusor contractions and decreasing the frequency of detrusor contractions. The suggested preparations are oxybutynin (immediate release), tolterodine (immediate release) and darifenacin (once-daily preparation). These medications can improve symptoms in many women, but can have unpleasant antimuscarinic side effects such as a dry mouth (Table 14.5). It is therefore advised to prescribe the lowest recommended dose when starting a new treatment.

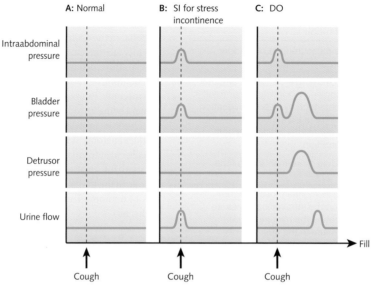

Fig. 14.5 Cystometry. (A) Normal bladder: no increase in detrusor pressure with filling or contraction with cough; (B) genuine stress incontinence – urine flow with cough seen and (C) detrusor overactivity (DO) – detrusor contracts after cough and urine flows with detrusor contraction.

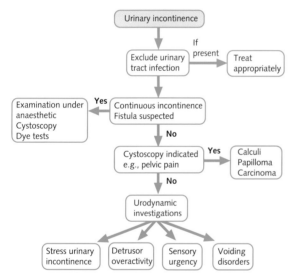

Fig. 14.6 Algorithm for diagnosis of urinary incontinence.

Transdermal medications can be offered to women unable to tolerate oral medication.

- **Mirabegron** (second-line therapy) is recommended as an option for treating the symptoms of overactive bladder only for people in whom antimuscarinic drugs are contraindicated or clinically ineffective, or have unacceptable side effects.
- **Duloxetine** is an inhibitor of serotonin and noradrenaline reuptake and increases the tone of the urethral sphincter. It

Table 14.5 Antimuscarinic (atropine-like) side effects

Type of side effect	Description
Peripheral	Dry mouth
	Reduced visual accommodation
	Constipation
	Glaucoma
Central	Confusion

is not recommended as a first-line treatment of SUI, but can be offered as a second-line therapy if women prefer pharmacological to surgical treatment or are not suitable for surgical treatment.

- **Topical oestrogen replacement** can improve the symptoms of stress incontinence in postmenopausal women.

Surgical

Many patients with SUI can be cured by surgery. Surgery aims to lift and support the bladder neck and urethra, restoring the normal intraabdominal position.

- **Tension-free vaginal tape** can be inserted through a small vaginal incision over the mid-urethra. Long-term success rates are up to 90%, comparable to **colposuspension** (see earlier discussion).
- Invasive options for improving DO include bladder wall **injections with botulinum toxin A** with good chance of a large reduction in symptoms. However, it is a treatment

that wears off over time and has a risk of requiring temporary clean intermittent catheterization in 10% to 15% of patients

- **Bulking agents** can be injected to add bulk to the urethra and reduce leaking with coughing and sneezing. These also may require repeat injections and carry a risk of intermittent self-catheterization.
- **Presacral nerve stimulation** with an implant. Risks include infection and migration of prosthesis.
- **Posterior tibial nerve stimulation** can be provided by specialist nurses, which has been shown to be successful in 48% to 72% of cases.
- Major surgical procedures include **augmentation cystoplasty** or **urinary diversion**, but these interventions carry serious potential complications and life-long follow-up, therefore decision to proceed with these should be carefully considered.

Acute urinary retention requires catheterization to both relieve the retention and avoid permanent bladder injury. Post-operative or postpartum retention usually resolves with free bladder drainage for 48 hours or so. If the bladder has an over-distension injury, then free bladder drainage is required until normal function returns. Chronic retention may require intermittent self-catheterization, a long-term indwelling catheter or a suprapubic catheter. However, there is an ongoing risk of infection and sepsis with these methods.

If a patient has a large fistula, closure by an experienced surgeon is required. However, it is possible for small fistulae to close spontaneously by continence-free drainage of the bladder.

Complications

Although incontinence itself is not life-threatening, it does cause major psychosocial problems. Changes in lifestyle are common and occasionally symptoms are so severe to render the woman housebound. Continence pads can be a financial burden for patients. Excoriation and soreness of the vulva can cause great discomfort, and risk fungal infection and recurrent UTI with potential for damage to renal function. Chronic overdistension of the bladder can cause denervation of the detrusor muscle and worsen ongoing voiding difficulties.

RED FLAGS

Urgent referral for review is warranted in patients with macroscopic haematuria, microscopic haematuria over the age of 50 years, recurrent urinary tract infection with haematuria and suspected pelvic mass arising from the urinary tract, to exclude malignancy.

RECURRENT UTIs

UTIs are a common type of bacterial infection with up to 50% experiencing them as adults. Recurrent UTI is defined as three or more episodes of symptomatic UTI within a 12-month period, ideally culture-proven infections.

Recurrent infections suggest an underlying anatomical or functional pathology, therefore should be investigated. Renal tract ultrasound should be arranged and computed tomography (CT) scan of the kidneys, ureters and bladder should be considered with a history of renal colic. If there is any voiding dysfunction, urodynamics should be considered. Flexible cystoscopy should also be considered, as up to 8% of women >50 years of age with recurrent infection will have significant abnormalities detected at cystoscopy, such as chronic inflammation.

Prophylactic low-dose antibiotic regimen treatment can be commenced for 6 months, as data indicate that this can reduce rate of UTI. The choice of antibiotic used should be based on the most recent sensitivities when available, but it is important to remember that long-term antibiotic prophylaxis is strongly associated with the development of antimicrobial resistance.

PAINFUL BLADDER SYNDROME

Painful bladder syndrome (PBS) is a relatively new terminology (replacing the diagnosis of 'interstitial cystitis' in many patients). It is defined as pelvic pain, pressure or discomfort perceived to be related to bladder filling, lasting at least 6 months, and accompanied by at least one other urinary symptom, e.g., persistent urge to void/frequency in the absence of other identifiable infection or pathology. It most commonly affects those aged 40 to 60 with a 9:1 female predominance. Patients should be advised to keep a bladder diary, food diary, have an MSU (Midstream urine) performed and be asked about the psychological impact this disorder has on their quality of life. Cystoscopy can be performed to rule out other causes. Urodynamics may play a role if the patient has concurrent OAB Overactive bladder, SUI or voiding dysfunction symptoms. A multidisciplinary team approach must be taken before considering surgical management options.

CONSERVATIVE MANAGEMENT

- Dietary: Avoid caffeine/alcohol, acidic foods/carbonated drinks
- Stress management and exercise
- Analgesia
- Support groups
- Consider referral to physiotherapy, pain team specialists and or a clinical psychologist

MEDICAL MANAGEMENT

- Amitriptyline or cimetidine (off-licence specialist treatment) have been shown to be beneficial if conservative measures have failed.

SURGICAL MANAGEMENT

- Intravesical injections, e.g., lidocaine, hyaluronic acid or botox.

- Cystoscopic fulguration and laser treatment and transurethral resection of lesions (if Hunner lesions present).
- Neuromodulation treatment, e.g., posterior tibial nerve stimulation or sacral neuromodulation.
- Oral cyclosporins.
- Cystoscopy with or without hydrodistension.
- Major surgery is reserved for refractory cases of Painful bladder syndrome (BPS) and carries significant risks as discussed above for incontinence.

● Chapter Summary

- Pelvic floor organ prolapse is a common condition caused by weakening of the pelvic floor. Risk factors include pregnancy and childbirth, postmenopausal atrophy and causes of raised intraabdominal pressure.
- Urinary incontinence is the complaint of any involuntary leakage of urine. It is a common symptom that can affect women of all ages with a wide range of severity.
- Urogynaecological symptoms should be thoroughly investigated to achieve the correct diagnosis and to aid management options.
- It is important that treatment is determined by the underlying condition, the severity of the symptoms and crucially by the effect on the patient's quality of life.
- Painful bladder syndrome is a diagnosis of exclusion and a multidisciplinary team approach should be taken for managing patients with this condition.

UKMLA Conditions
Menopausal problems
Urinary incontinence

UKMLA Presentations
Urinary incontinence
Urinary symptoms
Vaginal prolapse
Vulval/vaginal lump

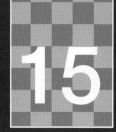

Gynaecological endocrinology

BACKGROUND

Monthly menstruation for those of reproductive age is a manifestation of cyclical higher brain/ovarian activity. Many external and internal factors may affect this careful hormonal balance, thus resulting in disruptions to the menstrual cycle.

AMENORRHOEA

Definition

Amenorrhoea is the absence of menstruation. This may result as part of a normal physiological process, e.g., in prepubescent children, during pregnancy or lactation and after the menopause, or this may be pathological due to an underlying disease or condition. Amenorrhoea can be defined as either being primary or secondary in nature (Table 15.1).

Diagnosis

History

History is crucial in diagnosing the cause of amenorrhoea as the aetiology can be so varied. By definition, menarche will not have occurred in women with primary amenorrhoea. Important areas to cover include:

- Menstrual and pubertal history
- Full gynaecological and obstetric history
- Preexisting medical conditions and symptoms
- General health
- Psychological wellbeing
- Family history

Key additional questions to ask when assessing a patient with amenorrhoea:

- How old were you when you went through puberty? The timing of any pubertal development will establish whether this is normal, precocious or delayed
- Do you have regular periods? Menstrual irregularity or oligomenorrhoea may suggest conditions such as polycystic ovarian syndrome. Cyclical pain may suggest a congenital or acquired outflow obstruction to menstrual fluid.
- Do you have any known gynaecology conditions, e.g., polycystic ovarian syndrome (PCOS), prior pelvic surgery or sexually transmitted infections? *Procedures such as*

cervical surgery, e.g., Large loop excision of the transformation zone (LLETz) or cone biopsy) can cause cervical stenosis.
- Have you had any previous pregnancies? What was the outcome of each of those pregnancies? Pituitary failure can occur after massive postpartum haemorrhage (Sheehan syndrome). Any cause for uterine curettage, such as surgical management of miscarriage or termination, can result in intrauterine adhesions (Asherman syndrome).
- Do you have any medical problems? Some chronic medical conditions such as thyroid dysfunction or diabetes mellitus can affect menstruation.
- Do you take any regular medications? A full drug history should identify medications that can cause amenorrhoea. Antipsychotics can cause increased prolactin levels and illicit drug use such as cocaine and opiates can cause hypogonadism (Table 15.2).
- Have you noticed any leaking of milk from your breasts, headache or loss of vision? *Pituitary tumour, e.g., prolactinoma.*
- Do you suffer from excessive hair on your face/acne? Hirsutism and virilism can be due to congenital adrenal hyperplasia, PCOS or an androgen-secreting tumour.
- Do you suffer from hot flushes and vaginal dryness? How old was your mother/grandmother when they went through menopause? *Symptoms and risk factors for premature ovarian insufficiency.*
- Is there any family history of delay in puberty or genetic disorders? *Hereditary changes.*
- What is your current height and weight (in order to calculate BMI)? Any significant changes in your weight recently? *Low BMI can cause amenorrhoea particularly in cases of anorexia and bulimia.*
- Are you under a lot of stress? Excessive stress may disrupt menstruation.

HINTS AND TIPS

Hirsutism is the excessive growth of terminal hair in androgen-dependent areas (face, chest, linea alba). It can be due to increased androgen levels, but can be idiopathic. Hirsutism can be very distressing to patients and therefore should be dealt with sensitively and professionally.

Table 15.1 Subtypes of amenorrhoea

Type of amenorrhoea	Definition	Prevalence	Causes
Primary	When menstruation has not yet started by the age of 16 years in the presence of normal secondary sexual characteristics, or 14 years in the absence of other evidence of puberty.	Rare (0.3% of female population)	Normal secondary sexual characteristics: **Genitourinary malformations**, e.g., imperforate hymen, vaginal septum, absent vagina or absent uterus. Absent secondary sexual characteristics: **Underlying chromosomal** or **hormonal cause**, e.g., Turner syndrome (45,XO) or hypothalamic–pituitary dysfunction.
Secondary	Absent periods for at least 6 months in a woman who has previously had regular periods, or 12 months if she has had oligomenorrhoea (bleeds less frequently than 6 weekly).	Common (4% of female population)	**Physiological**, e.g., prepubescent children, pregnancy/lactation and postmenopause. **Iatrogenic**, e.g., hormonal contraception, radiotherapy or illicit drug use. **De novo genitourinary malformations**, e.g., cervical stenosis or Asherman syndrome. **Intrinsic hormonal disruption**, e.g., hypothalamic dysfunction, premature ovarian insufficiency, pituitary and thyroid causes.

Table 15.2 Prescribed drugs that can cause hyperprolactinaemia[a]

Types of drug	Drug class
Antipsychotic drugs	Phenothiazines Haloperidol
Antidepressants	Tricyclic antidepressants
Antihypertensive drugs	Methyldopa Reserpine
Oestrogens	Combined oral contraceptive pill
H$_2$ receptor antagonists	Cimetidine Ranitidine Metoclopramide and domperidone

[a]Do not forget chemotherapy for malignancy or immunological disorders.

Examination

A general examination should be performed. Measure height and body weight, and calculate body mass index (BMI). The examination should be top-to-toe.

Hair and face: Look for signs of excess androgens such as hirsutism, acne, weight gain and male pattern balding. Assess visual fields if a pituitary tumour is suspected. Asses for anosmia (Kallman syndrome).

Neck and body: Assess for signs of thyroid disease, diabetes and Cushing syndrome such as striae, buffalo hump and significant central obesity. Typical features of Turner syndrome include short stature, a webbed neck, shield chest with widely spaced nipples, wide carrying angle and scoliosis. Examine for secondary sexual development using the Tanner system (Fig. 15.1).

Abdomen: Examine the abdomen for any pelvic masses. Assess for groin nodes, hernias or undescended testes.

Genitalia: Pelvic inspection should be performed with the patient's consent (if able to consent), chaperone and parent present if indicated. This should be performed with particular sensitivity in young patients as this may cause much embarrassment or provoke anxiety. Often only inspection is indicated if the patient has not been sexually active previously. Assess for clitoromegaly, a sign of virilization and for vaginal patency if appropriate. If a haematocolpos is present, you may see a bulging blue-coloured bulge at the introitus . In those not sexually active, abdominal ultrasonography should be performed to assess pelvic anatomy.

Investigations

Target investigations for amenorrhoea to a specific cause as highlighted by the history if possible. All patients of childbearing age must have a urine pregnancy test to exclude pregnancy as the cause. A summary of investigations is shown in Figs. 15.2 and 15.3.

Pelvic ultrasound

This can identify polycystic ovaries if suspected with typical appearance of enlarged ovaries and multiple peripheral follicles. It can also be used to identify anatomical abnormalities (such as an absent uterus caused by androgen insensitivity) or outflow obstruction such as haematometra (blood within the uterus).

Blood tests

- **Serum gonadotrophins** (luteinizing hormone (**LH**) and follicle-stimulating hormone (**FSH**)): In polycystic ovarian syndrome (PCOS) the LH-to-FSH ratio is usually greater

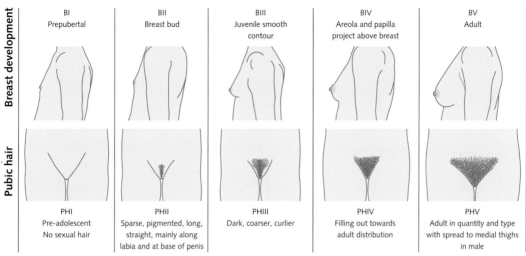

	BI Prepubertal	BII Breast bud	BIII Juvenile smooth contour	BIV Areola and papilla project above breast	BV Adult

	PHI Pre-adolescent No sexual hair	PHII Sparse, pigmented, long, straight, mainly along labia and at base of penis	PHIII Dark, coarser, curlier	PHIV Filling out towards adult distribution	PHV Adult in quantity and type with spread to medial thighs in male

Tanner stage	Breast development (B)	Pubic hair (PH)
1	Prepubertal – no breast tissue	Prepubertal – no pubic hair
2	Breast bud stage with elevation of breast and papilla; enlargement of areola	Sparse growth of long, slightly pigmented hair, straight or curled along labia
3	Further enlargement of breast and areola; no separation of their contour	Darker, coarser and more curled hair, spreading sparsely over the junction of pubis
4	Areola and papilla form a secondary mound above level of breast	Hair adult in type, but covering smaller area than in adult; no spread to medial surface of thighs
5	Mature stage: projection of papilla only, related to recession of areola	Adult in type and quantity, with horizontal distribution

Fig. 15.1 Tanner staging of puberty for females. (https://www.clinicalkey.com/student/search/tanner%20staging%20in%20females?source=home&page=1.) Macleod's Clinical Examination 15th Edition - April 11, 2023 **Editors:** Anna R Dover, J. Alastair Innes, Karen Fairhurst. Chapter 15.

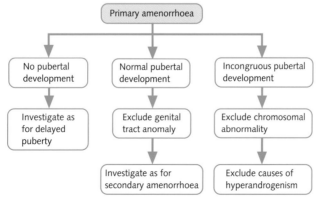

Fig. 15.2 Algorithm for primary amenorrhoea.

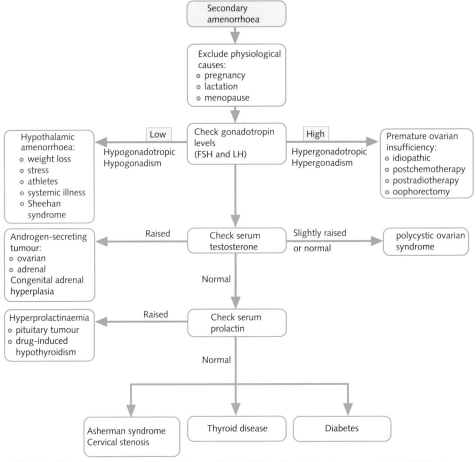

Fig. 15.3 Algorithm for secondary amenorrhoea. *FSH,* Follicle-stimulating hormone; *LH,* luteinizing hormone.

than 2.5. Levels of both are greatly raised with ovarian insufficiency and both are usually at the lower limit with hypothalamic amenorrhoea and hypogonadotropic hypogonadism.

- **Serum testosterone**: May be normal or raised with PCOS, although free testosterone is usually raised. With very high testosterone levels an androgen-secreting tumour should be suspected.
- **Sex hormone binding globulin** (SHBG): In PCOS, SHBG levels may be low, resulting in a higher presence of unbound testosterone in the blood. High levels may be seen in anorexia, liver disease, pregnancy, hyperprolactinaemia and hyperthyroidism.
- **Serum prolactin**: *Important to exclude hyperprolactinaemia.* However, this should be interpreted with caution as prolactin levels may temporarily be raised for other reasons, such as a response to stress or following a breast examination. It may also be falsely elevated by medications, as described above.

- **Thyroid-stimulating hormone (TSH)** and free thyroxine **(fT4)**: If hypo- or hyperthyroidism are suspected.

Specialist tests

- **Karyotyping** (chromosomal analysis) should be performed in unexplained primary amenorrhoea, primary ovarian insufficiency or if there is suspicion of a chromosomal abnormality such as Turner syndrome (XO).
- **MRI head** should be performed if there is galactorrhoea, persistently high prolactin levels, visual field defects or severe persistent headache to exclude a pituitary or central nervous system (CNS) tumour.
- If chronic illness is suspected, investigations should be guided by clinical history and examination.

Summary

A summary of the management of primary amenorrhoea can be found in table 15.3.

Table 15.3 Management of primary amenorrhoea

Underlying cause	Management
Gonadal dysgenesis secondary to congenital developmental disorder of the reproductive system (androgen insensitivity syndrome, Turner syndrome, Rokitansky-Kustner-Hauser syndrome, late-onset congenital adrenal hyperplasia)	An example of this is Turner syndrome (45,XO): Management involves hormone replacement therapy (HRT) to stimulate secondary sexual development in those not yet exposed to oestrogen and to protect against cardiac disease and osteoporosis. Women who carry a Y chromosome should have both gonads removed, because of the risk of malignancy.
Hypothalamic dysfunction: Low BMI, eating disorders, high levels of stress, excessive exercise	Patients should receive adequate psychological and dietician support to achieve a BMI of >18 and manage lifestyle stresses.
Haematocolpos or transverse vaginal septum	Surgical excision of the persistent vaginal membrane.
Congenital abnormalities, e.g., absent vagina	Referral to tertiary centre for consideration of vaginal reconstruction.
Constitutional delay	Refer to tertiary paediatric and adolescent specialist for consideration of sex steroid replacement.
Hyperprolactinaemia	Pituitary microadenomas are tumours less than 10 mm in diameter that can secrete hormones, but most are clinically inactive. Treatment is advised to reduce risk of osteoporosis. Dopamine agonists such as bromocriptine and cabergoline should be used and will lower serum prolactin levels. A pituitary macroadenoma >10 mm may require surgical in addition to medical intervention, but medication alone can cause improvement of symptoms and tumour shrinkage. A transsphenoidal resection can be performed but has a risk of diabetes insidious, cerebrospinal fluid leak and tumour reoccurrence. If hyperprolactinaemia is medication induced, then stopping the medication will resolve the prolactin levels and symptoms. However, if it is not suitable to stop the treatment, additional oestrogen may be advised to protect from osteoporosis.
Androgen-secreting tumours	Ovarian and adrenal hormone-secreting tumours should be surgically removed, preserving maximal ovarian tissues.
Premature ovarian insufficiency (POI)	Hormone replacement therapy to minimize risks of hypo-oestrogenic state, e.g., osteoporosis and cardiovascular risks.

COMMUNICATION

It is important to appreciate the psychosocial and psychosexual aspects of a diagnosis of conditions such as gonadal dysgenesis and absence of female reproductive organs. Patients receiving these diagnoses must be adequately supported and counselled. Patients and their families should be informed of support groups such as https://dsdfamilies.org/.

RED FLAG

As per NICE 2022 guidance, alternate causes of hyperandrogenism, e.g., late-onset congenital adrenal hyperplasia, Cushing syndrome or an androgen-secreting tumour) must be excluded if:

1. Signs of virilization, e.g., deep voice, reduced breast size, increased muscle bulk and clitoral hypertrophy.
2. Rapidly progressing hirsutism (less than 1 year between hirsutism being noticed and seeking medical advice).
3. Total testosterone level >5 nmol/L or more than twice the upper limit of normal reference range)

SECONDARY AMENORRHOEA

Secondary amenorrhoea is defined as the absence of periods for 6 months or more if the patient previously had regular periods or 12 months without a period, if previously they had oligomenorrhea. Causes of secondary amenorrhoea may either be ovarian, hypothalamic or uterine in origin. A summary of its management can be found in Table 15.4.

PRECOCIOUS PUBERTY AND DELAYED PUBERTY

Definition

Precocious puberty occurs when pubertal characteristics occur before the age of 9 years.

Delayed puberty is considered when there are no signs of pubertal development by age 14 years.

Prevalence

The overall prevalence of precocious puberty is estimated to be 1:5000 to 1:10,000 children. The exact prevalence of children with delayed puberty is unclear due to many variable factors such as variation in the mean pubertal age between different ethnic groups and genetic influence on the onset of puberty.

Causes

Aetiology of precocious puberty and delayed puberty are both varied and with multiple systemic causes. The majority of cases of precocious puberty have idiopathic causes, followed by ovarian causes such as oestrogen-secreting tumours. Delayed puberty has predominantly CNS-related aetiology, such as infection, tumours and head trauma, followed by idiopathic causes. Rarer causes include genetic and chronic illness (Figs. 15.4 and 15.5).

Diagnosis

History
History is very important to establish the cause of delayed (Fig. 15.6) or precocious puberty as the aetiology for both can be so varied. Your history and examination should be part of a comprehensive medical and gynaecological review, as outlined earlier in this chapter for amenorrhoea.

Investigations

Ultrasound pelvis and adrenals
This can identify features such as polycystic ovaries and congenital anomalies. If tumours are suspected, computed tomography (CT) or MRI scans are the gold-standard investigations.

Blood tests
A full endocrine profile should be performed including serum gonadotrophins LH and FSH, oestradiol, testosterone, sex hormone-binding globulin (SHBG), androstenedione, progesterone and dehydroepiandrosterone sulphate. This will highlight endocrinological causes.

Specialist tests
If other tests have not highlighted aetiology, bone age studies, chromosomal analysis and CT/MRI should be performed in unexplained precocious or delayed puberty. If chronic illness is suspected, investigations should be guided by clinical findings.

Management

Management of delayed puberty is aimed at treating the underlying cause. A multidisciplinary approach with the paediatric and genetic team should be taken.

Endocrine precious puberty is by suppression of oestrogen and androgen production by gonadotropin-releasing hormone analogues to reverse the physical changes.

If the diagnosis is congenital adrenal hyperplasia (CAH), the treatment is with steroid replacement.

XY gonadal dysgenesis may predispose to gonadal malignancy, therefore removal of gonads may be required.

Chronic illness or hypothyroidism needs the appropriate medical team input for treatment.

Hormone-secreting tumours will need surgical excision.

HINTS AND TIPS

Psychological support and counselling are essential as these children and teenagers will likely feel different from their peers, which could cause long-term psychological issues.

VIRILISM

Definition

Virilism is a severe form of androgen excess characterized by hirsutism, voice deepening, temporal balding, amenorrhoea, clitoromegaly and breast atrophy. It can be due to excessive endogenous or exogenous androgens, with endogenous production by the ovary being the most common source.

Table 15.4 Management of secondary amenorrhoea

Underlying cause	Management
Polycystic ovarian syndrome (PCOS) PCOS is a common condition affecting 2–26 in every 100 women. Short-term effects include oligomenorrhoea or secondary amenorrhoea, subfertility, acne and hirsutism. Long-term risks include diabetes, sleep apnoea, hypertension, stroke, depression and anxiety and endometrial hyperplasia or malignancy. Diagnosis is achieved by performing the following investigations:	• Weight loss (even a 5% reduction of weight can lead to spontaneous ovulation again). • Ensure patient has at least four menstrual bleeds per year or continual endometrial protection (Mirena coil). Withdrawal bleeds can be medically induced with hormonal contraception or progesterone therapy to reduce the risk of endometrial hyperplasia and cancer. A COCP with antiandrogen and progestogenic effect of cyproterone acetate or additional antimineralocorticoid activity (Dianette, Yasmin) works particularly well to induce withdrawal bleeds and treat acne. • Metformin may assist with weight loss and fertility. • Topical and systemic acne treatments. • Topical eflornithine (antiprotozoal drug that inhibits the enzyme ornithine decarboxylase in hair follicles) for hirsutism or laser hair removal. • Artificial reproductive therapies for assisted conception.
Total testosterone	Normal to moderately elevated
SHBG	Normal to low (marker of degree of hyperinsulinaemia)
Free androgen index	Normal or elevated
LH, Prolactin, TFTs	To exclude POI, hypothyroidism and hyperprolactinaemia.
TVUS (request scan unless diagnosis of PCOS is obvious on clinical and biochemical grounds)	Twelve or more follicles in at least one ovary (measuring 2–9 mm in diameter) or increased ovarian volume >10 cm³. Polycystic ovaries do not have to be present to make the diagnosis of PCOS and the finding of polycystic ovaries on scan does not alone establish the diagnosis. Ultrasound should not be used in the diagnosis of PCOS in adolescents.
Hyperprolactinaemia	As per primary amenorrhoea.
Asherman syndrome	Hysteroscopic division of adhesions and temporary insertion of an intrauterine contraceptive device can help prevent redevelopment of adhesions.
Cervical stenosis	Surgical cervical dilatation.
Sheehan syndrome	Sheehan syndrome is a postpartum infarction of the pituitary gland, triggered due to massive obstetric haemorrhage. Oestrogen replacement would be required as COCP or HRT. In addition, replacement of all pituitary hormones may be required.
Androgen secreting tumours	As per primary amenorrhoea
Premature ovarian insufficiency	Hormone replacement therapy to minimize risks of hypo-oestrogenic state, e.g., osteoporosis and cardiovascular risks.

Prevalence

Approximately 10% of healthy normal women have some degree of hirsutism, but without signs of virilism. True virilism is rare.

Causes

See Figs. 15.7 and 15.8 for summary.

Ovarian androgens

PCOS is the most common cause of ovarian androgens and hirsutism (90%), and occurs in up to 20% of women. Characteristically there are raised levels of circulating LH and sex steroids. Pituitary production of LH is raised in PCOS, causing increased ovarian androgen production and increased LH-to-FSH ratio. This leads to a reduced production of SHBG by the liver, and, as SHBG binds to circulating androgens, free testosterone levels increase (Fig. 15.9).

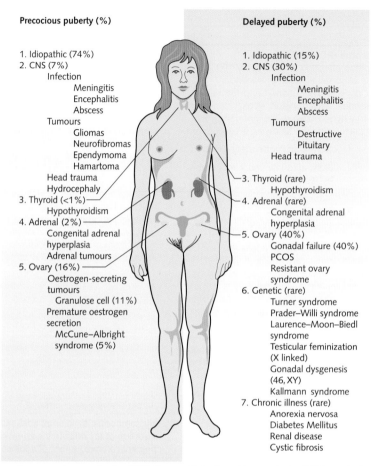

Precocious puberty (%)

1. Idiopathic (74%)
2. CNS (7%)
   Infection
      Meningitis
      Encephalitis
      Abscess
   Tumours
      Gliomas
      Neurofibromas
      Ependymoma
      Hamartoma
   Head trauma
   Hydrocephaly
3. Thyroid (<1%)
   Hypothyroidism
4. Adrenal (2%)
   Congenital adrenal
   hyperplasia
   Adrenal tumours
5. Ovary (16%)
   Oestrogen-secreting
   tumours
      Granulose cell (11%)
   Premature oestrogen
   secretion
      McCune–Albright
      syndrome (5%)

Delayed puberty (%)

1. Idiopathic (15%)
2. CNS (30%)
   Infection
      Meningitis
      Encephalitis
      Abscess
   Tumours
      Destructive
      Pituitary
   Head trauma
3. Thyroid (rare)
   Hypothyroidism
4. Adrenal (rare)
   Congenital adrenal
   hyperplasia
5. Ovary (40%)
   Gonadal failure (40%)
   PCOS
   Resistant ovary
   syndrome
6. Genetic (rare)
   Turner syndrome
   Prader–Willi syndrome
   Laurence–Moon–Biedl
   syndrome
   Testicular feminization
   (X linked)
   Gonadal dysgenesis
   (46, XY)
   Kallmann syndrome
7. Chronic illness (rare)
   Anorexia nervosa
   Diabetes Mellitus
   Renal disease
   Cystic fibrosis

Fig. 15.4 Aetiology for precocious puberty. *CAH,* Congenital adrenal hyperplasia; *CNS,* central nervous system.

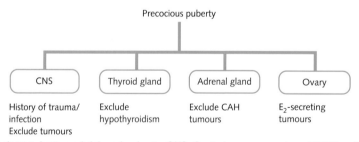

Fig. 15.5 Causes of precocious puberty and delayed puberty. *CNS,* Central nervous system; *PCOS,* polycystic ovarian syndrome.

Androgens are converted to oestrogen in adipose tissue, raising oestradiol levels, which further stimulates pituitary production of LH. Obesity increases insulin levels, which stimulates further ovarian androgen production, but also reduces SHBG levels and increases the peripheral conversion of androgens to oestrogen.

Androgen-secreting tumours of the ovary are rare and include arrhenoblastomas and hilar cell tumours. Pregnancy luteomas are a rare source of excess ovarian androgen secretion that develop due to an exaggerated response by the ovarian storm to human chorionic gonadotropin.

Adrenal androgens

CAH describes a group of rare inherited disorders caused by mutations in genes that code for enzymes involved in

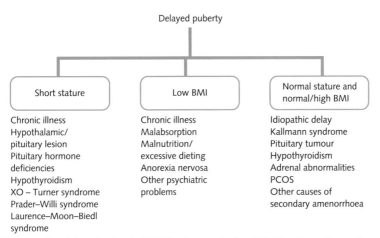

Fig. 15.6 Aetiology for delayed puberty. *BMI,* Body mass index; *PCOS,* polycystic ovarian syndrome.

Delayed puberty

Short stature	Low BMI	Normal stature and normal/high BMI
Chronic illness	Chronic illness	Idiopathic delay
Hypothalamic/ pituitary lesion	Malabsorption	Kallmann syndrome
Pituitary hormone deficiencies	Malnutrition/ excessive dieting	Pituitary tumour
Hypothyroidism	Anorexia nervosa	Hypothyroidism
XO – Turner syndrome	Other psychiatric problems	Adrenal abnormalities
Prader–Willi syndrome		PCOS
Laurence–Moon–Biedl syndrome		Other causes of secondary amenorrhoea

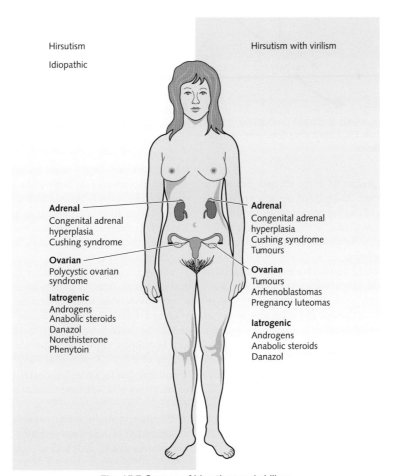

Hirsutism

Idiopathic

Hirsutism with virilism

Adrenal
Congenital adrenal hyperplasia
Cushing syndrome

Ovarian
Polycystic ovarian syndrome

Iatrogenic
Androgens
Anabolic steroids
Danazol
Norethisterone
Phenytoin

Adrenal
Congenital adrenal hyperplasia
Cushing syndrome
Tumours

Ovarian
Tumours
Arrhenoblastomas
Pregnancy luteomas

Iatrogenic
Androgens
Anabolic steroids
Danazol

Fig. 15.7 Causes of hirsutism and virilism.

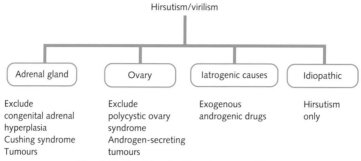

Fig. 15.8 Algorithm for hirsutism and virilism.

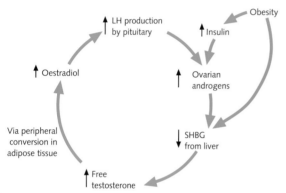

Fig. 15.9 Mechanism of increased androgen production in polycystic ovarian syndrome. *LH,* Luteinizing hormone; *SHBG,* sex hormone-binding globulin.

hydroxylation of cortisol precursors in the adrenal glands. The most common enzyme defect, 21-hydroxylase deficiency, leads to excess circulating levels of cortisol precursors and androgens. These precursor steroids are similar to the male hormone testosterone, therefore there can be development of male characteristics and precocious puberty.

Excessive stimulation of the adrenal cortex, such as with an adrenal adenoma causes raised cortisol levels and is often associated with excess androgen production, as seen with endogenous Cushing syndrome. Adenoma and adenocarcinoma of the adrenal gland produce high levels of androgens but are rare.

Exogenous androgens

Androgens, like most hormones, have a normal concentration range with a circadian rhythm. Additional androgens and anabolic steroids can cause hirsutism and virilism depending on the amount and length of time taken. Certain medications have androgenic properties that can lead to these side effects, including norethisterone, phenytoin and danazol.

Diagnosis

History

A full medical and gynaecology history as discussed earlier in this chapter should be taken and emphasis should be on the following questions to assess likely causation:

- Onset of symptoms
- Menstrual history
- Medical history
- Family history of similar presentations

Examination

Examination should be a full physical examination as described in examination for 'amenorrhoea' as above.

Levels of hirsutism can be objectively scored using scoring systems such as the visual scale Ferriman–Gallwey, which assesses nine areas of the body, and a nonaffected woman would usually score under 8. Women with idiopathic hirsutism usually have no other abnormal findings on examination. Signs of virilism such as temporal balding and breast atrophy should also be assessed. Marked symptoms of virilism suggest an androgen-secreting tumour.

Obesity is associated with increased androgen production and clearance rates. A pattern of fat distribution of truncal obesity associated with cervical fat pad, purple striae, thin skin and facial plethora indicates that Cushing syndrome should be considered. Obesity without cushingoid features and acanthosis nigricans (pigmented raised patches) is suggestive of PCOS. Severe CAH will have been diagnosed in childhood due to ambiguous external genitalia; milder late-onset forms of CAH have similar presentations to those of PCOS.

Palpation of an abdominal or pelvic mass in a hirsute woman is suggestive of androgen-secreting neoplasia, although the tumours are usually too small to cause palpable masses.

Investigations

Degree of necessary investigation is determined by the degree of symptoms experienced by the woman. For example, rapid onset of symptoms is more likely to suggest a serious pathology.

Pelvic ultrasound

This can identify polycystic ovaries if suspected with typical appearance of enlarged ovaries and multiple peripheral follicles, or be suggestive of an ovarian androgen-secreting tumour.

Blood tests

Serum gonadotrophins LH and FSH should be measured. With very high serum testosterone levels an androgen-secreting tumour should be suspected.

Specialist tests

It is possible for small tumours to be missed with ultrasound scanning, so if there is a level of suspicion, CT scanning should be performed. Investigations for CAH and Cushing syndrome should be performed if symptoms and clinical signs suggest these diseases.

Idiopathic hirsutism is a diagnosis made by excluding other pathology.

Management

Hirsutism and virilism generally respond well to medical treatments, but sometimes there is a need to perform genital reconstructive surgical procedures.

Idiopathic hirsutism can be treated cosmetically using electrolysis or bleaching, as described earlier in this chapter.

Androgen-secreting tumours should be surgically removed.

Treating the cause of excess cortisol production in Cushing syndrome should normalize circulating androgen levels.

Glucocorticoid and mineralocorticoid replacement is the mainstay of treatment for CAH.

● Chapter Summary

- Regular monthly periods in women of reproductive age are a good predictor of regular ovulation resulting from cyclical ovarian activity.
- The hormones in the reproductive system are carefully balanced. Intrinsic and extrinsic disruption to this balance can have a multitude of systemic effects, both in the short term and longer term.
- It is important to exclude pathological causes for abnormal menstrual patterns, particularly underlying malignancies, which may require urgent treatment.
- When discussing gynaecological endocrine disorders with patients, a sensitive and caring approach should be taken, given the impact that some diagnoses may have on patients' lives and relationships.

UKMLA Conditions
Menopausal problems
Menstrual problems

UKMLA Presentations
Amenorrhoea
Menopause
Subfertility

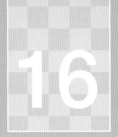

BACKGROUND

Definition

Fertility problems are estimated to affect one in seven couples in the UK. Referral for clinical assessment and investigations for subfertility should be considered for women of reproductive age who have not conceived after 1 year of regular unprotected vaginal sexual intercourse, in the absence of any known cause of infertility.

Primary subfertility refers to couples who have never had any previous pregnancies, and secondary subfertility is if there has been previous gravidity.

In certain cases, it may be suitable for earlier referral for specialist assessment, such as a known clinical cause of infertility or a history of predisposing factors for infertility, e.g., previous pelvic inflammatory disease (PID).

Prevalence

Couples should be informed that over 80% of the general population will conceive successfully within 1 year if under 40 years of age and they are having regular unprotected vaginal sexual intercourse.

Of those who do not conceive in the first year, about half will go on to conceive within the second year, giving a cumulative pregnancy rate of over 90%.

Causes

There are multiple factors that can affect fertility, either from the male partner, female partner or both (Fig. 16.1). There are also many cases of unexplained subfertility in up to 25% of couples who cannot conceive spontaneously.

Natural conception requires XX and XY partners who have intercourse resulting in male ejaculation. The sperm must be of sufficient volume, count, progression and normal form to pass through the cervical mucus, uterine cavity and into the fallopian tube. The female must be able to ovulate, and the ovum be picked up by the fimbrial end of a patent fallopian tube and transported to meet the sperm, after which the fertilized embryo implants within the endometrium. Conception occurs in the 4 days around ovulation, sperm can survive for around 7 days and an egg can be fertilized for up to 1 day after ovulation.

Female fertility decreases with age, and factors such as body mass index (BMI), alcohol and smoking can also have a negative effect.

DIAGNOSIS

History

For heterosexual couples, a fertility history should be taken at the same time from the couple. Questions should be asked sensitively and so as to not attribute blame to either of the partners, should a male or female factor cause be identified.

History from the female partner

- How long have you been actively trying to conceive for?
- How often are you having unprotected intercourse?
- Do you have any problems having intercourse? Current guidelines recommend intercourse every 2 to 3 days. Any issues with intercourse including vaginismus, dyspareunia or male erectile or ejaculatory dysfunction are relevant.
- Have you had any previous pregnancies? Take a full obstetrics history of pregnancy outcomes and mode of delivery, also ensuring you ask about previous miscarriages and the gestation at which these occurred and any ectopic pregnancies which could suggest a tubal problem.
- Do you have any gynaecology conditions? Ask about any known gynaecology diagnosis such as polycystic ovary syndrome (PCOS), prior pelvic surgery, sexually transmitted infections and check smear tests are up-to-date.
- Are your periods particularly heavy or painful? Menorrhagia could suggest fibroids, dysmenorrhoea could indicate endometriosis and oligo-amenorrhoea could suggest anovulation. Dyspareunia could also suggest PID or endometriosis.
- Do you have any medical conditions? Poorly controlled chronic diseases such as diabetes, renal disease or hypothyroidism may cause subfertility.
- Do you take any regular medications? Take a full drug history to identify any potentially teratogenic medications. Encourage women to take folic acid supplements from 3 months prior to trying to conceive.
- Do you smoke or drink alcohol? Smoking can reduce the motility of the fallopian tube cilia. Heavy drinking may also impact fertility rates.

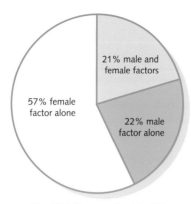

Fig. 16.1 Causes of subfertility.

Table 16.1 Female factor causes for subfertility

Problem	Cause
Ovulatory dysfunction	Chronic systemic illness Eating disorders Polycystic ovary syndrome (PCOS) Hyperprolactinaemia Hypo/hyperthyroidism Cannabis use Nonsteroidal antiinflammatory drugs (NSAIDs)
Tubal factor	Pelvic inflammatory disease Previous tubal surgery Previous ectopic pregnancy/salpingectomy Endometriosis Smoking
Uterine problems	Fibroids Uterine septum Congenital anomaly, e.g., absent uterus Asherman syndrome (intrauterine adhesions)
Coital dysfunction	Vaginismus Vulvodynia Dyspareunia

A summary of the female factor causes of subfertility can be found in Table 16.1.

History from the male partner

- Have you ever fathered any pregnancies? If the answer is yes, this will suggest female factor infertility.
- Have you ever had any injury or operations on your groin or testicles? Procedures such as inguinal hernia repairs, orchidopexy for undescended testes, previous testicular torsion and bladder neck surgery can all affect male fertility.
- Do you have any medical conditions? Chronic conditions such as renal disease and diabetes can affect

spermatogenesis, and cystic fibrosis can have agenesis of the vas deferens. Infections such as mumps orchitis and epididymo-orchitis can also cause obstruction or poor-quality sperm.

- Do you take any regular medications? Some medications/oncology treatments may affect spermatogenesis.
- Do you smoke, drink alcohol or use any illicit drugs? Smoking, alcohol and drug use all reduce fertility and negatively affect sperm quality and quantity.
- What is your occupation? Occupations that cause raised testicular temperature such as prolonged driving, or exposure to heavy metals, solvents or agricultural chemicals can lead to oligospermia.

A summary of the male factor causes of subfertility can be found in Table 16.2. These can be broken down in three categories; pretesticular, testicular or posttesticular.

COMMUNICATION

A couple's fertility journey can be an emotional rollercoaster, which can put much strain on their relationship. As well as providing the couple with clear clinical advice for investigation and management, it is important to ask about their psychological well-being and whether they require any further support with this. Couples should be signposted to the HFEA website which has information on emotional support and can be accessed for free https://www.hfea.gov.uk/treatments/explore-all-treatments/getting-emotional-support/.

Examination

- General observations are important in the assessment – what is the patient's BMI? *BMI <19 or >30 can significantly impact fertility.*
- Do they have appropriate secondary sexual characteristics? Evidence of hirsutism or acanthosis nigricans may suggest PCOS.
- On abdominal examination, are there any scars from previous surgery? Is the uterus palpable? *An enlarged uterus may suggest fibroids or adenomyosis.*
- Is the uterus fixed and/or retroverted? This may suggest pelvic adhesions or endometriosis.
- Are there any palpable adnexal masses? *Large ovarian cysts will be palpable.*
- A Cusco's speculum should be used to examine the patient vaginally following obtaining consent and a chaperone. Is there an imperforate hymen or vaginal membrane visible? Does the cervix appear normal? Is there vaginal discharge

Table 16.2 Male factor causes for subfertility

Problem	Cause
Pretesticular	Kallmann syndrome Prader-Willi Treatment is with gonadotrophins
Testicular	**Congenital** Klinefelter syndrome XX male syndrome Noonan syndrome Cryptorchidism **Acquired** Varicocele Testicular tumours Testicular injury Chemotherapy/radiotherapy Idiopathic
Posttesticular	**Congenital** Cystic fibrosis Congenital absence of the vas deferens (need to perform a renal ultrasound – 30% will have concurrent renal abnormality) Young syndrome **Acquired** Vasectomy Infection **Sexual dysfunction** Erectile dysfunction Timing or frequency of sexual intercourse Diabetes/spinal injury/multiple sclerosis **Sperm motility/function** Immotile-cilia syndrome Immunological infertility

suggestive of PID? *Triple swabs should be taken regardless to exclude underlying STIs.*

- In males, is there evidence of prior inguinal hernia repair? Are there visible varicocoeles? An orchidometer can be used to assess testicular size and the vas deferens should be palpated.

INVESTIGATIONS

Target investigations for subfertility to a specific cause as highlighted by the history if possible (Table. 16.3).

Treatment

Treatment for subfertility should be aimed at the specific cause as identified by the investigations. However, many couples suffer from unexplained infertility and may go on to require in vitro fertilization (IVF) treatment.

HINTS AND TIPS

Clomifene citrate is an antioestrogen that occupies oestrogen receptors in the hypothalamus, increasing gonadotropin hormone-releasing hormone (GnRH) release, which leads to increased release of luteinizing hormone (LH) and follicle-stimulating hormone (FSH). This induces follicular development and ovulation and should be given on days 2 to 6 of the cycle. Ovulation can be suggested by ovulation kits and raised day 21 progesterone. The dose can be titrated, but treatment should not be continued for longer than 6 months. There is a risk of multiple pregnancies while inducing ovulation; ultrasound follicle tracking can monitor for multiple follicles to ensure they are taking a dose that minimizes the risk of multiple pregnancy.

ETHICS

Inform women who are offered ovulation induction or ovarian stimulation that there is no direct association between this treatment and invasive cancer or adverse outcomes (including cancer) in children born from ovulation induction. However, information about long-term health outcomes in women and children is still awaited.

ASSISTED REPRODUCTION THERAPY

Recent data suggest that just over 2% of all the babies born in the UK are conceived through IVF treatment. The number of IVF cycles performed each year has increased steadily since 1991. For people with unexplained infertility, mild endometriosis or mild male factor infertility, they should be advised to try to conceive for a total of 2 years prior to having assisted reproduction therapy (ART).

Intrauterine insemination

Intrauterine insemination (IUI) is a technique where sperm are selected and introduced into the uterine cavity directly. The female partner can have stimulated ovulation or spontaneous. It is a technique option considered as an alternative to vaginal sexual intercourse in the case of physical disability or psychosexual problem, severe vulvodynia/vaginismus, people in same-sex relationships or those using donor sperm. IUI is also used in cases when unprotected sexual intercourse is not recommended, such as with a human immunodeficiency virus (HIV) positive male partner, after 'sperm washing'.

Intracytoplasmic sperm injection

Intracytoplasmic sperm injection (ICSI) is an assisted fertility technique in which a single sperm is injected directly into an egg. This technique is beneficial in patients with severe deficits in semen quality of low count. It should also be considered for couples in whom a previous IVF treatment cycle has resulted in failed or very poor fertilization.

In vitro fertilization

IVF involves inducing ovulation followed by harvesting the oocytes from either the female partner or an egg donor and allowing them to fertilize in a laboratory using sperm from the male partner or a sperm donor. The embryo is then transferred back into the patient in

Table 16.3 Investigations and treatment for couples with subfertility

Type of investigation	Interpretation	Treatment
Blood tests	Serum progesterone in the midluteal phase of the cycle (day 21 of a 28-day cycle) can confirm ovulation. Serum gonadotrophins: follicle-stimulating hormone (FSH) and luteinizing hormone (LH) if irregular cycles. Antimüllerian hormone (AMH) assessment of ovarian reserve. Prolactin if the patient has irregular cycles or galactorrhoea, visual field loss and headache to asses possible prolactinoma. Thyroid function tests if signs of thyroid disease. Testosterone levels can be performed in both males and females, for example if the man appears hypoandrogenic (nonhirsute, small soft testes) or if the woman is overly hirsute.	If PCOS anovulation diagnosed: 1) Weight loss (to achieve a BMI <30) 2) Ovarian stimulation with either metformin or clomifene citrate (*first line*) 3) Ovarian stimulation with both metformin and clomifene citrate or laparoscopic ovarian drilling (*second line*) Lifestyle changes: Stopping smoking, reduce alcohol and caffeine intake Premature ovarian insufficiency: IVF with egg donor often required If hyperprolactinaemia: Treat with dopamine agonists or surgery if indicated
Semen analysis	This should be the first investigation to be performed, prior to any invasive female investigations, as it may identify the cause of subfertility and prevent unnecessary tests which carry risks. The male partner should provide a specimen after 3 days of abstinence after a period of good health (systemic illness can reduce sperm quality). The examination should take place within 1 hour of production and is assessed for sperm volume, count, motility, progression and morphology. If the result of the first semen analysis is abnormal, a repeat confirmatory test should be offered ideally 3 months after the initial analysis to allow time for the cycle of spermatozoa formation to be completed (see Fig. 16.2). If sperm analysis reveals azoospermia (no sperm) or severe oligozoospermia (<3000/mL), an immediate repeat sample should be analyzed.	Conservative: Advise to wear loose underwear, reduce alcohol intake and smoking cessation. In hypogonadotropic hypogonadism, offer gonadotrophin drugs to improve fertility. Ejaculatory failure: Surgical correction of epididymal blockage, sperm recovery, e.g., urine collection with retrograde ejaculation, percutaneous epididymal aspiration, testicular sperm aspiration or open testicular biopsy. If semen persistently abnormal, assisted fertility should be considered, such as intrauterine insemination (IUI) or intracytoplasmic sperm injection (ICSI).
Transvaginal US (TVUS)	This can identify structural abnormalities of the pelvic organs such as fibroids, congenital abnormalities of the uterus and hydrosalpinx. It can also identify bulky ovaries with multiple peripheral follicles seen with polycystic ovaries. Total antral follicle count can give an impression of ovarian reserve, together with AMH result.	Operative hysteroscopy if TVUS highlights abnormality such as endometrial polyps or submucosal fibroids; this can be investigated and surgically resected using hysteroscopy. If there is history of previous uterine surgery (such as surgical management of miscarriage), this may identify uterine adhesions (Asherman syndrome) or uterine septum which can be excised hysteroscopically.

Table 16.3 Investigations and treatment for couples with subfertility—cont'd

Type of investigation	Interpretation	Treatment
Tubal investigations	If there is a high suspicion of symptomatic endometriosis the gold standard would be for these patients to have a laparoscopy (where pathology can be treated at the same time, e.g., excision of endometriosis, adhesiolysis and removal of ovarian endometriomas) and tubal dye test to assess tubal patency (see Chapter 3, Common investigations). If patients have no known risk factors for tubal disease, a hysterosalpingography (HSG) is an appropriate investigation (which avoids surgery). Radiopaque dye is introduced via the cervix through the uterus and an X-ray is taken to look for passage of the dye. Blockage can be caused by internal or external tubal factors or tubal spasm (Fig. 16.3). Hysterosalpingo-contrast-ultrasonography (HyCoSy) is an alternative to HSG performed using Doppler ultrasound to monitor the passage of fluid via the cervix through the uterus and tubes. It is crucial to ensure the patient is not pregnant prior to tubal patency investigations, therefore they are usually performed at the beginning of the menstrual cycle. Antibiotic cover with metronidazole and doxycycline is routinely used to prevent dissemination of any existing STIs.	If hydrosalpinges are identified, offer either salpingectomy or tubal clipping, as this improves the chance of a live birth with IVF and reduces the risk of ectopic pregnancy. If there are proximal tubal blockages, salpingography plus tubal catheterization, or hysteroscopic tubal cannulation can be considered. However, tubal potency does not guarantee function and these patients are at risk of ectopic pregnancy.

	WHO 2010	WHO 2021
Semen volume (mL)	1.5 (1.4–1.7)	1.4 (1.3–1.5)
Total sperm number (10^6 per ejaculate)	39 (33–46)	39 (35–40)
Total motility (%)	40 (38–42)	42 (40–43)
Progressive motility (%)	32 (31–34)	30 (29–31)
Non progressive motility (%)	1	1 (1–1)
Immotile sperm (%)	22	20 (19–20)
Vitality (%)	58 (55–63)	54 (50–56)
Normal forms (%)	4 (3–4)	4 (3.9–4)

Fig. 16.2 Updated World Health Organization (WHO), 6th edition, 2021. Normal reference ranges for sperm analysis. (From Boitrelle F, Shah R, Saleh R, et al. The Sixth Edition of the WHO Manual for Human Semen Analysis: A critical review and SWOT analysis. Life (Basel). 2021 Dec 9;11(12):1368. doi: 10.3390/life11121368.)

the hope of an ongoing pregnancy. The patients must be adequately educated about potential long-term health outcomes including the consequences of multiple pregnancy as well as potential small increased risk of borderline ovarian tumours. The absolute risks of long-term adverse outcomes in children born as result of IVF are low.

IVF techniques and protocols can vary, but generally involve the following steps:

1. Downregulation of woman's own hormones using gonadotropin hormone-releasing hormone (GnRH) agonists to avoid premature luteinizing hormone (LH) surges in IVF (*Switching off the natural cycle to artificially 'take control'*).

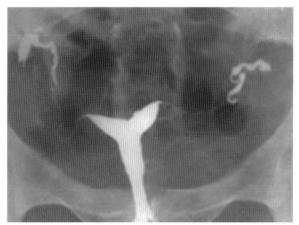

Fig. 16.3 Hysterosalpingogram. (From Letterie GS. Management of congenital uterine abnormalities. *Reprod Biomed Online* 2011;23:40–52. Elsevier, with permission.)

2. Controlled ovarian stimulation in IVF using an individualized starting dose of follicle-stimulating hormone (FSH) for the lowest effective dose and duration of use *(To minimize the risk of ovarian hyperstimulation syndrome (OHSS).*
3. Using human chorionic gonadotrophin to trigger ovulation with ultrasound monitoring of ovarian response.
4. Oocyte retrieval using transvaginal US (TVUS) under sedation and sperm retrieval (methods described in Table 16.3).
5. IVF of the oocytes with sperm and embryo transfer strategies.
6. Luteal phase support with progesterone.

Donor sperm

It is appropriate to use donor semen and insemination in some cases, such as azoospermia or severe deficits in semen quality in those who do not wish to undergo ICSI. It can be considered if there is a high risk of transmitting a genetic or infectious disorder to the offspring.

Donor oocyte ('Egg donor')

In some cases it is appropriate to use a donor oocyte, for example, in premature ovarian insufficiency, gonadal dysgenesis such as Turner syndrome, bilateral oophorectomy and ovarian failure following chemotherapy or radiotherapy. It can be considered if there is a high risk of transmitting a genetic disorder to the offspring or in cases of IVF treatment failure.

CLINICAL NOTES

There has been a substantial increase in the number of patients freezing their eggs 'socially' for future treatment; however, it still represents a small fraction of patients undergoing IVF. The most common reason was having no current partner, with the most common age being 37 to 39 years. Success is affected by the age of the woman at the time of freezing and the live birth rate is lower than using fresh eggs or thawed frozen embryos. Recent developments of vitrification techniques, the use of a hyaluronan-enriched embryo transfer medium as a 'glue' to help embryo implantation and the use of time-lapse videography to monitor the cell division pattern of the embryos to select the embryos with the best potential are improving the success rates for ART.

COMPLICATIONS

IVF has an association with multiple pregnancy and the high complication rate associated with this. Since 2009 the Human Fertilisation and Embryology Authority (HFEA) has introduced regulations to promote single embryo transfer only to minimize the risk of multiple births from IVF treatment.

- **Multiple pregnancy**: In IVF clinics the current regulated maximum multiple birth rate should be 10%.
- **Ovarian hyperstimulation syndrome (OHSS)**: A serious systemic disease that occurs as a result of high levels of oestrogen during IVF treatment. The subsequent increased vascular permeability causes accumulation of fluid in the 'third space', such as the abdomen and chest, and intravascular fluid depletion. In its mild form it can cause mild abdominal pain, but can lead to pronounced painful ascites and pleural effusions, hepatorenal failure and respiratory distress syndrome (Table 16.4). If during IVF too many follicles have developed, it is safer to abandon the cycle than risk developing OHSS.
- **Ovarian torsion:** Multifollicular ovaries can have a dramatic increase in size during IVF treatment, and therefore there is a high risk of ovarian torsion.

Table 16.4 Grading of severity of ovarian hyperstimulation syndrome (OHSS) according to the management of OHSS (Green-top guideline no. 5)

Classification	Features	Management
Mild	Bloating Mild abdominal pain Ovary <8 cm^3	Outpatient Review in 2–3 days Most resolve spontaneously 7–10 days
Moderate	Moderate bloating Nausea and vomiting US evidence of ascites Ovaries 8–12 cm^3	Outpatient Review in 2–3 days Most resolve spontaneously within 7–10 days
Severe	Ascites clinically Occasional hydrothorax Oliguria Hct >0.45 Na <135 Low osmolality <282 K >5 Low alb <35 Ovaries >12 cm^3	Most require inpatient Urine pregnancy test Daily weight Daily abdominal girth Input/output chart Drink to thirst Bloods: FBC, Hct, U+Es, Osm, LFTs + CRP ABG CXR ECG (K changes/low voltage) Inform HEFA + centre where the IVF was performed at Give LMWH
Critical	Tense ascites Large hydrothorax Hct >0.55 WCC >25 Oliguria VTE ARDS	HDU/ITU As above + consider paracentesis if persistent oliguria secondary to increased abdominal pressure → reduced renal perfusion or respiratory compromise. Give LMWH

ABG, Arterial blood gas; Alb, albumin; ARDS, adult respiratory distress syndrome; CRP, C-reactive protein; CXR, chest X-ray; Hct, haematocrit; HDU, high dependency unit; HFEA, Human Fertilisation and Embryology Authority; ITU, intensive care unit; K, potassium; LFTs, liver function tests; LMWH, low-molecular-weight heparin; Na, sodium; U+Es, urea and electrolytes; VTE, venous thrombus embolism; WCC, white cell count.

ETHICS

Individual National Health Service (NHS) Clinical Commissioning Groups make the final decision about who can have NHS-funded in vitro fertilization (IVF) in their local area. Common criteria to qualify for NHS funding include age <40 years, both partners are nonsmokers, no previous children to either couple from current or previous relationships and body mass index <30 kg/m^2. It is important that when counselling your patients, you advise them early whether they may or may not qualify for NHS IVF if required.

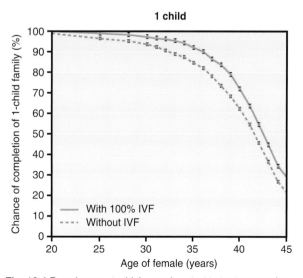

Fig. 16.4 Female age at which couples start to try to conceive vs. the chance of having one child, with and without use of in vitro fertilization (IVF). (From Habbema JDF, Eijkemans JC, Leridon H, te Velde ER. Realizing a desired family size: when should couples start? *Hum Reprod.* 2015;30(9):2215–2221.)

PROGNOSIS

The age of the oocyte is the most important prognostic factor in predicting IVF success (Fig. 16.4). The chance of a live birth following IVF treatment falls significantly with rising female age.

Current data show that pregnancy rates per embryo transfer for patients receiving IVF treatment using their own eggs is over 44% under 35 years of age, but only up to 20% at age 40 years, and 2% if over 45 years of age. The chance of a live birth falls if the woman has never had a pregnancy or live birth and with the number of unsuccessful cycles.

● Chapter Summary

- Multiple factors can affect fertility from the male partner, female partner or both.
- No clear cause (unexplained subfertility) is found in up to 25% of patients who cannot conceive spontaneously.
- Causative factors should be carefully investigated through a target history, examination and appropriate investigations.
- Lifestyle factors impact greatly on fertility. Partners should be strongly advised to optimize BMI, stop smoking and reduce alcohol and caffeine intake.
- The age of the oocyte (either from the female partner or an oocyte donor) is the most important prognostic factor in predicting IVF success.

UKMLA Presentations
Amenorrhoea
Endometriosis
Pelvic inflammatory disease
Subfertility

Menopause 17

BACKGROUND

Definition

'Menopause' is derived from the Greek words *Men* (month) and *Pausis* (cessation) and refers to a person's final menstrual period. Menopause can only be diagnosed retrospectively after 12 months of absent menstruation without the influence of hormonal contraception. Almost 90% of patients will experience menopausal symptoms, while 20% will suffer from severe symptoms. The time leading up to the menopause is referred to as the 'climacteric' or 'perimenopausal' period. During this phase, patients may experience irregular or heavier menstrual bleeding than normal due to anovulatory cycles, as well as menopausal symptoms.

The menopause generally occurs between the ages of 45 and 55 years with the average age in the UK of 51 years. 'Premature menopause' occurs in women under aged 40 years and may be due to multiple factors such as surgical menopause (bilateral oophorectomies), impact of chemoradiotherapy or premature ovarian insufficiency (POI) (see Chapter 16).

SYMPTOMS

In addition to absent menstrual cycles, a variety of systemic symptoms can occur. These include vasomotor symptoms, such as hot flushes and night sweats, as well as musculoskeletal symptoms such as joint and muscle pain. It can cause fluctuations in mood, including low mood and low libido and urogenital symptoms such as vaginal dryness (Fig. 17.1). Menopausal symptoms can have a significant impact on people's quality of life.

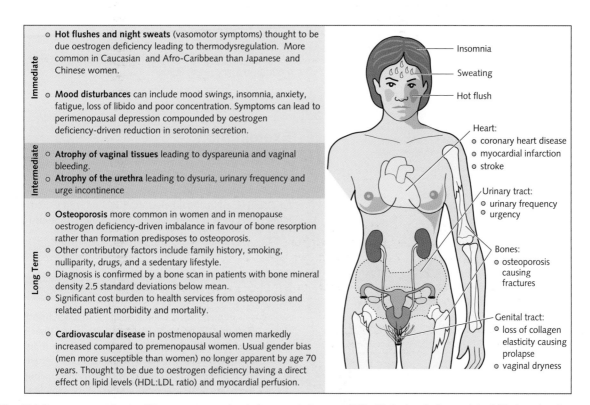

Immediate
- Hot flushes and night sweats (vasomotor symptoms) thought to be due oestrogen deficiency leading to thermodysregulation. More common in Caucasian and Afro-Caribbean than Japanese and Chinese women.
- Mood disturbances can include mood swings, insomnia, anxiety, fatigue, loss of libido and poor concentration. Symptoms can lead to perimenopausal depression compounded by oestrogen deficiency-driven reduction in serotonin secretion.

Intermediate
- Atrophy of vaginal tissues leading to dyspareunia and vaginal bleeding.
- Atrophy of the urethra leading to dysuria, urinary frequency and urge incontinence

Long Term
- Osteoporosis more common in women and in menopause oestrogen deficiency-driven imbalance in favour of bone resorption rather than formation predisposes to osteoporosis.
- Other contributory factors include family history, smoking, nulliparity, drugs, and a sedentary lifestyle.
- Diagnosis is confirmed by a bone scan in patients with bone mineral density 2.5 standard deviations below mean.
- Significant cost burden to health services from osteoporosis and related patient morbidity and mortality.
- Cardiovascular disease in postmenopausal women markedly increased compared to premenopausal women. Usual gender bias (men more susceptible than women) no longer apparent by age 70 years. Thought to be due to oestrogen deficiency having a direct effect on lipid levels (HDL:LDL ratio) and myocardial perfusion.

Insomnia
Sweating
Hot flush
Heart:
- coronary heart disease
- myocardial infarction
- stroke

Urinary tract:
- urinary frequency
- urgency

Bones:
- osteoporosis causing fractures

Genital tract:
- loss of collagen elasticity causing prolapse
- vaginal dryness

Fig. 17.1 Common symptoms of the menopause due to hormonal changes. *HDL,* High-density lipoprotein; *LDL,* low-density lipoprotein.

Pathophysiology

After 45 years of age, as a result of successive menstrual cycles, only a few thousand oocytes remain. The depletion of the oocytes combined with their increased resistance to pituitary hormones follicle-stimulating hormone (FSH) and luteinizing hormone (LH) causes the cessation of menstruation. FSH and LH lose the function to regulate oestrogen, progesterone and testosterone, alongside a natural decline of oestrogen levels during menopause, causing the menopausal symptoms. Table 17.1 outlines the hormonal changes during the menopause.

Table 17.1 Hormonal changes with the menopause

Hormone	Levels during menopause
Follicle-stimulating hormone	↑↑
Luteinizing hormone	↑↑
Oestrogen	↓↓
Progesterone	↓↓

DIAGNOSIS

History

The diagnosis of menopause can be made by history taking and examination due to the identifiable key features. However, it is important to not miss an alternative differential diagnosis as individual symptoms could be related to a different pathology. Questions should be asked with a sensitive and nonjudgemental approach.

HISTORY

- When was your last menstrual period?
- Do you experience hot flushes or night sweats? Differential diagnoses may include infections such as tuberculosis or malignancies such as myeloma, therefore a systematic systems review should be explored.
- Are you experiencing any changes to your mood? Oestrogen deficiency-driven reduction in serotonin levels can cause mood swings, insomnia, anxiety, poor concentration and loss of libido. Differential diagnoses include depression, anxiety and hypoactive sexual desire syndrome.
- Do you suffer from vaginal dryness? Differential diagnoses may include vaginal thrush.
- Do you have any pain when passing urine? Are you having to pass urine more frequently? These can be symptoms of vaginal tissue or urethral atrophy. However, it is important to exclude other causes for these such as urinary infection or vaginal pathology.
- Are you using any contraception? Women in the climacteric period can still have ovulatory cycles, therefore can become pregnant. Contraception is often continued until after confirmed menopause.
- Are you up-to-date with smear tests? In any woman with complaints of intermenstrual or postcoital bleeding it is crucial that her smear history is explored and referral for colposcopy is made if required.
- What impact is this having on your quality of life?

Examination

A general examination including body mass index (BMI) and blood pressure (BP) should be performed.

Examination should be tailored towards the history findings, for example, a bimanual pelvic examination, and Cusco's speculum performed if there are any urogenital symptoms (Table 17.2).

INVESTIGATIONS

A diagnosis of menopause should be made through history and clinical features. However, an elevated FSH level (30 or more) can be used to diagnose menopause in women aged 40 to 45 years with menopausal symptoms or change in menstrual cycle, or in women under 40 years of age with suspected menopause. If FSH levels are >30, a second confirmatory sample should be repeated 4 to 6 weeks later to confirm the diagnosis of menopause.

Table 17.2 Investigating menopausal symptoms

Symptoms	Investigations
Urinary symptoms (dysuria, frequency, urgency)	Urine dipstick ± Urine microscopy, culture and sensitivities ± Urodynamic testing
Intermenstrual/postcoital bleeding	Cervical smear ± Colposcopy Transvaginal ultrasound scan to assess for endometrial pathology ± hysteroscopy and endometrial biopsy
Low-impact fractures/ family history of osteoporosis	X-ray Dual-energy X-ray absorptiometry (DEXA) scan
Urogenital symptoms	Bimanual pelvic examination and speculum ± high and low vaginal swabs for sexually transmitted infections (STIs) or candida (thrush) Assess for vaginal atrophy

Table 17.3 Route of administration for hormone replacement therapy

	Advantages	Disadvantages
Oral	Cheap, effective	First-pass metabolism Variable plasma levels Higher doses required Increased risk of thromboembolism and strokes compared with transdermal preparations
Transdermal (patch/gel)	Avoids first-pass metabolism No increased risk of venous thromboembolism Continuous administration	Cost Skin reactions
Vaginal	Good for urogenital symptoms Minimal systemic absorption Licenced for 3 months' use without progesterone opposition (in the UK)	Unlikely to treat systemic symptoms
Mirena intrauterine system	Licenced for 4 years to provide the progesterone arm of hormone replacement therapy (HRT) Contraceptive	Only provides progesterone for endometrial protection Patients will still need oestrogen

MANAGEMENT

Optimal management of the menopause should be tailored and adapted to the individual patient and their particular symptoms. Options include hormone replacement therapy (HRT), nonhormonal treatments and nonpharmaceutical treatments.

Medical

Hormone replacement therapy

HRT reduces symptoms of the menopause and is the most effective and widely used treatment. It can contain oestrogen and progesterone, or oestrogen-only preparations. As oestrogen replacement alone can cause endometrial hyperplasia, it should only be used in women who have already undergone a hysterectomy. However, women who have a uterus must have progesterone added to protect the endometrium.

When prescribing HRT the lowest effective dose should be used. There are multiple routes of administration, which means treatment can be individually tailored to patients. These include oral tablets, transdermal patch, gels, implants, vaginal rings or pessaries. The Mirena intrauterine system can also be used as the progesterone component of HRT. Table 17.3 shows the advantages and disadvantages of different routes of administration. Patient should also be counselled regarding the risks of breast cancer associated with HRT (Fig. 17.2).

Preparations can be given continuously or in sequential preparations where patients will experience a monthly withdrawal bleed, however these must not be used for more than 5 years due to risk of endometrial hyperplasia. Fig. 17.3 outlines the HRT patient pathway.

RED FLAGS

Contraindications to hormone replacement therapy:
- Endometrial cancer
- Breast cancer
- Undiagnosed vaginal bleeding
- Undiagnosed breast lumps
- Severe active liver disease
- Pregnancy (always rule out before starting therapy)
- Personal history of venous thromboembolism – ORAL therapy is contraindicated but if benefits of treatment outweigh risks, then TRANSDERMAL preparations can be used.

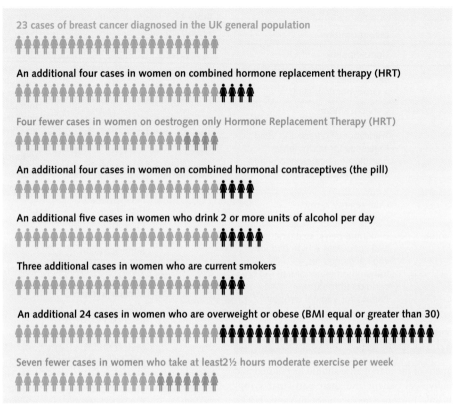

Fig. 17.2 A comparison of lifestyle risk factors versus hormone replacement therapy (HRT) treatment differences for developing breast cancer. Incidence displayed as number of women developing breast cancer over the next 5 years per 1000 women aged 50 to 59. *BMI,* Body mass index. (*Women's health concern infographic,* November 2015.)

Common side effects described with HRT include breast tenderness, leg cramps, nausea, bloating, irritability and depression. Unscheduled vaginal bleeding is common within the first 3 months of initiating treatment, but should be reported if ongoing. Review of patients on HRT should be made annually unless there are any clinical indications for an earlier review such as side effects. Patients presenting with persistent unscheduled bleeding while using HRT require an ultrasound scan to assess the endometrial thickness. If this is >4.0 mm a hysteroscopy and endometrial biopsy should be performed. Similarly, if an incidental finding of a thickened endometrium >7.0 mm is found in the absence of bleeding, a hysteroscopy and biopsy should also be performed to exclude endometrial hyperplasia or malignancy.

Vaginal oestrogen

Vaginal oestrogen preparations should be offered to women with urogenital atrophy, including those on systemic HRT to relieve symptoms. There is minimal systemic absorption and adverse effects are rare. Vaginal dryness can be helped with vaginal moisturizers and lubricants either in isolation or with vaginal oestrogen.

Nonhormonal pharmacological agents

If hormonal agents are contraindicated or not tolerated for vasomotor symptoms, nonhormonal treatments can be considered although they are not routinely offered. Options include selective serotonin reuptake inhibitors, selective norepinephrine reuptake inhibitors and clonidine.

Conservative

Lifestyle changes

Lifestyle changes such as regular aerobic exercise, reduction in alcohol consumption and smoking are all beneficial for symptom control. Menopausal patients often find that certain food substances can trigger hot flushes.

HRT – Patient Pathway

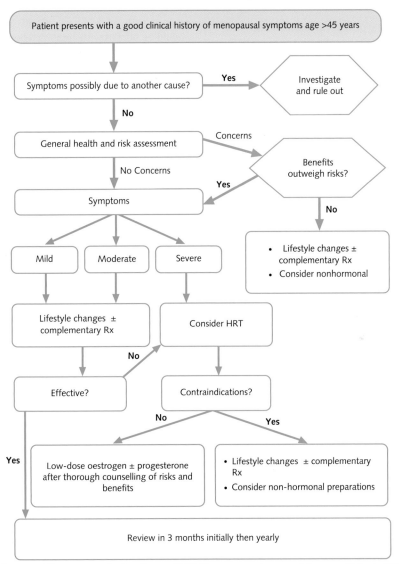

Fig. 17.3 Hormone replacement therapy – patient pathway. *HRT*, Hormone replacement therapy. (Adapted from Panay N. Menopause. In *Oxford Desk Reference: Obstetrics and Gynaecology*, Oxford, UK: Oxford University Press; 2011.)

Cognitive behavioural therapy

There is good evidence that cognitive behavioural therapy can alleviate low mood and anxiety as a result of the menopause.

Complementary therapy

There are a variety of complementary remedies believed to help menopausal symptoms. However, different preparations may vary, safety is not always certain and it is possible for medication interactions to occur. Isoflavones (phytoestrogens derived from beans) or black cohosh (a North American root) are thought to relieve vasomotor symptoms. There is evidence that St. John's Wort can relieve vasomotor symptoms in patients with a history of or at high risk of breast cancer. However, it has potentially serious interactions with other drugs including tamoxifen.

PREMATURE OVARIAN INSUFFICIENCY

Approximately 1% of women experience 'premature menopause' or 'POI'. It is diagnosed in women under the age of 40 years with cessation of periods and a history of menopausal symptoms. Taking a thorough history is crucial as causes can include surgery, chemotherapy or radiotherapy, chromosomal defects and autoimmune disease. Formal diagnosis can be made with elevated FSH levels on two separate occasions taken 4 to 6 weeks apart of >30. Sex steroid replacement should be offered with combined hormonal contraception or HRT, unless contraindicated, which can continue until the age of natural menopause. Advice should be given about bone, cardiovascular health and managing symptoms. It is important to remind patients that HRT does not act as a contraceptive and it is possible to have occasional ovulatory cycles with premature menopause, therefore natural conception can rarely occur. See Chapter 16 for management of subfertility for patients with POI.

Chapter Summary

- The menopause can have a range of systemic symptoms including vasomotor, psychological and urogenital. It typically occurs between the ages of 45 and 55 years.
- Hormone replacement therapy (HRT) reduces symptoms of the menopause and is the most effective and widely used treatment. Women should be fully educated about the benefits, potential risks and alternative treatments available.
- Common side effects with HRT include breast tenderness, leg cramps, nausea, bloating, irritability and depression.
- Conservative measures used to treat menopausal symptoms include cognitive behavioural therapy, lifestyle changes and complementary therapies such as isoflavones and St. John's Wort.
- 'Premature menopause' is a cessation of periods in women under 40 years old and occurs in approximately 1% of women.

UKMLA Conditions
Menopause

UKMLA Presentations
Loss of libido
Menopausal problems

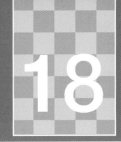

18

MISCARRIAGE

Definitions

In the UK, miscarriage is defined as the spontaneous loss of a pregnancy before 24 completed weeks of pregnancy. Miscarriages can be termed 'early' or 'late':

- An '**early**' miscarriage is one that occurs within the first 12 completed weeks of pregnancy.
- A '**late**' miscarriage refers to a pregnancy loss between 13 and 24 completed weeks of gestation.

A **stillbirth** refers to a baby that is born with no signs of life after 24 completed weeks of pregnancy.

Recurrent miscarriage is defined as the loss of three or more consecutive pregnancies.

Terminology commonly used to describe the type and stage of miscarriage are shown in Table 18.1.

Incidence

Spontaneous miscarriage is the most common complication of pregnancy. The overall incidence is between 15% and 20% of all clinical pregnancies, with the majority occurring in the first trimester. Recurrent miscarriage affects 1% of couples trying to conceive.

Aetiology

In the majority of cases, no definitive cause for miscarriage is found. Risk factors and conditions known to cause miscarriage and recurrent miscarriage are listed in Table 18.2.

Clinical presentation

Typically, patients present with a history of vaginal bleeding and lower abdominal pain. The amount of bleeding can vary from light spotting to heavy bleeding with the passage of clots or even pregnancy tissue/products of conception (POC). Women typically describe cramping, central lower abdominal pain 'like period pains' or 'like contractions'.

It is important to note that light vaginal spotting and abdominal pain are very common in early pregnancy and do not necessarily indicate a miscarriage or ectopic pregnancy. It is also important to emphasize that intercourse or exercise will not provoke a miscarriage. Bear in mind that an ectopic pregnancy can also present similarly with vaginal bleeding and abdominal pain, and so this differential diagnosis should always be excluded. Patients experiencing a missed miscarriage may be completely asymptomatic.

Retained products of conception (RPOC) within the uterine cavity can be a focus of infection, especially with spontaneous rupture of membranes in the second trimester, resulting in a septic miscarriage. Vaginal loss may be purulent and offensive smelling, and the patient may be pyrexial and tachycardic. Treatment involves antibiotics and prompt removal of the infective source, although this may mean a termination of pregnancy if a fetal heartbeat is still present.

Patients who present with life-threatening haemorrhage and haemodynamic instability/shock require urgent resuscitation and intervention, usually with an evacuation of retained products of conception (ERPC) to stop the bleeding.

RED FLAGS

Any woman presenting with lower abdominal pain (with or without vaginal bleeding) and a positive pregnancy test must be managed as an ectopic pregnancy until otherwise proven.

COMMUNICATION

Miscarriage can be very distressing for the woman and her partner. It is important to display sensitivity and empathy when counselling patients. Charities such as 'The Miscarriage Association' (www.miscarriageassociation.org.uk) provide information and support for those experiencing a miscarriage and it is good practice to signpost these resources to patients.

History

Good history taking is important to distinguish if the patient is experiencing a miscarriage or other differentials such as an ectopic pregnancy, or nonpregnancy-related conditions such as appendicitis or gastroenteritis. History taking has been covered in detail in Chapter 2. Important points to note are:

- **The presenting complaint**: Establish the presenting complaint focusing on any bleeding, pain and vaginal loss.

Table 18.1 Terminology of miscarriage

Terminology	Description	Clinical findings	Ultrasound findings
Viable intrauterine pregnancy	An ongoing pregnancy	No abdominal pain or vaginal bleeding. Cervical os is closed.	A gestational sac with fetal pole and cardiac activity within the uterine cavity
Complete miscarriage	All pregnancy tissue has been expelled from the uterus	Abdominal pain and vaginal bleeding initially but has now settled. Cervical os may be open or closed.	No pregnancy tissue remains within the uterine cavity (note that a diagnosis of complete miscarriage can only be made in the presence of a previous scan confirming an intrauterine pregnancy)
Incomplete miscarriage	Nonviable pregnancy with the passage of some but not all pregnancy tissue	Abdominal pain and vaginal bleeding that may be ongoing. Cervical os may be open or closed.	Nonviable pregnancy tissue remains within the uterus
Threatened miscarriage	A viable intrauterine pregnancy that is currently ongoing in a patient presenting with symptoms	Abdominal pain and/or vaginal bleeding. Cervical os is closed.	A gestational sac with fetal pole and cardiac activity within the uterine cavity
Inevitable miscarriage	A patient presenting with symptoms but with no passage of pregnancy tissue yet	Abdominal pain and vaginal bleeding. Cervical os is open.	Pregnancy tissue is low in the uterus or within the cervix
Missed/silent miscarriage	Nonviable pregnancy in an asymptomatic patient	No abdominal pain or vaginal bleeding. Cervical os is closed.	Nonviable pregnancy within the uterine cavity
Pregnancy of unknown location	Positive pregnancy test but no pregnancy tissue is seen	No abdominal pain or vaginal bleeding. Cervical os is closed.	No intrauterine or extrauterine pregnancy seen

Enquire about the location of abdominal pain – is it central or on one side (suggestive of an ectopic)? Quantify the amount of bleeding – size of the clots (5p, 50p, palm-size), number of pads used in a day, were they soaked through? This gives an idea about the likelihood of inevitable miscarriage.

- **Spontaneous conception or IVF pregnancy**: Although all women can be very affected by a possible miscarriage, it is often those who have undergone IVF who are most anxious and distressed. IVF is also a risk factor for ectopic pregnancy.
- **LMP**: This is required to calculate the estimated gestation. Establish whether the patient is sure of these dates and whether periods are regular. In an IVF pregnancy, gestation is calculated from the implantation date. The estimated gestation will help with interpreting a scan. For example, if the patient is 9 weeks pregnant by dates, you would expect to see a fetal pole and heartbeat on ultrasound. At 4 weeks gestation, you would only expect to see a gestational sac.

- **Previous ultrasound**: Establish whether the patient has had a scan in this pregnancy. This can confirm an intrauterine pregnancy and rule out an ectopic as a differential diagnosis.
- **Obstetric and gynaecological history**: Enquire about previous pregnancies, including miscarriages and ectopic pregnancies. Establish contraceptive use – note that use of the intrauterine contraceptive device carries a risk of ectopic pregnancy. Ask about previous pelvic inflammatory disease, endometriosis and pelvic surgery as these increase the risk of ectopic pregnancy due to adhesions.
- **Other symptoms**: Enquire about fever, shoulder tip pain, diarrhoea, dizziness/light-headedness and nausea/vomiting.

Examination

Firstly, observe from the end of the bed. Does the patient look well or unwell? Pale or shocked? Is there any bleeding externally? This first snapshot assessment will identify a patient who needs urgent attention.

Table 18.2 Aetiology and investigation of miscarriage

Aetiology	Examples	Investigation
Maternal age	Maternal age is an independent risk factor for miscarriage. The risk of miscarriage in women aged 20–24 is around 11%, rising to 25% in women aged 35–39 and doubling to 51% in women aged 40–44. Above the age of 45, the risk of miscarriage can be as high as 93%.	-
Previous miscarriage	The risk of further miscarriage increases after each successive pregnancy loss, reaching approximately 40% after three consecutive miscarriages.	-
Paternal age	Risk of miscarriage increases in couples where the man is over the age of 40.	-
Fetal abnormalities	Around 30%–57% of miscarriages can be attributed to fetal chromosomal abnormalities (e.g., autosomal trisomies, polyploidies and monosomy X), some of which are incompatible with life.	Cytogenetic analysis of pregnancy tissue. Parental karyotyping of both partners should be performed if cytogenetic analysis reveals an unbalanced structural chromosomal abnormality.
Endocrine factors	Women with poorly controlled diabetes mellitus at the time of conception have a 45% risk of miscarriage and fetal anomaly. Untreated thyroid disease is also associated with recurrent miscarriage.	Blood glucose levels. Thyroid function tests.
Maternal infection	Any severe febrile infection can predispose to sporadic miscarriage. Examples include syphilis, malaria, *Listeria, influenza* and *Toxoplasma* species. Additionally, certain organisms such as Zika virus, rubella, and cytomegalovirus can cause fetal congenital malformations. Bacterial vaginosis (BV) has been linked to second-trimester miscarriage and preterm delivery.	High vaginal swab to screen for BV. Toxoplasmosis, rubella, cytomegalovirus, herpes and other agents infection screen.
Autoimmune factors	Antiphospholipid antibodies (anticardiolipin antibodies, lupus anticoagulant) are present in 15% of women with recurrent miscarriage. They inhibit trophoblastic function and differentiation, can cause a local inflammatory response, and cause thrombosis of placental vasculature. Treatment with low-dose aspirin and low-molecular-weight heparin can improve outcomes.	Antiphospholipid antibody assays performed on two occasions at least 12 weeks apart to account for false-positive or false-negative results.
Thrombophilia	Thrombophilia has been implicated in recurrent miscarriage. This includes protein C and S deficiencies, factor II (prothrombin) gene mutation, factor V Leiden mutation and antithrombin III deficiency.	Screening for inherited thrombophilias.
Cervical weakness	Cervical weakness, commonly secondary to previous cone biopsies or large loop excision of the transformation zone (LLETZ), is a recognized cause of second-trimester miscarriage. The diagnosis is clinical, usually based on a history of second-trimester miscarriage preceded by spontaneous rupture of membranes or painless cervical dilatation.	Serial transvaginal monitoring of cervical length during pregnancy.
Uterine abnormalities	The reported prevalence of uterine structural anomalies such as bicornuate or septate uteri is between 2% and 38%. This appears to be higher in women with second-trimester miscarriages and preterm deliveries.	Transvaginal ultrasound to assess the uterine cavity. In suspected abnormality, hysteroscopy and laparoscopy can be used to confirm the diagnosis.
Lifestyle	Maternal cigarette smoking, alcohol intake and caffeine consumption have been associated with sporadic miscarriage in a dose-dependent manner.	

Examining the abdomen, you are likely going to feel a soft abdomen. In the first trimester, the uterus is unlikely to be palpable unless, for example, the patient is known to have fibroids.

A Cusco speculum should be used with the patient's consent, to examine the patient vaginally and with a chaperone present. Visualize the cervix and determine whether it is open or closed. Is there any ongoing bleeding? POC may be visible at the external os. Care should be taken to remove these during the examination as pregnancy tissue within the cervical canal can be a cause of cramping pain, bleeding and 'cervical shock', a vagal response to cervical dilatation. Cervical shock can cause syncope, hypotension and bradycardia. If there is any offensive discharge, swabs should be taken to assess for infection.

Investigations

a) **Urinary pregnancy test**: This should be performed to confirm pregnancy.
b) **Serum β-human chorionic gonadotropin (BHCG)**: This can be helpful in combination with a transvaginal ultrasound in distinguishing between early intrauterine pregnancies from a miscarriage or ectopic pregnancy. A pregnancy is usually visible on transvaginal ultrasound with serum BHCG levels >1000 IU. In an ongoing pregnancy, BHCG levels can be expected to double every 48 hours.
c) **Blood tests**: All patients presenting with bleeding in early pregnancy should have a baseline haemoglobin and group and save. Women who are Rhesus negative would require anti-D immunoglobulin should they undergo surgical intervention for a miscarriage or ectopic pregnancy, or in second trimester miscarriage.
d) **Transvaginal ultrasound**: This is essential to make a diagnosis. The uterus is examined, looking for a gestational sac, fetal pole and cardiac activity (fetal heartbeat). A fetal heartbeat is usually seen from approximately 6 weeks' gestation. RPOC may be seen within the uterine cavity in an incomplete miscarriage. If the uterine cavity is empty, this could mean a very early intrauterine pregnancy, ectopic pregnancy or complete miscarriage. The adnexa should be scanned to look for an ectopic mass and the Pouch of Douglas examined for free fluid.

Management

Conservative
Expectant management can be offered for up to 14 days to allow the miscarriage to happen naturally without any intervention. This is only an option in women who are haemodynamically stable without increased risk of bleeding and with no evidence of infection. Patients should be advised that the process of miscarriage may take several weeks for complete resolution, and

that there is a risk of prolonged bleeding, infection and RPOC ultimately requiring medical or surgical intervention. Patients should be counselled and given written information about what to expect throughout the process, including the likely duration and severity of bleeding, advice on analgesia and where and when to get help in an emergency.

Medical
Medical management of miscarriage involves the use of prostaglandin analogues to stimulate myometrial contraction and expulsion of pregnancy tissue. This avoids the potential risks associated with surgical intervention. Misoprostol is most commonly used, usually administered orally or vaginally. Success rates vary but can be as high as 96% depending on the type of miscarriage, gestational age, route of administration, duration and dose. Medical management can be undertaken as an inpatient or outpatient. Inpatient management is generally advised for patients at increased risk of bleeding, for example, second-trimester miscarriage, known coagulation disorders and haemodynamic compromise. Patients should be advised of the potential increase in pain and bleeding with medical management, along with greater analgesic needs, and failure requiring surgical intervention.

Surgical
Surgical management involves the removal of pregnancy tissue from the uterus usually by suction curettage. Surgical management of miscarriage (SMM) has now mostly replaced the term 'evacuation of retained products of conception' (ERPC). Surgical management is often advised in cases of persistent or excessive bleeding, haemodynamic instability, evidence of infection/septic miscarriage or suspected gestational trophoblastic disease (GTD). SMM has a high success rate but also the highest risk of complication among all three management options. Risks include anaesthetic complications, uterine perforation, haemorrhage, cervical trauma and intrauterine adhesions (Asherman syndrome). SMM is generally performed under general anaesthesia as a day-case procedure, and ultrasound guidance can be employed to minimize the risk of uterine perforation. Some units offer outpatient surgical evacuation techniques under local anaesthetic or sedation. This is known as manual vacuum aspiration (MVA) and is generally more suitable with earlier gestations or small amounts of RPOC.

Follow-up

As much as possible, pregnancy tissue should be sent for histological examination to confirm the diagnosis and exclude the presence of GTD. Following this, pregnancy tissue should be disposed of sensitively according to the patient's wishes and in accordance with local legislation.

No follow-up is required routinely following SMM unless the patient is being investigated for recurrent miscarriage. Follow-up should be arranged with expectant/medical management if the symptoms exceed the period of expectant management or if a pregnancy test remains positive after 3 weeks. It is crucial that women are given information of when and how to get help in an emergency.

Recurrent miscarriage

As mentioned, recurrent miscarriage is the loss of three or more consecutive pregnancies, and this affects 1% of couples. Poor reproductive history is an independent predictor of future pregnancy outcome, and a previous live birth does not prevent a woman from experiencing subsequent recurrent miscarriage. Risk factors and investigations have been discussed in Table 18.2. Couples should be assessed and counselled in a specialist recurrent miscarriage clinic.

It is important to remember that in the majority of patients, no cause for recurrent miscarriage will be identified despite detailed investigation. Patients should be cared for in a dedicated early pregnancy assessment unit, and reassured that the prognosis for a successful future pregnancy is around 75% with supportive care alone.

ECTOPIC PREGNANCY

Definitions

An ectopic pregnancy refers to any pregnancy occurring outside the uterine cavity.

Approximately 95% of ectopic pregnancies occur in the fallopian tubes, specifically the ampullae or isthmic portions. Around 2% to 3% occur as interstitial ectopic pregnancies. Rarer locations include the cervix, ovary, abdominal cavity and caesarean section scar (Fig. 18.1).

A heterotopic pregnancy is an extremely rare occurrence of an intrauterine pregnancy and co-existing ectopic pregnancy.

Prevalence

The incidence of ectopic pregnancies is approximately 1 in 100 pregnancies. Around a third of ectopic pregnancies occur spontaneously, but the majority are caused by conditions that damage the fallopian tubes or their ciliary lining. Risk factors for ectopic pregnancy include:

- Previous ectopic pregnancy (10%–20% risk of future ectopic)
- History of pelvic inflammatory disease

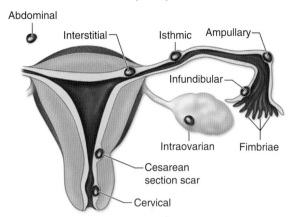

Sites of Ectopic Implantations

Fig. 18.1 Implantation sites of ectopic pregnancies. (Source: Parikh S, Patel NR. *Ferri's Clinical Advisor 2023.* Elsevier, 2023: 543–545.e1. © 2023.)

- Pregnancy in the presence of an intrauterine contraceptive device
- Subfertility and assisted conception techniques including IVF
- Previous pelvic/abdominal surgery or pelvic conditions (e.g., endometriosis) due to presence of adhesions
- Cigarette smoking
- Maternal age >40 years

Unfortunately, women can still die as a result of ectopic pregnancy; 0.2 per 100 cases lead to maternal death. Therefore, accurately diagnosing and appropriately managing the condition is crucial.

Clinical presentation

It cannot be emphasized enough that any presentation of lower abdominal pain (with or without bleeding) and a positive pregnancy test must be managed as an ectopic pregnancy until proven otherwise (such as with an intrauterine pregnancy seen on transvaginal ultrasound).

A high index of suspicion of ectopic pregnancy should be maintained with presentations of vaginal bleeding or lower abdominal pain with associated syncope, dizziness/light-headedness, diarrhoea or vomiting and shoulder tip pain following a period of amenorrhoea. Similar to the presentation of miscarriage, the most common symptom is lower abdominal pain, usually preceding the onset of vaginal bleeding, although some patients may be completely asymptomatic in an early ectopic pregnancy. Pain is usually localized to one side of the abdomen, usually in the right or left iliac fossa, and typically is insidious in onset and worsening. In cases of a ruptured ectopic it can cause generalized abdominal pain, and irritation of the inferior diaphragm from blood resulting in referred shoulder tip pain. Blood in the pelvis can also cause irritability of the bowel, and therefore diarrhoea and vomiting. Any history of syncope, dizziness or light-headedness may indicate haemodynamic instability. There have been cases of ectopic pregnancy presenting with only gastrointestinal symptoms. Vaginal bleeding, another common presenting symptom, can range from light loss or 'spotting' to heavy bleeding with large clots. It is important to note that having vaginal bleeding does not mean that the woman has an intrauterine pregnancy (IUP). As symptoms can be nonspecific, all women presenting to accident and emergency with these symptoms should undergo a pregnancy test.

Clinical examination may reveal signs of haemodynamic shock including hypotension and tachycardia. There may be signs of peritonism (rebound tenderness, guarding), abdominal/pelvic tenderness, cervical excitation and abdominal distension.

Management

Conservative

Conservative (expectant) management of ectopic pregnancy is an option available to clinically stable, asymptomatic patients with a confirmed ectopic pregnancy measuring <35 mm, no visible heartbeat on ultrasound, be willing and able to attend follow-ups, and a serum BHCG level <1500 IU/L. Lower initial BHCG and rapid decrease are significant predictors of spontaneous resolution. Patients should be advised that up to 29% will require additional medical or surgical management and that ectopic rupture can occur with decreasing BHCG levels. Any change in symptoms should prompt attendance to hospital. Follow-up involves serial measurements of serum BHCG in conjunction with transvaginal ultrasound according to local schedules. Women who may be suitable for conservative management should also be offered medical or surgical management if preferred.

Medical

Medical management of ectopic pregnancy involves the administration of methotrexate, a folic antagonist that interferes with DNA synthesis and destroys rapidly dividing cells including pregnancy tissue. It is suitable for haemodynamically stable women with minimal pain, an unruptured tubal ectopic pregnancy <35 mm with no visible heartbeat, serum BHCG levels <1500 IU/L, no intrauterine pregnancy and willingness for follow-up. Patients with a serum BHCG level between 1500 and 5000 IU/L can be offered either methotrexate or surgery. Methotrexate is administered as a single-dose intramuscular injection, with the dose measured based on the patient's body surface area. It is both a cytotoxic and teratogenic medication, and patients should be advised on the importance of attending regular follow-up appointments for serum BHCG monitoring

and the need for effective contraception to avoid pregnancy for at least 3 months following completion of treatment.

Patients receiving methotrexate commonly experience side effects, predominantly abdominal pain, photosensitivity, nausea and vomiting and diarrhoea. It can be difficult to distinguish between side effects of medication and tubal rupture. Patients should be made aware and given clear instructions on when to present to emergency services. Single-dose methotrexate has a similar efficacy to surgical treatment in stable patients. Success rates of up to 90% have been reported although around 15% of patients will require a second dose. About 5% to 10% of patients will require surgery due to rupture of the ectopic during follow-up.

COMMUNICATION

Women undergoing conservative and medical management of ectopic pregnancy must be aware of the ongoing risk of ectopic rupture even in the event of a falling β-human chorionic gonadotropin. They must be given clear verbal and written advice and contact details in the event of an emergency.

Surgical

The majority of tubal ectopic pregnancies are managed surgically. Laparoscopic surgery should be offered whenever possible as it is associated with lower analgesic requirements, reduced intraoperative blood loss, shorter hospital admission and quicker postoperative recovery. Laparotomy may be quicker and more appropriate in cases with haemodynamic instability, massive haemoperitoneum or dense adhesions.

Surgical management should be offered first-line to patients with confirmed ectopic pregnancy measuring >35 mm, visible fetal heartbeat, significant pain or serum BHCG >5000 IU/L. Salpingectomy (removal of the fallopian tube) on the affected side is preferred over salpingotomy (removal of the ectopic pregnancy via an incision within the fallopian tube) in the presence of a healthy contralateral tube (Fig. 18.2). Salpingotomy has higher rates of residual trophoblastic tissue compared to salpingectomy (8% vs. 4%) and requires serial BHCG monitoring to ensure resolution. Salpingotomy may be considered in patients with contralateral tube damage or an absent contralateral tube.

Anti-D prophylaxis should be offered to Rhesus-negative women who have surgical management of ectopic pregnancy.

Prognosis

Following an ectopic pregnancy, the risk of future ectopic pregnancy in subsequent pregnancies is between 10% and 20%, with up to a 76% chance of an intrauterine pregnancy. Even with only one

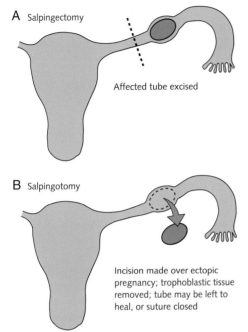

A Salpingectomy

Affected tube excised

B Salpingotomy

Incision made over ectopic
pregnancy; trophoblastic tissue
removed; tube may be left to
heal, or suture closed

Fig. 18.2 Surgical options for treatment of tubal ectopic pregnancy. (From Kay SE, Sandhu CJ. *Crash Course Obstetrics and Gynaecology*. Elsevier, 2019: 119–127. © 2019.)

fallopian tube, chances of conceiving are only slightly reduced. Due to the risk of recurrence, patients are advised to have an early scan in future pregnancies to locate the site of the pregnancy.

> **CLINICAL NOTES**
>
> Guidelines for managing ectopic pregnancy can be found in the Royal College of Obstetrics and Gynaecology 'Green-top guideline No. 21' published in 2016, 'Diagnosis and Management of Ectopic Pregnancy, and NICE guideline 'Ectopic Pregnancy and Miscarriage: Diagnosis and Initial Management' published in 2019.

PREGNANCY OF UNKNOWN LOCATION

A pregnancy of unknown location (PUL) means there are no signs of either intrauterine or extrauterine pregnancy, or RPOC in a woman with a positive pregnancy test. This may be due to very early pregnancy not yet visible on scan, following miscarriage or an undiagnosed ectopic pregnancy. Up to 69% of PULs resolve spontaneously, but as many as 28% are subsequently diagnosed with ectopic pregnancy.

A pregnancy is usually visible on transvaginal ultrasound with serum BHCG levels >1000 IU. Therefore, if no visible pregnancy is seen with BHCG levels above this, this should be managed as a potentially undiagnosed ectopic pregnancy. Serial BHCG measurements should be performed along with repeat transvaginal ultrasound at regular intervals.

GESTATIONAL TROPHOBLASTIC DISEASE

Definition

GTD comprises a group of conditions caused by abnormal fertilization and leading to abnormal formation of trophoblastic tissue. Persistence of GTD after primary treatment, commonly defined as a persistent elevation of BHCG, is referred to as gestational trophoblastic neoplasia (GTN).

Complete molar pregnancies arise as a result of duplication of a single sperm following fertilization of an 'empty' ovum, which contains no genetic material (Fig. 18.3). It can also arise following dispermic fertilization of an 'empty' ovum. They are therefore diploid and androgenic (all paternal genetic material), with no evidence of fetal tissue.

Partial molar pregnancies occur more commonly than complete molar pregnancies. They can contain fetal tissue, fetal red blood cells and even a foetus. Partial moles contain two sets of paternal haploid chromosomes and one set of maternal haploid chromosomes (Fig. 18.3). They usually occur due to dispermic fertilization of a normal ovum, and are therefore triploid.

Choriocarcinomas are BHCG-secreting tumours of trophoblastic cells that occur due to incomplete removal of a molar pregnancy. They behave like a cancer and can metastasize, particularly to the lungs, liver and brain.

> **SUMMARY BOX – GESTATIONAL TROPHOBLASTIC DISEASE**
>
> - Premalignant
>   - Hydatidiform moles: complete or partial molar pregnancies
> - Malignant (GTN)
>   - Choriocarcinoma
>   - Invasive mole
>   - Placental site trophoblastic tumour (PSTT)
>   - Epithelioid trophoblastic tumour (ETT)
>   - Atypical placental site nodules (PSNs)

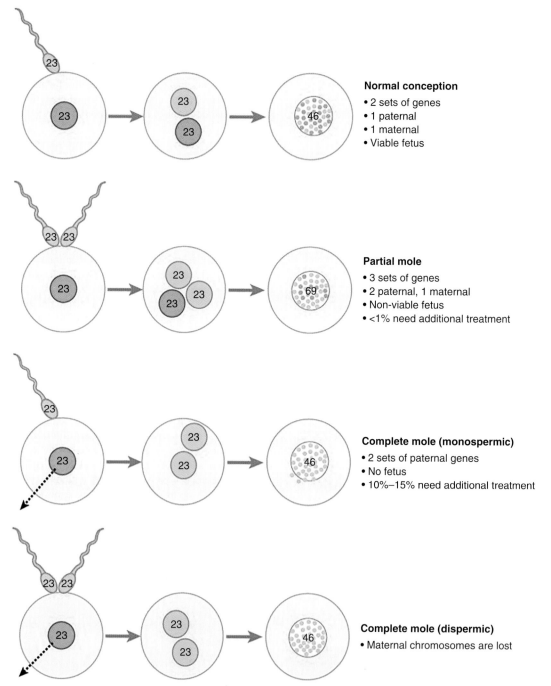

Fig. 18.3 Genetic make-up of normal pregnancy and partial and complete molar pregnancies. (From Tidy J. *Clinical Obstetrics and Gynaecology*. Elsevier, 2023: 166–173. © 2023.)

Prevalence

The incidence of GTD is uncommon – approximately 1 in 714 live births. Women at the extremes of reproductive age, and those of Asian ethnicity have a higher incidence. GTN can develop after any pregnancy event, such as following a molar pregnancy, nonmolar pregnancy (miscarriage, ectopic pregnancy) and term pregnancy (live birth). The incidence of GTN is rare, estimated at 1 in 50,000 live births.

In the UK, there are three GTD centres running a national registration and treatment programme. This has conferred a 98% to 100% cure rate for GTD, with only 5% to 8% of cases requiring chemotherapy. The need for chemotherapy with a complete mole is 13% to 16% and 0.5% to 1% after a partial mole. Patients with GTN and GTD should be registered and managed in dedicated GTD centres as this has been shown to improve overall outcomes.

Clinical presentation

Molar pregnancy tissues secrete BHCG, resulting in significantly higher serum BHCG levels. This classically leads to exaggerated symptoms of pregnancy such as excessive uterine enlargement or abdominal distension and severe hyperemesis gravidarum. Irregular/persistent vaginal bleeding is the most common presenting symptom. A urine pregnancy test may remain positive and serum BHCG levels may remain persistently elevated even more than 8 weeks after a pregnancy event.

Diagnosis

Definitive diagnosis of molar pregnancy can only be made with histologic examination of pregnancy tissue. Complete molar pregnancies develop into a multivesicular mass of trophoblastic tissue, which is described as having a classical 'bunch of grapes' or 'snowstorm' appearance on transvaginal ultrasound (Fig. 18.4). Serum BHCG levels greater than two multiples of the median are also highly suggestive.

Management

Surgical management is recommended in the management of molar pregnancies in order to remove the abnormal trophoblastic tissue. This is best performed by suction curettage under ultrasound guidance to minimize the risk of uterine perforation and ensure complete removal of tissue. Pregnancy tissue must be sent for histological assessment to confirm the diagnosis. Excessive vaginal bleeding can be associated with molar pregnancy and therefore the procedure should be supervised by a senior clinician. Medical management should be avoided if possible, due to the increased risk of developing GTN and requiring chemotherapy.

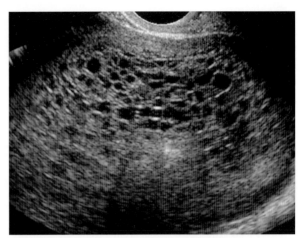

Fig. 18.4 Complete molar pregnancy: classic 'snowstorm' appearance. Transabdominal scan shows a vesicular echogenic mass distending the endometrium. The mass is filled with innumerable uniformly distributed cystic spaces that correspond to hydropic chorionic villi. (From Pfeuti C, Gomez Slagle, HB. *Ferri's Clinical Advisor 2023*. Elsevier, 2023: 993.e6-993.e11. © 2023.)

Patients with confirmed molar pregnancies as well as persistently elevated serum BHCGs should be urgently referred to national GTD centres for follow-up. Follow-up after GTD is individualized and monitored with serial serum BHCG measurements to ensure it is falling. If BHCG levels remain abnormal after 6 months, plateau or increase, chemotherapy is started. Patients may be treated either with single or multiagent chemotherapy depending on a risk scoring system (FIGO 2000 scoring system for GTN). Patients should be advised not to conceive until their follow-up is complete or from 1 year of completion of treatment. Recurrence rates are low (approximately 1%) and are more associated with complete rather than partial molar pregnancy.

HYPEREMESIS GRAVIDARUM

Definition

Nausea and vomiting in the first trimester is a common pregnancy symptom affecting 80% of pregnancies. Hyperemesis gravidarum affects up to 3.6% of pregnancies and is diagnosed by:

- Severe prolonged nausea and vomiting
- Associated weight loss of >5% prepregnancy
- Dehydration
- Electrolyte imbalance

The cause is thought to be due to rising BHCG levels, therefore trophoblastic or multiple pregnancies that are associated with higher BHCG levels can increase the severity of nausea and vomiting.

History and examination

Other causes of nausea and vomiting should be excluded by asking about symptoms of abdominal pain, urinary symptoms, infection, chronic *Helicobacter pylori* infection and drug history. A previous history of hyperemesis gravidarum should be sought as it can recur in subsequent pregnancy. Examine the patient and note the patient's general appearance, observations, weight and signs of dehydration.

Investigations

Urine dipstick: Assess the degree of ketonuria and if leucocytes or nitrites are present. Urine should be sent for microscopy, culture and sensitivities to rule out urinary tract infection.

Blood tests: A full blood count and urea and electrolytes should be performed to rule out infection, anaemia, measure haematocrit and assess electrolyte imbalances, especially hyponatraemia and hypokalaemia. There is a structural similarity between thyroid-stimulating hormone (TSH) and BHCG, which can cause abnormal thyroid function test results. Hyperemesis gravidarum can cause deranged liver function tests with raised transaminases and bilirubin. Abnormal thyroid function tests and liver function tests usually normalize with treatment and resolution of hyperemesis gravidarum.

Transvaginal ultrasound: An ultrasound scan should be arranged to confirm a viable intrauterine pregnancy and exclude multiple pregnancy or GTD as a cause for hyperemesis.

Management

Hyperemesis gravidarum can be managed as an outpatient, in an ambulatory day care unit or as an inpatient depending on the severity of the nausea and vomiting.

Woman with mild nausea and vomiting can be managed in the community with oral antiemetics, oral hydration and dietary advice. Those who are not tolerating oral fluids can attend an ambulatory day care unit for intravenous (IV) fluids, antiemetics and vitamins, thus avoiding admission to hospital. Inpatient management may be required if there is continued vomiting despite oral antiemetics, significant weight loss and ketonuria. The treatment involves IV antiemetics and fluids and replacement of B vitamins.

Initially, antiemetic treatment is with a single agent, but if nausea and vomiting are not controlled, then multiple agents can be used. Safe antiemetics to use in hyperemesis include cyclizine, metoclopramide (beware of extrapyramidal symptoms and oculogyric crisis as side effects) and ondansetron. IV fluid replacement should be with 0.9% saline and supplemental potassium if required. Dextrose infusions should not be used as they can precipitate Wernicke encephalopathy.

If symptoms do not resolve, then a course of corticosteroid therapy can be considered after consultant review. IV hydrocortisone 100 mg twice a day is started and then converted to oral prednisolone on a reducing regime to the lowest dose to control symptoms. Corticosteroid treatment for managing hyperemesis gravidarum should be continued until reaching the gestational age by which hyperemesis typically resolves.

Chapter Summary

- Lower abdominal pain and vaginal bleeding can be presentations of both miscarriage and ectopic pregnancy.
- All women presenting with lower abdominal pain (with or without bleeding) and a positive pregnancy test must be managed as an ectopic pregnancy until proven otherwise.
- Ectopic pregnancy can be a gynaecological emergency and patients may require urgent surgical management.
- Early pregnancy complications can cause distress to patients. Adequate support and information must be provided.

UKMLA Conditions
Hyperemesis

UKMLA Presentations
Acute abdominal pain
Acute and chronic pain management
Ectopic pregnancy
Shock

Antenatal booking and prenatal diagnosis
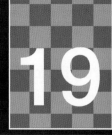

19

The antenatal booking appointment is of utmost importance as it identifies the patient's risk factors. Doing so could tailor care, and further investigations and referrals could be arranged. This visit takes place around the 10th week of pregnancy and is almost universally conducted by trained midwives or doctors. During this visit, it is paramount to:

- Take a thorough history to identify risk factors for the pregnancy
- Educate the patient about key 'do's and dont's' in pregnancy
- Discuss antenatal screening options

ANTENATAL BOOKING HISTORY

It is important to take the history confidentially as sensitive information may be disclosed.

Current pregnancy

An essential step in any booking visit is an accurate estimation of the gestational age. Most commonly, this is calculated using the first day of the patient's last menstrual period and an obstetric wheel/pregnancy calculator. The obstetric wheel/pregnancy calculator will give both the current gestational age and an estimated delivery date.

> **HINTS AND TIPS**
>
> Naegele's rule. If you do not have access to an obstetric wheel/pregnancy calculator, using Naegele's rule is an easy way of estimating the due date. The rule assumes the patient has a 28-day cycle, and the estimated date of delivery (EDD) is calculated by adding 7 to the first day of the last menstrual period (LMP) and deducting 3 from the month of the LMP. Finally, add 1 to the year; for example, if a patient's LMP was 3 May 2023, then the EDD would be 10 February 2024.
>
> However, national screening guidelines advise that all patients are offered an ultrasound scan between 11 and 14 weeks for **the most accurate EDD**, by measuring the fetal crown-rump length (CRL).

> **HINTS AND TIPS**
>
> An ultrasound scan between 11 + 2 and 14 + 0 weeks' gestation will:
> - confirm viability
> - measure the crown-rump length to calculate the estimated date of delivery
> - diagnose multiple pregnancy and check chorionicity
> - examine for major fetal anomalies
> - perform screening for trisomies (trisomy 21 (Down syndrome), 13 and 18)

> **HINTS AND TIPS**
>
> If a patient presents for their dating scan after 14 weeks of gestation, head circumference will be used to calculate the EDD instead of CRL.

The history includes whether or not it is a planned pregnancy and whether any fertility treatment was required to become pregnant. Patients undergoing fertility treatment are at risk of multiple pregnancy and/or may have had complications such as ovarian hyperstimulation syndrome (see Chapter 16).

Obstetric history

The risk assessment includes a thorough enquiry about previous pregnancies and outcomes. This allows interventions in the current pregnancy to reduce the risk of adverse outcomes. For example, commencing patients on aspirin if there is a history of preeclampsia in a previous pregnancy. Obstetric history is usually documented with the letters G (for gravida) and P (for parity) (see Chapter 2).

Medical history

Identification of coexisting medical problems is essential in pregnancy. Early management plans may reduce the risk of adverse fetal and maternal outcomes in some maternal medical conditions. Risk factors for venous thromboembolism should be identified. These will be discussed in detail in the medical disorders and pregnancy section (see Chapter 22).

Drug history and allergies

An enquiry should be made about the medications the patient is taking including over-the-counter supplements. Folic acid should be recommended in the first trimester, and specialist advice may be needed if the patient has been taking any potentially teratogenic medications. Any allergies must be highlighted.

Family history

Family history of hypertension, diabetes, genetic conditions and mental health issues should be screened as part of the risk assessment at the booking visit. For example, a family history of type 2 diabetes in a first-degree relative increases the risk for gestational diabetes mellitus (GDM) in the current pregnancy. Therefore, a glucose tolerance test should be planned for these patients.

The family origin questionnaire (FOQ) also is an integral part of antenatal screening. It aims to identify the population groups at the highest risk of sickle cell, thalassaemia and other haemoglobin variants.

Social history

Consideration should be given to the patient's occupation to minimize any risk they may be exposed to. For example, teachers are at risk of infectious diseases such as chicken pox.

Smokers should be offered a referral to a specialist smoking cessation clinic and educated about the risks to their pregnancy. They will also need to be referred for regular growth scans for the risk of growth restriction that may develop later in pregnancy.

In addition, alcohol abuse and illicit drug use should be identified with referral to the appropriate drug and alcohol service, and education about pregnancy risks should be made a priority. Domestic abuse, sexual abuse or female genital mutilation should be screened sensitively and appropriate follow-up needs to be planned.

HINTS AND TIPS

Women from some minority ethnic backgrounds and living in deprived areas have an increased risk of death. They may need closer monitoring and additional support based on the 2020 MBRRACE-UK reports on maternal and perinatal mortality. Compared with White women (8/100,000), the risk of maternal death during pregnancy and up to 6 weeks after birth is:

- Four times higher in Black women (34/100,000)
- Three times higher in women with mixed ethnic background (25/100,000)
- Two times higher in Asian women (15/100,000; does not include Chinese women)

At a booking visit, the examination will include the patient's blood pressure and recording their height and weight to calculate body mass index (BMI). In addition, carbon monoxide levels will be recorded to find out if the patient is exposed to harmful doses of second-hand smoke so that life style changes could be recommended to reduce the potential harm to placental function from smoking. A cardiovascular examination should be considered if the woman has immigrated to the UK; this excludes conditions such as rheumatic heart disease that are more common in some developing countries and may have a serious impact on health in pregnancy.

BOOKING INVESTIGATIONS

A nationally agreed set of investigations should be offered to patients to allow screening for certain conditions to minimize their risk to the mother and foetus if present. These are:

- Full blood count
- Haemoglobin electrophoresis
- Blood group and antibody screen
- Infections (syphilis, hepatitis B and human immunodeficiency virus (HIV))
- Urine dip/culture

Full blood count

A full blood count is an important investigation as it allows for the detection of anaemia and platelet disorders. There is a lower normal range for haemoglobin in pregnancy due to the normal physiological changes that occur with an increased circulatory volume (see Chapter 22).

Haemoglobin electrophoresis

Haemoglobinopathies are disorders of haemoglobin structure and are more common in certain ethnic groups. Thalassaemia and sickle cell disease are screened for to allow the identification of foetuses at risk of having the condition. Both conditions are autosomal recessive, so for the individual to be affected, they need to have two defective copies of the gene. Patients can be asymptomatic carriers of the condition without knowing. During pregnancy, if the mother is found to be a carrier, her partner should also be screened.

Both conditions can render the patient anaemic, and supplementation with iron and folate may be required if these levels are proven to be low. It is important not to iron overload these patients.

Blood group and antibody screen

Certain antibodies can cause haemolytic disease of the foetus and newborn. Therefore, blood is screened at booking and again at 28 weeks to ensure antibodies have not developed. Patients with these particular antibodies will need regular blood tests to quantify the levels and may require close surveillance in a fetal medicine unit depending on the levels. This is to monitor fetal anaemia caused by haemolysis.

The most common antibodies causing haemolytic disease of the foetus and newborn are the rhesus (Rh) antibodies. Those who are rhesus negative will be offered anti-D prophylaxis.

HINTS AND TIPS

RHESUS BLOOD GROUP SYSTEM AND ANTI-D

In pregnancy, if an Rh-negative patient has a partner who is Rh-positive, their offspring may be Rh-positive. During the pregnancy, fetal blood may enter maternal circulation and cause antibodies to develop to the D antigen. Suppose in a subsequent pregnancy the foetus is Rh-negative, these antibodies may cross the placenta and attack fetal red cells, causing anaemia and subsequent fetal hydrops with or without stillbirth.

Recently, patients who are found to be Rh-negative at booking can be offered noninvasive prenatal testing – fetal DNA can be isolated from a maternal blood sample, and therefore the fetal rhesus status can be determined. If the foetus is Rh-negative, no treatment is needed. However, if the foetus is Rh-positive, the patient should be offered anti-D immunoglobulin at 28 weeks.

HINTS AND TIPS

Indications for anti-D if the foetus is Rh-positive:
- Prophylaxis at 28 weeks.
- Postnatally.
- If a potentially sensitizing event has occurred, that is, any event that may cause the passage of fetal cells into the maternal circulation, such as abdominal trauma, bleeding in pregnancy after 12 weeks and invasive procedures.

SCREENING FOR INFECTIONS

This involves a blood test for syphilis, hepatitis B and HIV. Women are also screened for urinary tract infections during pregnancy.

Syphilis (*Treponema pallidum*)

Syphilis is a sexually transmitted infection that can be easily treated. Fetal infection can lead to nonimmune hydrops and stillbirth. The risk of transmission to the foetus can be dramatically reduced by treating the mother. Patients identified with syphilis should be referred to a genitourinary medicine clinic for:

- Treatment with benzylpenicillin injections
- Screening of other sexually transmitted infections
- Contact tracing, including the partner

Hepatitis

Hepatitis B is a viral infection transmitted:

- sexually
- vertically (mother to foetus)
- via blood

The patient should be referred to a hepatologist if she has not been seen previously. Her liver function tests should be monitored during pregnancy and postnatally due to the chronic nature of the infection. Again, partner testing is recommended as well as testing any existing children she may have. They can be offered vaccination if found to be negative.

Postnatal vaccination of the foetus has been shown to reduce the risk of transmission. Patients with the hepatitis E antigen (HBeAg) carry the highest risk of transmitting the infection to the foetus.

Hepatitis C is also a viral illness that is transmitted sexually, vertically (mother to foetus) or via blood. Current guidelines, however, **do not recommend routine screening**.

Human immunodeficiency virus

HIV is a blood-borne virus transmitted sexually, vertically and by blood. Although incurable, modern advances in management have increased the life expectancy of affected individuals and significantly reduced the vertical transmission rate (see Chapter 22).

Screening for HIV allows patients to commence treatment if required and decide the mode of delivery depending on antigen levels. All cases should be managed by a multidisciplinary team involving obstetricians, HIV specialists and specialist midwives.

HINTS AND TIPS

Since April 2016, antenatal screening for rubella **is no longer advised** by the National Screening Committee, because rubella infection in the UK is rare and MMR (measles, mumps and rubella) vaccine uptake is high. Women born outside of the UK are advised to discuss the MMR vaccine with their general practitioner before planning a pregnancy so that they can receive the live vaccine if they are nonimmune.

Urinary tract infections

Urinary tract infections may be symptomatic or asymptomatic. In untreated asymptomatic cases, there is a significant risk of pyelonephritis and preterm birth. Current guidelines recommend screening for asymptomatic bacteriuria in all pregnant women using a urine dipstick at every midwife and consultant appointment. Symptomatic patients should start the treatment and choice of antibiotic should be reviewed once the urine culture result is available.

ANTENATAL EDUCATION

Pregnancy can be a daunting time for some patients, especially for those embarking on their first pregnancy or those very young. Therefore, education during the booking visit is a vital step, and providing clear (often written) information can be an invaluable tool to put patients at ease. Increasingly, online information is available through phone apps, for example.

Topics that should be covered include:

- Common symptoms in pregnancy (see Box 19.1).
- Maternity benefits.
- Working during pregnancy.
- Dietary information – advise a mixed diet with fruit, vegetables, fibre, lean meat, fish, lentils, starchy foods (bread/pasta, etc.) and dairy; foods to avoid and why are shown in Table 19.1.
- Smoking – discussion about smoking cessation is essential, plus referral to specialist services if accepted.
- Alcohol consumption –avoided entirely in the first trimester and throughout pregnancy. Those who choose to drink should be advised to drink no more than 1 to 2 units a week and to avoid binge drinking.
- Medications, vitamins and supplements – important to emphasize that most medications have insufficient data to

BOX 19.1 COMMON SYMPTOMS IN PREGNANCY

Mild symptoms usually resolve by 16 to 20 weeks and can be managed by eating little and often and with oral antiemetics.
If excessive and causing dehydration, it is called 'hyperemesis gravidarum' (see below).

HEARTBURN
Avoid large meals and lying supine soon after food.
Reduce caffeine and foods with high fat content.
Antacid preparations.

CONSTIPATION
Increase fibre in diet, avoid dehydration.

HAEMORRHOIDS
Haemorrhoid creams, avoidance of constipation.

VARICOSE VEINS
Compression stockings can be helpful.
Elevation of legs.
Avoid prolonged periods of standing.

BACKACHE
Advice on posture, massage and water exercising can help.

SYMPHYSIS PUBIS DYSFUNCTION
Physiotherapy referral for advice and consideration of pelvic support devices.

Table 19.1 Dietary precautions in pregnancy

Food product	Potential risks
Soft cheeses, unpasteurized milk/cheese, raw fish (sushi)	Infection with *Listeria,* which can lead to miscarriage and stillbirth
Unwashed salad, fruit, vegetables, raw meats	Toxoplasmosis infection, which can lead to miscarriage, stillbirth or disability
Shellfish (oysters), raw eggs	Food poisoning (vibrio, *Salmonella* bacteria)
Caffeine	Limit intake to 300 mg per day

be deemed 100% safe in pregnancy. Therefore, their use should be limited to occasions when they are necessary. Complementary medicines, again have little or no safety data.

- Folic acid (400 mcg od or 5 mg od in higher risk groups) – during the first 12 weeks to reduce the risk of neural tube defects.
- Driving – appropriate positioning of the seatbelt, i.e., wearing it above and below the bump NOT over.
- Flying – flights more than 4 hours are independently associated with an increased risk of venous thromboembolism. Therefore, unless travel is essential, it may be advisable to avoid it, especially when there are other risk factors such as raised BMI. Compression stockings have been shown to reduce this risk.
- Exercise – moderate exercise is safe in pregnancy, although patients should be informed of the risks with contact sports and other forms of vigorous exercise.
- Pets – there is a risk of toxoplasmosis from cat faeces and contaminated soil. Therefore avoidance of handling cat litter and wearing gloves when gardening, as well as handwashing, should be advised.

ONGOING ANTENATAL CARE AND RISK ASSESSMENT

Depending upon the classification of risk, ongoing antenatal care in pregnancy may be delivered by general practitioners, midwives, obstetricians or a combination of all three. Generally, low-risk patients in their first pregnancy will have around 10 visits spread throughout their pregnancy, and those who have had a baby before and are low-risk will have 7 visits.

Patients should be screened at each visit for any new risk factors. These could be related to various aspects of care such as medical, surgical, mental health, obstetric (maternal and/or fetal) and social circumstances. In patients with issues that have been identified, the care schedule will need to be modified, and appropriate referrals will need to be arranged according to their individual needs.

Venous thromboembolism

Risk factors for venous thromboembolism should be assessed at the booking appointment and after any hospital admission or significant health event during pregnancy. Consultant obstetrician referral should be done if risk factors are present, such as history of a previous deep vein thrombosis, thrombophilia and medical comorbidities increasing the risk of thrombosis (see Chapter 22).

Gestational diabetes

At booking appointment, a woman's risk factors for GDM should be assessed. An oral glucose tolerance test should be booked according to NICE guidelines on diabetes in pregnancy if one of the following risk factors is present:

- BMI above 30 kg/m^2.
- Previous macrosomic baby weighing 4.5 kg or more.
- Previous GDM.
- Family history of diabetes (first-degree relative with diabetes).
- An ethnicity with a high prevalence of diabetes (including people of African, black Caribbean, South Asian, Middle Eastern and Chinese family origin).

Preeclampsia and hypertension in pregnancy

At the booking appointment and again in the second trimester, risk factors for preeclampsia are assessed such as hypertensive disorder in previous pregnancy, chronic maternal renal disease and diabetes (see Chapter 21). Those at risk need to be advised to take low-dose aspirin (75–150 mg). In addition, a woman's blood pressure must be checked and recorded at every routine face-to-face antenatal appointment using a validated device.

Monitoring fetal growth and well-being

A risk assessment for fetal growth restriction at the booking appointment, and again in the second trimester is offered. Appropriate growth scans are requested depending on the risk factors. Patients with previous growth restriction, hypertension, diabetes need to have growth scans (see Chapter 23 for other risk factors). For patients not having regular growth scans, symphysis fundal height measurement at each antenatal appointment is offered after 24 + 0 weeks of gestation.

SCREENING FOR CHROMOSOMAL ABNORMALITIES

National Screening Committee guidelines recommend offering all patients a screening test for Down syndrome (trisomy 21), Edward syndrome (trisomy 18) and Patau syndrome (trisomy 13). These three conditions increase in incidence with increasing maternal age. Informed consent must be obtained before testing, including the options for further testing and continuing care in pregnancy if the result is high risk.

COMMUNICATION

Patients must understand the difference between a screening test and a diagnostic test. The combined, quadruple and noninvasive prenatal tests are all screening tests. Screening tests help determine how likely it is that foetus has one of the trisomies. They are not diagnostic tests, like chorionic villus sampling (CVS) and amniocentesis, which give a definite result as to whether the baby is affected or not. Patients should also be aware that a positive diagnostic test result for a trisomy could decide whether a patient wants to continue or end the pregnancy.

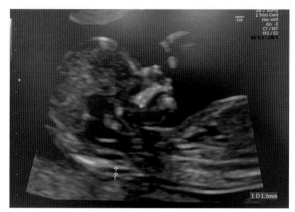

Fig. 19.1 Nuchal translucency measurement.

Combined screening test

The combined screening test includes a blood test with an ultrasound scan. This is performed between 11 and 14 + 0 weeks of gestation, and nuchal translucency (NT) (Fig. 19.1) is measured during the ultrasound scan. The blood test involves measuring maternal serum levels of βHCG and pregnancy-associated plasma protein A.

NT is an ultrasound observation which is the measurement of the fluid behind the foetus' neck. This appears as a black space on ultrasound. The width of this space is measured – on average, foetuses affected with Down syndrome have an increased NT. Increased NT could be a normal variant. However, it could be related to trisomies and cardiac abnormalities as well.

If the result shows that the chance of having a baby with trisomy 21, 13 or 18 is lower than 1 in 150, this is a lower-chance result. If the risk is between 1 in 2 and 1 in 150 – this is called a higher chance result. Patients with higher chance results will be offered further prenatal testing.

Triple or quadruple test

For those patients who book late or have missed the cut-off for combined screening, a second-trimester screening in the form of the triple or quadruple test can be offered. These are also blood tests for placental hormones, after which a risk score is generated. The triple test consists of α-fetoprotein, oestriol and βHCG. The quadruple test is the same with the addition of inhibin-A.

Noninvasive prenatal testing

Also known as cfDNA (cell-free DNA) screening, it is a blood test that looks for DNA in maternal blood. Noninvasive prenatal testing (NIPT) is more accurate than the combined and triple/quadruple tests, especially for trisomy 21; its sensitivity is more than

99%. However, it is a screening test and not 100% accurate. This is because the cfDNA is derived from the placenta, not the baby itself.

Most patients with a higher chance of the first-line screening test for chromosomal abnormalities – combined or quadruple test – can have NIPT as a second-line test. If the NIPT result is a lower chance no further prenatal testing is recommended. Patients who have a higher chance result from NIPT are offered a diagnostic test (chorionic villous sampling (CVS) or amniocentesis).

NIPT has been added to the existing NHS screening pathway for screening of trisomies as part of an evaluative rollout. The test will be offered in the NHS if:

- The first-line screening test performed in the NHS and shows a higher chance result (some of the patients in this group may need a diagnostic test, each case should be reviewed individually).
- Singleton and twin pregnancies.
- Until 21 weeks plus 6 days of gestation.

FETAL ANOMALY SCREENING PROGRAMME (FASP)

According to National Screening Committee guidelines, all pregnant women in England should be offered an ultrasound scan between 18+0 and 20+6 weeks to diagnose fetal defects (see further reading for the abnormalities screened). If abnormalities are detected, it may be appropriate to offer invasive testing and prenatal diagnosis with referral to a fetal medicine centre (e.g., if a cardiac anomaly is seen, amniocentesis is offered for chromosomal abnormalities). In some situations, the woman will need follow-up scans and discussion with the neonatal team for delivery planning and a postnatal plan for the baby (e.g., gastrointestinal abnormalities such as gastroschisis involve scanning for fetal growth and planning delivery in a unit with neonatal surgery facilities).

PRENATAL DIAGNOSIS

The introduction of screening programmes and increased awareness of certain genetic conditions have led to the option of prenatal diagnosis becoming a common diagnostic tool. It is estimated that around 5% of pregnant patients are offered invasive prenatal diagnostic tests (30,000 patients in the UK).

Screening tests are NOT diagnostic and only offer a risk score. In individuals who are deemed high risk, prenatal diagnosis provides a way of establishing a diagnosis as to whether the foetus does indeed have the condition suspected by the screening. In addition, parents who are carriers for certain conditions (e.g., sickle cell disease) may wish to know whether or not their child is affected by the condition. Undergoing prenatal diagnosis allows the couple to be prepared for the child's needs if they choose to continue with the pregnancy or, indeed opt for a termination of pregnancy. Furthermore, it allows medical teams to modify antenatal care and prepare for the baby's delivery and needs once born.

Ultrasound

As mentioned above, ultrasound is used at several stages in pregnancy. The early scan at 11 to 14 weeks allows for the measurement of NT, and later, the anomaly ultrasound scan (18–20 weeks) provides for a more detailed assessment of any structural anomaly. Although often not realized by patients, this is a form of prenatal diagnosis. Some anomalies will prompt further diagnostic interventions such as amniocentesis or fetal blood sampling (FBS).

Chorionic villous sampling and amniocentesis

Obtaining sample

CVS is a technique used to obtain a sample of chorionic villi from the fetal placenta. It can be carried out via the transabdominal route or, less commonly, the transcervical route under continuous ultrasound guidance (Fig. 19.2).

Amniocentesis aims to obtain a sample of amniotic fluid from which fetal cells can be harvested. Under ultrasound guidance, a needle is passed through the anterior abdominal wall into the amniotic cavity. Amniotic fluid is then aspirated, and the needle is withdrawn (Fig. 19.3).

Testing the sample

The fetal cells are then cultured and undergo testing to establish the fetal karyotype (the number and visual appearance of the chromosomes in the cell). Results come back in 2 to 3 days using the polymerase chain reaction technique and up to 2 weeks from a culture. The amniotic fluid sample could also

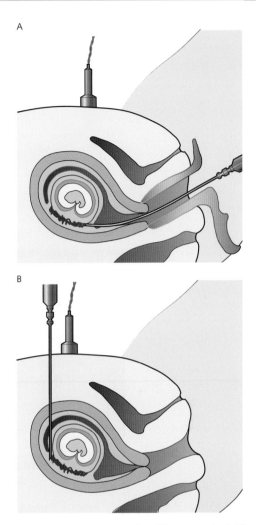

Fig. 19.2 Chorionic villous sampling: (A) transcervical; (B) transabdominal.

help diagnose suspected fetal infection where samples tested for infection such as cytomegalovirus.

Timing of the procedure

CVS is usually performed between 11 weeks and 13 weeks + 6 days and should not be performed before 10 weeks due to concerns about increased loss rates and limb abnormalities.

Amniocentesis is carried out after 15 weeks of pregnancy; procedures done before this gestation are associated with a higher risk of fetal loss and limb abnormalities.

Risks

As with any medical procedure, there are associated risks; therefore before undergoing the procedure, it is essential that

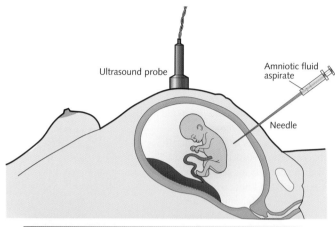

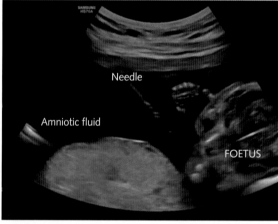

Fig. 19.3 Amniocentesis.

patients understand the risks and the benefits. Women should be informed that the additional risk of miscarriage following amniocentesis or CVS performed by an appropriately trained operator is likely below 0.5%. In twin pregnancies, this risk is around 1%.

HINTS AND TIPS

As CVS is performed earlier than amniocentesis, the patient has the choice of an earlier termination if an abnormal result is confirmed, which patients may find more acceptable. However, the risk of placental mosaicism can yield an inconclusive result requiring further testing.

HINTS AND TIPS

- Amniocentesis and chorionic villus sampling can sensitise rhesus-negative mothers, hence, anti-D immunoglobulin is advised.
- Before any invasive test, review blood-borne virus screenings, viral loads, and antigen tests to discuss the specific risk of viral transmission.

Fetal blood sampling

FBS in prenatal diagnosis involves the aspiration of fetal blood using a transabdominal approach under ultrasound guidance. It is important to recognize that this is very different from the FBS performed in labour when a blood sample is obtained from the fetal scalp. The technique can be used to detect fetal anaemia or fetal thrombocytopoenia. However, the use of middle cerebral artery (MCA) Doppler assessment has largely replaced FBS for diagnosing anaemia. MCA Doppler assesses blood flow dynamics– if the flow is faster than usual, this could be because the baby is anaemic. FBS also allows the transfusion of blood or platelets if required. However, the need for the procedure must be balanced against a miscarriage risk of 1% to 2% in counselling a patient.

● Chapter Summary

- The booking visit allows identification of the risk factors in the pregnancy and the planning of optimal management strategies.
- Women will be offered the following screening programmes in NHS at the booking visit: infectious diseases (HIV, syphilis and hepatitis B), sickle cell and thalassaemia and fetal anomaly.
- Antenatal screening tests – combined test, triple or quadruple test or noninvasive prenatal testing – are offered to women to identify those at high risk of having a baby with a chromosomal abnormality.
- Women who have a higher chance result from a screening test are offered diagnostic testing with chorionic villus sampling or amniocentesis.
- At booking visits, women are risk assessed for venous thromboembolism (VTE), gestational diabetes mellitus (GDM), preeclampsia, hypertensive disorders and growth restriction. Appropriate follow-up is then arranged depending on the severity of the risk factors.
- High-risk pregnancies are managed in a consultant-led clinic or have shared care with midwives and obstetricians.

MLA Conditions
Urinary tract infection

MLA Presentations
Abnormal urinalysis
Normal pregnancy and antenatal care
Pregnancy risk assessment

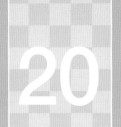

Antepartum haemorrhage | 20

DEFINITION

Antepartum haemorrhage (APH) is defined as any bleeding from the genital tract that occurs after 24 + 0 weeks' gestation and before the birth of the infant.

HINTS AND TIPS

Antepartum haemorrhage (APH) is an important cause of maternal and perinatal morbidity and mortality. Up to 20% of preterm infants are born in association with APH.

INCIDENCE

The incidence of APH is 3% to 5%.

AETIOLOGY

A summary is shown in Table 20.1. Placenta praevia combined with placental abruption accounts for about 50% of the causes of an APH. The source of the bleeding is the mother in both of these conditions. (i.e., it is not fetal blood).

RED FLAGS

With any bleeding in pregnancy, mothers should be resuscitated first before assessing the foetus. Do not forget **ABC** – **A**ssess the patient's airway, **B**reathing and **C**irculation.

HISTORY

When taking a history, it is important to elicit certain points including:

- Amount of bleeding
- Association with abdominal pain and/or contractions
- Association with mucoid discharge

- Presence of trigger events (sexual intercourse, trauma to abdomen)

The presence or absence of constant abdominal pain is particularly important to differentiate between placenta praevia and placental abruption. With the latter, there may also be painful uterine contractions as the myometrium is infiltrated with blood that makes the uterus irritable.

If patients present with bloody mucoid vaginal loss on a single occasion, this may be the 'show' or cervical mucus plug coming away, which is associated with the onset of labour. There may be an obvious trigger event, for example, recent sexual intercourse can cause bleeding from a cervical ectropion or severe bleeding following a car accident would highly suggest a placental abruption.

COMMON PITFALLS

Do not forget to ask about the patient's smear history: when was the last smear? Was the result normal? Although rare, cervical disease can present for the first time in pregnancy.

HINTS AND TIPS

The presence of abdominal pain typically distinguishes placental abruption from placenta praevia.

EXAMINATION

The aim is to assess maternal and fetal well-being. This includes the following:

Maternal well-being:
- Pulse/blood pressure/respiratory rate
- Pallor
- Abdominal palpation for uterine tenderness/contractions
- Speculum examination for cervical abnormalities
- Digital examination in the presence of contractions to assess cervical change, but only if placenta praevia has been excluded

171

Table 20.1 Aetiology of antepartum haemorrhage

Source of haemorrhage	Type of haemorrhage
Uterine source	Placenta praevia Placental abruption Vasa praevia Circumvallate placenta
Lower genital tract source	Cervical ectropion Cervical polyp Cervical carcinoma Cervicitis Vaginitis Vulval varicosities
Unknown origin (approximately 50%)	

Fetal well-being:
- Abdominal palpation for lie/presentation/engagement
- Auscultation of fetal heart to determine viability
- Cardiotocograph (CTG) if >26 + 0 weeks' gestation to confirm fetal well-being

INVESTIGATIONS

Box 20.1 lists the investigations appropriate for the patient with an APH.

Blood tests

Blood should be cross-matched if the bleeding is significant and ongoing (e.g., major placenta praevia). Blood group must be checked – anti-D immunoglobulin should be given if the patient is rhesus negative, to prevent haemolytic disease of the foetus or newborn in a future pregnancy (see Chapter 19). A Kleihauer test examines the maternal blood film for the presence of fetal blood cells, suggesting fetomaternal haemorrhage. This can be seen with placental abruption.

If the patient also presents with hypertension, then liver and renal function tests can be performed and if they are deranged, preeclampsia should be considered as a cause (see Chapter 21). A Clotting profile also should be performed as patients with severe bleeding could have disseminated intravascular coagulation.

Fetal monitoring

A CTG should be done to confirm fetal well-being after 26 + 0 weeks' gestation. It may also show uterine irritability or established contractions.

BOX 20.1 INVESTIGATIONS FOR A PATIENT WITH AN ANTEPARTUM HAEMORRHAGE

- Full blood count
- Group and save/cross-match
- Coagulation profile
- Kleihauer test
- Renal function tests
- Liver function tests
- Cardiotocograph
- Ultrasound scan

Ultrasound scan

The placental site is checked at the routine 20-week anomaly scan. If it is low lying, a diagnosis of placenta praevia is suspected and a repeat scan should be arranged around 32 weeks.

A normal ultrasound scan does not exclude the diagnosis of the abruption as small clots may not be seen on the scan. Therefore, ultrasound is not essential when diagnosing placental abruption.

HINTS AND TIPS

- Risk assessment is essential at each visit. Women who present with recurrent unexplained antepartum haemorrhage (APH) should be classified as high risk and transferred to consultant-led care. Serial ultrasound assessment for fetal growth should be performed as these pregnancies are at risk of intrauterine growth restriction.
- Health professionals should be aware that domestic violence in pregnancy may result in APH. Women with repeated presentations that may include APH should be asked about this.

PLACENTA PRAEVIA

Definition

The placenta is wholly or partially attached to the lower uterine segment. The degree of attachment is classified as either minor, where the leading edge of the placenta is in the lower uterine segment but not covering the os, or major, where the placenta lies over the internal os (Fig. 20.1).

Placenta praevia

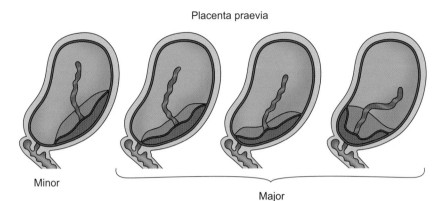

Fig. 20.1 Placenta praevia

Minor

Major

Incidence

Placenta praevia occurs in 1 in 200 pregnancies; this figure has altered with routine use of ultrasound scanning. The incidence is increased with the following risk factors:

- Previous caesarean section including previous placenta praevia
- Advanced maternal age
- Multiparity
- Multiple pregnancy
- Presence of a succenturiate placental lobe
- Smoking

It is associated with a maternal mortality rate of about 0.03% in the developed world. However, both maternal and fetal morbidity are substantially higher in developing countries due to complications such as haemorrhage and prematurity.

Particularly with increasing numbers of caesarean sections, there is an increased incidence of placenta accreta. This is a condition found in up to 15% of those with placenta praevia, in which the placenta is morbidly adherent to the uterine decidua and may even penetrate through the myometrium to invade surrounding organs. Magnetic resonance imaging (MRI) scan is thought to be helpful to aid diagnosis.

> **HINTS AND TIPS**
>
> Placenta praevia usually presents as painless vaginal bleeding.

History

Bleeding from a placenta praevia is usually unprovoked and occurs in the third trimester, in the absence of labour.

Examination

General observations including maternal pulse and blood pressure must be performed to ensure that mother is hemodynamically stable. On abdominal palpation, the uterus is soft and nontender. The low-lying placenta may displace the presenting part from the pelvis so that a cephalic presentation is not engaged, or there is a malpresentation.

With a minor degree of bleeding, a speculum can be passed to exclude a lower genital tract cause for the APH. A digital examination should be avoided because it may provoke massive bleeding.

> **RED FLAGS**
>
> Do not perform a digital examination to assess cervical dilatation unless you have excluded placenta praevia as this could cause major bleeding.

Diagnosis

Placenta praevia was originally defined as a placenta developing within the lower uterine segment and graded according to the relationship between the lower placental edge and the internal os of the uterine cervix by transabdominal scan (TAS). Classified as minor if the lower edge is within the lower segment but not reaching the internal os and major when the lower reaches/covers the internal os.

The use of transvaginal scanning (TVS) has allowed more precise evaluation of the distance between the placental edge and the internal os. The American Institute of Ultrasound in Medicine (AIUM) has recommended the term 'placenta praevia' be used when the placenta lies directly over the internal os. For pregnancies greater than 16 weeks of gestation, the placenta should be reported as 'low lying' when the placental edge is less than 20 mm from the internal os, and as normal when the placental edge is 20 mm or more from the internal os on TAS or TVS.

If a low-lying placenta is suspected, a follow-up scan in the third trimester is usually performed to make the diagnosis of placenta praevia. The diagnosis of placenta praevia should be confirmed by transabdominal and transvaginal ultrasound scans. Most of the time placenta moves up away from the cervical os, as the lower segment begins to form and the upper segment enlarges upwards.

HINTS AND TIPS

For the diagnosis of placenta praevia or a low-lying placenta, TVS is superior to transabdominal and transperineal approaches, and is safe.

Investigations

These are outlined in Box 20.1. Blood should be sent for haemoglobin, and group and save. Anti-D is indicated if the patient is rhesus negative. If the bleeding is heavy, cross-matching blood for transfusion is indicated and a baseline clotting screen is performed. Renal function tests are important if the urine output is poor secondary to hypovolaemia. A CTG should be performed to check fetal well-being. An ultrasound scan should be performed if the placental location is unknown. An MRI scan may be indicated if there is a high index of suspicion about placenta accreta.

Management

Asymptomatic women with a persistent low-lying placenta or placenta praevia at 32 weeks of gestation should have an additional TVS at around 36 weeks of gestation to confirm the diagnosis and have a discussion about mode of delivery.

If patients present with bleeding, management depends on the severity of the bleeding and gestation of the foetus. Immediate delivery by caesarean section may be appropriate if there is maternal or fetal compromise whereas the majority of preterm pregnancies with light bleeding are managed expectantly.

If the placenta remains at or over the cervical os, massive bleeding is likely to occur if the patient goes into labour and the cervix starts to dilate. Therefore, inpatient management is appropriate towards the end of the third trimester with immediate recourse to caesarean section if necessary. Steroids to improve fetal lung maturity should be considered following liaison with the paediatricians, in case preterm delivery is needed. Caesarean section is usually advised if the placenta is

encroaching within 2 cm of the internal cervical os. A consultant obstetrician and consultant anaesthetist should be present at delivery.

HINTS AND TIPS

Placenta praevia carries a higher risk of massive obstetric haemorrhage and hysterectomy. Therefore, delivery should be arranged in a unit with on-site blood transfusion services and access to critical care

Complications

Placenta praevia is associated with an increased risk of postpartum haemorrhage (PPH; see Chapter 31) regardless of the mode of delivery. The lower uterine segment where the placenta is sited is less efficient at retraction following delivery of the placenta compared to the upper segment. Thus occlusion of the venous sinuses is less effective, resulting in heavier blood loss. This may be further complicated by the presence of placenta accreta. Therefore, preparations should be in place for potential PPH. This includes cross-matching blood and both consultant obstetrician and anaesthetist input. The patient should be given adequate counselling regarding the possible need for medical and surgical measures to control bleeding including hysterectomy.

Future pregnancy

Placenta praevia has a recurrence rate of 4% to 8% with an increased risk of placenta accreta in each pregnancy.

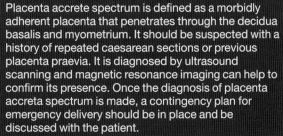

RED FLAGS

Placenta accrete spectrum is defined as a morbidly adherent placenta that penetrates through the decidua basalis and myometrium. It should be suspected with a history of repeated caesarean sections or previous placenta praevia. It is diagnosed by ultrasound scanning and magnetic resonance imaging can help to confirm its presence. Once the diagnosis of placenta accreta spectrum is made, a contingency plan for emergency delivery should be in place and be discussed with the patient.

Delivery for women with placenta accreta spectrum should be in a specialist centre with logistic support for immediate access to blood products, and adult and neonatal intensive care unit by a multidisciplinary team with expertise in complex pelvic surgery.

PLACENTAL ABRUPTION

Definition

Placental abruption is defined as the separation of the normally located placenta from the inner wall of the uterus before birth. The placental attachment to the uterus is disrupted by haemorrhage as blood dissects under the placenta, possibly extending into the amniotic sac or the uterine muscle. Abruption could be:

- Overt or concealed: As maternal blood escapes from the placental sinuses, it tracks down between the membranes and the uterus and escapes via the cervix; this is known as a 'revealed haemorrhage'. Sometimes, the blood remains sealed within the uterine cavity such that the degree of shock is out of proportion to the vaginal loss; this is known as a 'concealed haemorrhage' (Fig. 20.2).
- Partial or total: Abruption may be partial, affecting only part of the placenta, or total, involving the entire placenta.

Incidence

Placental abruption occurs in about 1% of pregnancies in the UK. In the majority of cases, the cause is unknown, but it is associated with:

- previous abruption
- advanced maternal age
- multiparity
- maternal hypertension or preeclampsia
- abdominal trauma (e.g., assault, road traffic accident)
- cigarette smoking
- cocaine use
- lower socioeconomic group
- external cephalic version

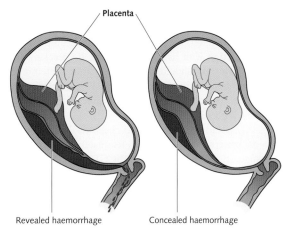

Placenta

Revealed haemorrhage · Concealed haemorrhage

Fig. 20.2 Types of placental abruption.

> **HINTS AND TIPS**
>
> Preeclampsia is associated with placental abruption, so the patient should be asked if she has experienced symptoms including headache, blurred vision, nausea, epigastric pain and oedema. Patients should have their blood pressure measured and urinalysis performed to exclude proteinuria.

> **HINTS AND TIPS**
>
> Placental abruption usually presents with vaginal bleeding associated with abdominal pain.

Examination

The general maternal condition, including pulse and blood pressure, should be assessed. On abdominal palpation, the uterus is typically tender. As bleeding extends into the uterine muscle, a contraction can occur, making the uterus feel hard. Fetal parts are therefore difficult to palpate. If the placental site is known (i.e., if placenta praevia has been excluded) a digital examination is appropriate in the presence of uterine contractions to diagnose the onset of labour.

Maternal hypertension and proteinuria must be checked due to the association between abruption and preeclampsia (see Chapter 21).

History

The patient can present at any stage of pregnancy with a history of bleeding and constant abdominal pain, which is usually unprovoked. There may be associated uterine contractions. Risk factors such as smoking or cocaine use should be checked.

Investigations

These are outlined in Box 20.1. Blood should be sent for haemoglobin, and group and save. Anti-D is indicated if the patient is rhesus negative. If the bleeding is heavy or if the patient is shocked, cross-matching units of blood for transfusion is indicated and a baseline clotting screen is performed. A Kleihauer test should be requested to diagnose fetomaternal haemorrhage, which occurs in an abruption.

Renal function tests are necessary if the urine output is poor or in conjunction with liver function tests if preeclampsia is suspected. Urinalysis should be done to exclude proteinuria; if present, a protein-to-creatinine ratio or a 24-hour urine protein level may be helpful to determine the degree of renal involvement (see Chapter 21).

A CTG should be performed to check fetal well-being. A sinusoidal pattern can be seen with fetomaternal haemorrhage and is suggestive of fetal anaemia. The CTG will also monitor uterine activity, either contractions or a uterus that might simply be irritable with irregular activity.

Diagnosis

An abruption is usually diagnosed on clinical grounds. Small retroplacental clots may not be seen on an ultrasound scan, therefore a normal scan does not exclude the diagnosis. A large retroplacental clot that can be seen on scan is likely to be obvious clinically, with abdominal pain and bleeding.

Management

As for placenta praevia, management of a placental abruption must start with assessment of the severity of the symptoms and prompt resuscitation. Immediate delivery of the foetus may be necessary as a life-saving procedure for the mother, regardless of gestation.

In a situation where the patient is clinically well and the foetus is not compromised, expectant management might allow the symptoms to resolve. Again, steroids should be considered to aid fetal lung maturity if preterm delivery is required.

Complications

Accurate assessment of blood loss is necessary to assess the risks of developing disseminated intravascular coagulation and renal failure. PPH occurs in 25% of cases, which rarely leads to Sheehan syndrome (pituitary necrosis secondary to hypovolaemic shock – see Chapter 31).

Future pregnancy

Women who have had a previous placental abruption are at increased risk in their next pregnancy. The risk of recurrence is about 8%. Low-dose aspirin (75–150 mg) should be considered to reduce the risk in the next pregnancy, especially if the placental abruption is associated with preeclampsia.

VASA PRAEVIA

This is a rare cause of APH, 1 in 2000 to 6000 pregnancies. There is a velamentous insertion of the cord and the vessels lie on the membranes that cover the internal cervical os, in front of the presenting part. When the membranes rupture, either spontaneously or iatrogenically, the vessels can be torn and vaginal bleeding occurs. Unlike placenta praevia and placental abruption, this blood is fetal blood and the foetus must be delivered urgently before it exsanguinates.

If the diagnosis is unclear, a Kleihauer test can be performed on the vaginal blood loss to test for the presence of fetal red blood cells. However, this may delay delivery inappropriately and should only be considered if the CTG is normal.

HINTS AND TIPS

Placenta should be examined histologically to confirm the diagnosis of vasa praevia, especially when stillbirth has occurred or where there has been acute fetal compromise during delivery with APH.

CIRCUMVALLATE PLACENTA

This type of placenta develops secondary to the outward proliferation of the chorionic villi into the decidua, beneath the ring of attachment of the amnion and chorion. This does not interfere with placental function, but it is associated with antepartum and intrapartum haemorrhage.

UNEXPLAINED ANTEPARTUM HAEMORRHAGE

In up to 50% of cases of APH, no specific cause is found. Overall, perinatal mortality with any type of APH is double that of a normal pregnancy, suggesting that placental function might be compromised. Therefore, with recurrent APH, it is appropriate to perform serial ultrasound scans to monitor fetal growth and to consider delivery at term, by inducing labour.

Chapter Summary

- There are many causes of antepartum haemorrhage, and by taking a good history and performing an examination a diagnosis can be made.
- Commonest causes of antepartum haemorrhage are placenta praevia and placental abruption.
- First resuscitate pregnant women present with bleeding – use an airway, breathing, circulation (ABC) approach when assessing.
- Placenta praevia usually presents with painless vaginal bleeding.
- Placental abruption usually presents with abdominal pain with or without bleeding.

UKMLA Conditions
Placenta praevia
Placental abruption
Vasa praevia

UKMLA Presentations
Bleeding antepartum

Hypertension in pregnancy 21

INTRODUCTION

High blood pressure is the most common medical problem that occurs during pregnancy, noted in 10% to 15% of all pregnancies with preeclampsia complicating 3% to 5%. Accurate diagnosis with prompt treatment is essential to ensure a good outcome for both mother and foetus as hypertensive disorders are a leading cause of fetal and maternal morbidity. Maternal mortality from hypertensive disorders is reducing in the UK, with fewer than one death for every million women giving birth (see Chapter 32). On the other hand, 1 in 20 (5%) of stillbirths are associated with preeclampsia (see Chapter 30; Box 21.1).

HINTS AND TIPS

To reduce the risk of preeclampsia:

Advise pregnant women with one high risk factor or more than one moderate risk factor to take aspirin 75 to 150 mg aspirin once a day. 150 mg is the recommended dose, however, if patients cannot tolerate it due to side effects, a 75 mg daily dose is considered. Aspirin should be commenced at 12 weeks and continued until the delivery.

Definition and classification

Hypertension is defined as blood pressure >140/90 mmHg in pregnancy. Hypertensive disorders fall into three main categories:

- **Preexisting or chronic hypertension**: Patients may have a known history of hypertension or be found to be hypertensive at booking or at < 20 weeks. Prepregnancy counselling allows a review of medications that may cause fetal morbidity. Fetal monitoring for growth and maternal monitoring to enable prompt treatment of raised blood pressure are important.
- **Gestational or pregnancy-induced hypertension (PIH)**: Hypertension presenting after 20 weeks of the pregnancy with no proteinuria.
- **Proteinuric hypertension or preeclampsia (preeclamptic toxaemia (PET)**: hypertension presenting after 20 weeks

with significant proteinuria. The aetiology of PET is still not fully understood, but it is thought that failure of the normal trophoblastic invasion of myometrial spiral arteries leads to a high-resistance circulation and uteroplacental under perfusion. This process then results in the release of antiangiogenic factors into the maternal circulation causing vasoconstriction (hence hypertension) and endothelial damage causing morbidity such as proteinuria. It is therefore a multisystem disorder.

HINTS AND TIPS

If pregnant women with chronic hypertension are suspected of developing preeclampsia, PIGF (placental growth factor) could be offered to rule out preeclamptic toxaemia (PET). PIGF is a biochemical marker recently introduced in the NHS that helps to rule out preeclampsia on the same day.

HISTORY

Presenting complaint

Hypertensive patients may be asymptomatic and a high blood pressure reading might only be picked up as part of the routine antenatal check. Therefore, accurate blood pressure measurement is essential.

Symptoms and signs of preeclampsia are shown in Fig. 21.1. However, it is important to ask specifically about:

1. Headache (secondary to cerebral oedema)
2. Visual disturbance (typically in the form of flashing lights)
3. Right upper quadrant or epigastric pain (due to oedema of the liver capsule)
4. Vomiting
5. Sudden onset swelling of the face, hands or feet

Gynaecological history

A history of high blood pressure when taking the oral contraceptive pill indicates susceptibility to high blood pressure in pregnancy.

BOX 21.1 RISK FACTORS FOR PREECLAMPSIA

HIGH RISK

- Hypertensive disease during a previous pregnancy
- Chronic kidney disease
- Diabetes (type I and type II)
- Autoimmune disease such as systemic lupus erythematosus, antiphospholipid syndrome
- Chronic hypertension

MODERATE RISK

- Nulliparity
- Age 40 years or older
- Body mass index of 35 kg/m² or more at first visit
- Family history of preeclamptic toxaemia (PET)
- Multifoetal pregnancy

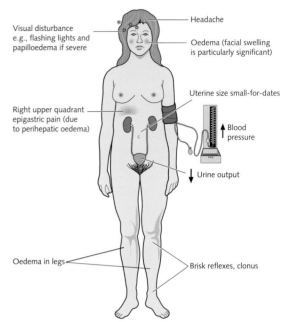

Fig. 21.1 Signs and symptoms of preeclampsia.

Obstetric history

Hypertensive episodes in previous pregnancies should be discussed as this will increase the risk in the current pregnancy (see Chapter 2). Features of the history that are of significance include the gestation period during which hypertension was diagnosed if treatment was required and the duration of treatment postnatally. Preeclampsia does not always recur with every pregnancy; it is more common in primigravidae or in the first pregnancy with a new partner.

Medical history

Those with a history of preexisting hypertension are very unlikely to have normal blood pressure in pregnancy and may even have evidence of end-organ damage at the start of pregnancy if it has previously been poorly managed. Conditions that predispose to hypertension include diabetes, renal and cardiac disease. These patients should be offered low-dose aspirin to prevent preeclampsia.

Family history

Preeclampsia is familial, with the strongest association being a sister affected in her pregnancy. The more severe the preeclampsia and the earlier it occurs in pregnancy, the more likely it is to be familial.

Drug history

Patients with preexisting hypertension might already be on medication. Common antihypertensives, such as diuretics,

angiotensin-converting enzyme inhibitors and angiotensin II receptor blockers are contraindicated. If a woman conceives while taking these medications, they should be discontinued as soon as possible and an alternative drug should be started, as there is an increased risk of congenital abnormalities if taken in the first trimester.

EXAMINATION

The examination begins with a general inspection. Any facial oedema should be noted and if it is not obvious to the physician, the patient or her partner may be asked to confirm its presence. Blood pressure should be checked and recorded.

HINTS AND TIPS

Blood pressure should be measured with the patient sitting or lying at 45 degrees. The arm should be at the same level as the heart. It is essential that the correct size of cuff is used; if a small cuff is used for an obese woman, the blood pressure will be artificially (and worryingly) high and vice versa for large cuffs in small women.

Abdominal palpation should then be performed to elicit liver tenderness followed by palpation of the uterus to ascertain if the symphysis fundal height is appropriate for the gestational age.

A small-for-dates foetus may be a sign of intrauterine growth restriction as a result of poor placental function in preeclampsia.

Brisk reflexes should be assessed and the presence of any clonus noted as these can be a sign of preeclampsia. Fundoscopy should be performed to look for papilloedema, which can occur in preeclampsia, or retinopathy, which is a complication of severe preexisting hypertension.

INVESTIGATIONS

Investigating hypertension in pregnancy is aimed at establishing which of the three categories the patient falls into and the severity of the disease.

RED FLAGS

When seeing a pregnant woman with raised blood pressure, one of your first questions must be 'Is there any proteinuria?' The presence of proteinuria should always raise suspicion of preeclampsia.

Urinalysis

The presence of proteinuria is very important when differentiating between PIH and PET. Therefore, in all cases, the urine should be tested using a urinary dipstick to provide a rapid bedside assessment.

The presence of protein may be due to PET, but may also be the result of contamination with blood, liquor (if the membranes have ruptured), vaginal discharge or a urinary tract infection (UTI). A UTI should be suspected if the proteinuria is associated with the presence of nitrites, leucocytes and/or blood. However, PET must still be suspected until a UTI is excluded by sending a mid-stream sample for microbiology testing.

Proteinuria assessed as ≥1+ on a urine dipstick should be quantified by sending samples to the laboratory for evaluating protein-to-creatinine ratio (PCR) or 24-hour urinary protein collection. These will help to distinguish between contaminants giving false positive and true proteinuria. A PCR >30 mg/mmol or a level of more than 0.3 g of protein in 24 hours should be regarded as significant.

Blood tests

In patients with preexisting hypertension, baseline investigations (full blood count, urea and electrolytes and liver function tests) should be performed at booking, as they will be an important reference point later in the pregnancy if hypertension gets worse and/or the patient develops PET. During pregnancy, hypertension is investigated with blood tests shown in Table 21.1.

COMMON PITFALLS

Because of the physiology of pregnancy, the normal ranges of some blood tests will change. For example, due to an increased glomerular filtration rate in pregnancy, there is a higher creatinine clearance. Hence a normal serum creatinine level in pregnancy will be lower than that of the normal adult range. Therefore, a creatinine level that would be considered normal in an average adult can be significantly abnormal in pregnancy. Another example of this is the liver enzyme alkaline phosphatase, which is raised in pregnancy due to placental production. Therefore, a high level in pregnancy does not usually indicate liver disease, which may be seen in preeclamptic toxaemia.

Table 21.1 Blood tests in the patient with hypertension

	Chronic hypertension	Pregnancy-induced hypertension	Preeclamptic toxaemia
Full blood count	Normal	Normal	↓ Platelets ↑ Haematocrit
Urea and electrolytes	Normal[a]	Normal	↑ Creatinine
Liver function tests	Normal	Normal	↑ Alanine aminotransferase (ALT)/aspartate aminotransferase (AST)
Clotting screen[b]	Normal	Normal	Can be deranged
Lactate dehydrogenase[b]	Measured if there are concerns regarding haemolysis[c]		

[a]Chronic hypertensive patients may have an element of preexisting renal impairment and therefore baseline renal function tests should be sent at booking to compare with later tests in pregnancy.
[b]Done only if indicated by clinical picture or low platelets.
[c]HELLP syndrome – haemolysis elevated liver enzymes and low platelets is a severe variant of preeclamptic toxaemia, which is named after its features.

Ultrasound

Essential hypertension, if poorly controlled, may affect fetal growth. Therefore, in these cases, serial ultrasound scans for fetal growth, liquor volume and Dopplers should be requested at 28, 32 and 36 weeks' gestation. Some units offer ultrasound assessment of uterine artery Dopplers at around 22 weeks in an attempt to predict those who may go on to develop preeclampsia. A renal tract ultrasound scan may also be considered antenatally for those women with chronic hypertension to assess end-organ damage.

PET may cause intrauterine growth restriction, oligohydramnios and abnormal Dopplers secondary to placental insufficiency. Therefore, ultrasound scans for fetal growth, liquor volume and Dopplers are also indicated at the aforementioned gestations.

TREATMENT

Preexisting/essential hypertension

Those with preexisting hypertension should ideally be seen prepregnancy and have their blood pressure optimized with a drug safe for pregnancy such as labetalol (Table 21.2). Any potentially teratogenic medications should be changed (see the 'Drug history' section).

HINTS AND TIPS

In a young person who is being diagnosed with hypertension for the first time, it is important to exclude an underlying disease such as coarctation of the aorta, renal artery stenosis, Conn syndrome, Cushing syndrome or a phaeochromocytoma.

The aim of treatment in this group is to maintain blood pressure readings below 150/100 mmHg. Those with evidence of end-organ damage (renal or retinal) may need even tighter control, below 140/90 mmHg. The risks of uncontrolled hypertension in this group are cerebral haemorrhage and other end-organ damage.

Pregnancy-induced hypertension

PIH presents after 20 weeks of pregnancy in patients with no history of hypertension and in the absence of proteinuria. The risks of uncontrolled blood pressure are those described earlier, and therefore monitoring with blood pressure measurement, urine dipstick testing and blood tests is very important:

Table 21.2 Antihypertensives

Drug	Description
Labetalol	α- and β-blockers – regarded as first-line treatment. Has direct cardiac effects and also lower peripheral vascular resistance. Should be avoided in asthmatics.
Nifedipine	Calcium channel blocker which causes arterial vasodilatation. Can cause headaches.
Methyldopa	α-Agonist which prevents vasoconstriction. It has been used for many years with a good safety profile. Should be stopped within 2 days of delivery and changed to another agent due to the risk of postnatal depression.
Hydralazine	Intravenous drug which causes vasodilatation. Can cause rapid hypotension, so is often given after a bolus of colloid.

- Mild hypertension (i.e., between 140/90 and 149/99 mmHg) does not always require treatment; blood pressure and urine should be checked weekly.
- Moderate hypertension (i.e., between 150/100 and 159/109 mmHg) should be treated (Table 21.2) and monitored twice weekly.
- Severe hypertension (i.e., >160/110 mmHg) requires inpatient treatment and close monitoring.

Both preexisting hypertensives and those with PIH are at an increased risk of developing preeclampsia, so continued monitoring is very important. Early delivery before 37 weeks of gestation is not usually indicated unless the blood pressure is very difficult to control or there are signs of fetal compromise. In those who require delivery before 37 weeks a course of steroids should be administered to aid fetal lung maturity.

Preeclampsia

Preeclampsia is defined as new hypertension developing after 20 weeks with significant proteinuria. The pathophysiological process of PET can only be ended by delivery of the placenta. Therefore, when treating PET, there is a fine balance between continuing pregnancy (to allow more time for fetal maturity) and risks to the mother (of worsening liver and/or renal symptoms or risk of cerebral haemorrhage).

Again, the severity of hypertension will influence whether or not antihypertensives are commenced:

- Mild PET (140/90–149/99 mmHg) does not always require antihypertensives.
- Moderate PET (150/100–159/109 mmHg) requires treatment (Table 21.2).
- Severe PET >160/110 mmHg requires urgent treatment and if not responsive to first-line oral treatments, may require intravenous antihypertensives.

BOX 21.2 CALCULATION OF MEAN ARTERIAL BLOOD PRESSURE (MAP)

Mean arterial pressure (MAP) can be estimated using the following formula:

$$MAP = \frac{(2 \times \text{diastolic BP}) + \text{systolic BP}}{3}$$

Or

$$MAP = \frac{\text{systolic BP} - \text{diastolic BP} + \text{diastolic BP}}{3}$$

In severe cases where there is a risk of eclampsia (seizures), intravenous magnesium sulphate ($MgSO_4$) has been shown to be beneficial as prophylaxis. It is usually used if the mean arterial pressure (Box 21.2) remains above 125 mmHg despite initial treatment, as well as other features including:

- headaches
- visual disturbance
- epigastric pain
- brisk reflexes or clonus (>3 beats)
- deranged blood tests such as low platelets, rising alanine aminotransferase (ALT) or creatinine

Blood tests (Table 21.1) should be performed frequently to assess any deterioration when a woman requires $MgSO_4$. Strict fluid input/output measurement is essential, with fluid restriction to prevent fluid overload. This is accepted as 1 mL/kg/h, and therefore 85 mL/h is used unless the patient is very underweight or overweight. Using $MgSO_4$ generally means the clinical picture necessitates delivering the baby once the mother is stable and/or steroids have been given (if required; see Chapter 25). The $MgSO_4$ should continue for 24 hours postdelivery as the woman is still at high risk for eclampsia.

HINTS AND TIPS

Preeclampsia is only cured by delivery of the foetus/es.

Eclampsia

Eclampsia is defined as the occurrence of seizures in pregnancy on a background of PET. Eclampsia affects 1 in 2000 pregnancies with around 40% of seizures occurring postnatally (usually within 48 hours of delivery). Seizures presenting for the first time in pregnancy should always be assumed to be eclamptic seizures until proven otherwise. The differential diagnosis includes:

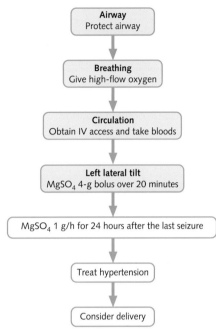

Fig. 21.2 Management of eclampsia. *IV,* Intravenous; *MgSO₄,* magnesium sulphate.

- epilepsy
- meningitis
- cerebral thrombosis
- intracerebral bleed
- intracerebral tumour

The management of eclampsia is detailed in Fig. 21.2. As always, the initial management of eclampsia should always follow the airway, breathing, circulation (ABC) approach. Stabilization of the mother is paramount and should be ensured before any consideration is given to the foetus.

HELLP

HELLP syndrome is a life-threatening disorder thought to be a severe variant of preeclampsia.

It is characterized by:

Haemolysis
Elevated **L**iver enzymes (raised ALT)
Low **P**latelet count

Patients may present with the symptoms of preeclampsia (see Fig. 21.1). Investigations include a lactate dehydrogenase level and reticulocyte count to assess for haemolysis (see Table 21.1). The treatment for HELLP syndrome is delivery in a timely manner for mother and baby, as with PET. The complications of HELLP syndrome include subcapsular liver haematoma, liver rupture and disseminated intravascular coagulation.

For the treatment of hypertension:

- Labetalol, nifedipine and methyldopa are preferred **in pregnancy.**
- Nifedipine, amlodipine, atenolol and enalapril are the drugs of choice in **postnatal period.**

POSTNATAL CARE

Following delivery, women need to have a period of monitoring for up to 4 to 5 days in hospital, as blood pressure levels may reduce and medications may need to be amended accordingly. Those on methyldopa antenatally should be changed to an alternative drug due to the association with postnatal depression (Table 21.2). Antihypertensive drugs should be continued on discharge if required and follow-up in the community with the general practitioner should be arranged including a medical review at the 6-week postnatal check. This should include advice on a yearly blood pressure check, as PET patients have been shown to be at increased risk of hypertension in later life.

FUTURE PREGNANCIES

In women with hypertensive disorders of pregnancy, the overall risk of recurrence in a future pregnancy is 20%. Aspirin should be advised from 12 weeks.

● Chapter Summary

- Preexisting/chronic hypertension is defined as hypertension of >140/90 mmHg diagnosed at booking or <20 weeks' gestation.
- Gestational/pregnancy-induced hypertension is defined as hypertension >140/90 mmHg diagnosed after 20 weeks' gestation without proteinuria.
- Preeclampsia is defined as hypertension >140/90 mmHg associated with proteinuria (PCR >30 mg/mmol or protein >0.3 g in 24 hours).
- PIGF is a new biomarker that helps to diagnose or rule out preeclampsia, especially in pregnant women who have chronic hypertension.
- Treatment includes antihypertensives to control the blood pressure and in severe cases of preeclampsia treatment is with magnesium sulphate and planning of delivery.
- Preeclampsia can present in the postnatal period and women are at risk of eclampsia for up to 5 days postnatally.
- Methyldopa should be avoided in postpartum period because of the risk of depression.
- Women with a history of preeclampsia are more likely to develop hypertension, cardiovascular, cerebrovascular and chronic kidney disease in later life.

UKMLA Conditions
Essential or secondary hypertension
Preeclampsia
Gestational hypertension

UKMLA Presentations
Hypertension

Medical disorders in pregnancy 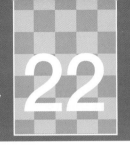 22

INTRODUCTION

Early optimization of medical disorders (ideally prepregnancy) can help to minimize the adverse effects and ensure a good outcome for both mother and foetus.

HAEMATOLOGY

Anaemia

The normal physiological changes in pregnancy cause an increased plasma expansion resulting in a decrease in the concentration of haemoglobin (Hb). Despite an increase in gastrointestinal iron absorption during pregnancy as iron requirements increase almost threefold, anaemia is a common condition for pregnant women. Therefore, a full blood count is routinely performed for all the patients at booking and at 28 weeks of gestation.

> **HINTS AND TIPS**
>
> Normal Hb levels show a variation in pregnancy compared to nonpregnant women due to physiological changes. Treatment should be advised if Hb:
> - ≤110 g/L in the first trimester
> - ≤105 g/L in the second and third trimesters
> - ≤100 g/L in the postpartum period

Following the detection of a low Hb in pregnancy oral iron treatment is recommended as the first-line diagnostic test for normocytic or microcytic anaemia. An increase in Hb must be demonstrated in 2 weeks which would support the diagnosis. If there is no response recorded to iron treatment then patient compliance should be checked and further investigations such as haematinics need to be considered.

All women should be counselled regarding diet during pregnancy and factors that may inhibit or promote iron absorption especially if they are on oral iron treatment. Vitamin C has been shown to increase its absorption from the gut and patients should be advised to take orange juice or a similar vitamin C-containing juice. Tannins found in tea and coffee reduce absorption so they should be avoided.

During pregnancy patients who complain about fatigue, dizziness or collapsing should be investigated for anaemia in addition to the routine screening.

> **RED FLAGS**
>
> Correction of anaemia is essential as it has been linked with low birth weight and preterm delivery. In addition, patients with adequate haemoglobin levels are less likely to need a blood transfusion following delivery.

Haemoglobinopathies

Haemoglobinopathies are recessively inherited disorders which affect the Hb component of blood. More than 1000 mutations are defined which result in haemoglobin variants or thalassaemias. In the UK, sickle cell screening is offered to all pregnant women in high-prevalence areas and in low-prevalence areas FOQ is used (Chapter 19). All pregnant women are offered screening for thalassemia.

> **HINTS AND TIPS**
>
> Serum ferritin should be checked prior to starting iron in patients with known haemoglobinopathy as treatment is only indicated when ferritin levels are low.

Thromboembolism

Venous thromboembolism (VTE) is one of the leading direct causes of maternal death and so all clinicians must be alert to the signs, symptoms, investigations and treatment.

The normal physiological adaptations to pregnancy mean that it is a prothrombotic state, increasing the risks of VTE by sixfold. These include:

- Increase in
  - clotting factors – FVIII, FIX, FX
  - fibrinogen
  - venous stasis in lower limbs (left > right)
- Decrease in
  - fibrinolytic activity
  - protein S
  - antithrombin

Risk factors

Risk factors for VTE are given in Box 22.1. Risk assessment for VTE should be performed at the booking appointment and at each visit with a midwife or a doctor.

Thromboprophylaxis

Prophylactic anticoagulation should be given depending on the risk assessment. For example, women with a previous deep vein thrombosis (DVT) should have prophylactic anticoagulation during the whole pregnancy whereas women with active ulcerative colitis without any other risk factors commence on prophylactic anticoagulants from 28 weeks of gestation.

A key point to remember is that the risk of VTE is not abolished once the foetus is delivered, but remains high until 6 weeks post-delivery. Therefore, any prophylactic measures should continue up until this point. (see Chapter 31 for postnatal risk assessment and thromboprophylaxis).

Symptoms and signs

DVT may present with pain, swelling and redness of the calf. Pulmonary embolism (PE) can present with shortness of breath, chest pain (pleuritic), collapse, cough or haemoptysis.

Patients found to be tachypnoeic, tachycardic, dyspnoeic or hypoxic (reduced saturations on pulse oximetry or low partial pressure of oxygen (PO_2) on arterial blood gas (ABG)) need to have a PE ruled out.

> **RED FLAGS**
>
> In all cases of suspected deep vein thrombosis or pulmonary embolism, a high index of suspicion is advised and treatment must be initiated until the diagnosis is ruled out.

Investigations

Investigation of a DVT usually starts with a clinical examination followed by venous Dopplers. It is important to bear in mind that the thrombosis may be located higher than the calf (propensity for iliofemoral DVT in pregnancy compared with femoral-popliteal DVT), and therefore imaging should include this area. This kind of DVT can present with abdominal pain.

PE investigations usually begin again with a thorough examination followed by an electrocardiogram (ECG), ABG, FBC and chest X-ray (CXR). On the ABG the patient may be hypoxic and hypercapnic, the ECG may reveal a sinus tachycardia and the CXR is important to rule out other potential causes of the symptoms, such as infection or pneumothorax.

If the CXR is normal, the patient may proceed to a ventilation/perfusion (V/Q) scan. This may identify an area of under perfusion indicating a PE. If the CXR is abnormal, a computed

> **BOX 22.1 RISK FACTORS FOR VENOUS THROMBOEMBOLISM IN PREGNANCY**
>
> - Thrombophilia (factor V Leiden, protein C deficiency, antiphospholipid syndrome)
> - Age >35 years
> - Body mass index >30 kg/m²
> - Parity ≥3
> - Smoker
> - Immobility (surgery, disability, admission to hospital)
> - Gross varicose veins
> - Multiple pregnancies
> - Active medical disease (inflammatory bowel disease, nephrotic syndrome, systemic lupus erythematosus)
> - Systemic infection

tomographic pulmonary angiogram (CTPA) may be indicated. This is very sensitive at diagnosing a PE but involves high doses of radiation. Therefore, V/Q scans are preferred as first line to protect maternal breasts from irradiation, which increases the risk of breast cancer.

> **COMMON PITFALLS**
>
> A D-dimer test is not performed as part of the investigations as its levels are usually high in pregnancy. However, a negative D-dimer would be very reassuring in ruling out a deep vein thrombosis or pulmonary embolism.

Treatment

With a confirmed DVT or PE, patients require anticoagulation with therapeutic doses of low molecular weight heparin (LMWH). Warfarin is generally avoided as it crosses the placenta and is known to be teratogenic, as well as carrying the risk of fetal intracranial bleeding. Postnatally, patients can be switched to warfarin even if they are breastfeeding as it is regarded as safe. Treatment should continue until the end of the pregnancy and for at least 6 weeks postnatally and until at least 3 months of treatment has been given in total.

Cerebral vein thrombosis

Cerebral vein thrombosis is an uncommon yet fatal problem encountered by obstetricians. It is more common in the puerperium and presents with headaches, seizures, vomiting, photophobia, reduced consciousness or even focal neurology. It is usually diagnosed with a magnetic resonance imaging (MRI) venous angiogram and treatment is usually with hydration and anticoagulation.

RESPIRATORY

Asthma

Asthma is frequently encountered in antenatal clinics and affects up to 7% of females of childbearing age. Usually, pregnancy does not influence the severity of the disease.

New diagnoses of asthma in pregnancy, although not common, should be considered in patients complaining of cough, shortness of breath, wheezing or chest tightness. See Table 22.1 for differential diagnosis of shortness of breath in a pregnant patient for differential diagnosis of shortness of breath in pregnancy. Classically these symptoms will be worse at night or associated with certain triggers like dust, exercise or pollen.

For known asthma sufferers, a detailed enquiry should include:

- current treatments
- peak flow record
- previous hospital admissions (especially those requiring admission to intensive care)

The peak expiratory flow rate trend will form an important part of monitoring in pregnancy, and therefore its importance should not be underestimated.

Some patients may discontinue their therapy due to fears over the effect they may have on the foetus. They can be reassured and encouraged to continue, to prevent any deterioration in their condition as poorly controlled asthma could pose more risk to the pregnancy.

ENDOCRINE

Hypertension in pregnancy is covered in Chapter 21.

Diabetes

Diabetes affects 2% to 5% of all women in pregnancy. Most units have a specialist joint multidisciplinary diabetic antenatal clinic, including obstetricians, endocrinologists, diabetic specialist nurses/midwives and dieticians, to optimize care. Patients can either have preexisting diabetes (15%) or develop gestational diabetes (GDM; 85%) which, left untreated, can have severe ramifications for both mother and foetus.

Glucose metabolism is altered during pregnancy such that pregnancy itself is a state of impaired glucose tolerance,

Table 22.1 Differential diagnosis of shortness of breath in pregnancy

Condition	Key characteristics	Investigations
Physiological	Common in third trimester.	Exclusion of other conditions
Anxiety/ hyperventilation	Underlying mental health concerns.	Hypocapnia without hypoxaemia on blood gas
Anaemia	Most of the patients are asymptomatic until it is severe. They may experience palpitations, headaches, tiredness.	Full blood count (FBC)
Pulmonary embolism	This condition ALWAYS needs to be considered, as pregnancy is a high-risk state for clotting. It could be associated with sudden onset pleuritic or central chest pain. Tachycardia is also a supporting finding. Risk factors should be reviewed (see risk factors for venous thromboembolism (VTE)).	Electrocardiogram (ECG) Chest X-ray Arterial blood gases V/Q* lung scan or CTPA**
Respiratory causes	1. Wheezy breathing and history are helpful in reaching the diagnosis of asthma. 2. Productive cough is common in pneumonia. 3. Subcutaneous emphysema, sudden onset pleuritic chest pain suggests pneumothorax.	Chest X-ray Sputum culture Swab for viral culture Full blood count Blood culture CRP
Cardiac causes	Breathlessness can be a result of pulmonary oedema in pregnant patients with mitral stenosis (MS). Orthopnoea, paroxysmal nocturnal dyspnoea and haemoptysis – should be asked about when there is a suspicion of MS. Peripartum cardiomyopathy (PPCM) is one of the common cardiac causes. Advanced maternal age, multiparity, black ethnicity, multiple pregnancy, preeclampsia and hypertension are risk factors for PPCM.	ECG Echocardiogram Chest X-ray Brain natriuretic peptide (BNP)

*Ventilation (V) Perfusion (Q) scan.
**CT pulmonary angiogram.

especially as it advances towards term. A major contribution to this is made by hormones secreted by the placenta:

- glucagon
- cortisol
- human placental lactogen

These effects are to some extent offset by increased insulin secretion. However, those who have an insufficient response will develop GDM. For the same reason, patients with preexisting type 1 diabetes will require an increase in the amount of insulin they administer. Those with type 2 diabetes may need conversion to insulin from oral hypoglycaemics as pregnancy progresses.

Preexisting diabetes

Preconception

Care of patients with preexisting diabetes, either type 1 or type 2, should ideally start well before conception, including:

- optimizing glycaemic control by monitoring glucose premeals and postmeals
- educating the patient about diabetes in pregnancy and the risks (Box 22.2)
- educating the patient about the risks of hypoglycaemia
- prescribing high-dose folic acid (5 mg) daily (preconception until 12 weeks)
- screening for nephropathy and retinopathy

HINTS AND TIPS

- The optimal is HbA1c below 48 mmol/mol (6.5%) in the preconception period.
- If the HbA1c level is above 86 mmol/mol (10%) women should be advised not to become pregnant due to risks to mother and foetus.

Ultrasound scans

Patients with preexisting diabetes have a higher rate of miscarriage, and therefore may request an early ultrasound scan. In addition, there is an increased risk of congenital anomalies, so nuchal translucency and a detailed anomaly scan including detailed assessment of the fetal heart should be arranged. Poor glycaemic control can lead to fetal macrosomia and increased liquor volume (see Chapter 23), therefore diabetic patients are advised to have serial growth scans in the third trimester.

Antenatal care

Patients should be seen more frequently than the suggested antenatal care pathway with reviews occurring every 2 to 3

BOX 22.2 RISKS OF DIABETES IN PREGNANCY

- Miscarriage.
- Congenital anomalies, in particular, cardiac.
- Fetal macrosomia and/or polyhydramnios.
- Induction of labour.
- Caesarean section.
- Birth trauma.
- Shoulder dystocia.
- Stillbirth.
- Neonatal hypoglycaemia.
- Obesity/diabetes in the baby (later in life).

---

weeks in a multidisciplinary diabetic antenatal clinic. Patients are encouraged to self-monitor their capillary blood glucose levels regularly to allow good glycaemic control. Target blood glucose levels are ≤5.3 mmol/L when fasting and ≤7.8 mmol/L 1 hour post meals.

Both diabetic retinopathy and diabetic nephropathy can worsen during pregnancy. Patients should have their eyes checked at booking and at 28 weeks, as well as undergo regular blood pressure checks and assessment of proteinuria. Aspirin 75 to 150 mg daily is advised because of the increased risk of preeclampsia.

Diabetic patients with preeclampsia or growth restriction may require early delivery and steroid injections for augmentation of fetal lung maturation. This commonly requires admission and an insulin sliding scale because the administration of steroids will worsen glycaemic control.

RED FLAGS

The mortality rate for ketoacidosis during pregnancy is 50%, so it should be diagnosed and treated immediately if it occurs during pregnancy.

Delivery and postnatal care

In the absence of complications, the timing of delivery needs to be carefully planned with the risks of prematurity and induction of labour against the risk of stillbirth (the rate of which is increased in diabetic mothers). Glucose control with a sliding scale is usually needed in labour. In addition, macrosomic babies have an increased risk of shoulder dystocia, therefore, senior assistance must be available at delivery.

Immediately following delivery, the foetus will be at risk of hypoglycaemia as it is no longer in a hyperglycaemic environment, although fetal insulin levels will still be high. Close monitoring and early feeds are important. Furthermore, once the placenta has been delivered, maternal requirements of insulin will fall and the doses of insulin should return to prepregnancy levels or slightly less than prepregnancy levels if breastfeeding.

Gestational diabetes

GDM is described as diabetes that develops for the first time in pregnancy. Pregnancy induces insulin resistance as part of normal physiology. GDM develops in women who are unable to respond to the increased demand for insulin during pregnancy.

Not all the cases diagnosed in pregnancy are GDM as screening for GDM can identify undiagnosed type 2 DM or preclinical type 1 diabetes.

Diagnosis

As per NICE guideline 75-g oral glucose tolerance test (OGTT) is used for diagnosis. The World Health Organization (WHO) defines frank diabetes as a fasting glucose level of >7 mmol/L or a 2-hour level of >11.1 mmol/L. GDM is diagnosed as a fasting glucose level of >5.6 mmol/L or a 2-hour level of >7.8 mmol/L. When undergoing an OGTT the patient is asked to starve the night before the test and will then have a venous blood glucose level measured. Following this they will be asked to drink a glucose load (75 g) and have a second glucose level taken 2 hours later.

Screening for GDM is offered to 'at-risk' groups. Risk factors for GDM are shown in Box 22.3 and patients with one or more risk factors should be offered an OGTT at around 26 to 28 weeks. Patients who have had GDM in a previous pregnancy will be offered an earlier OGTT (usually 16–18 weeks), and if this is negative, it will be repeated at 28 weeks.

Antenatal care

Risks of GDM to both the mother and foetus are similar to pregnancies in patients with preexisting diabetes (Box 22.2) with the exception of miscarriage and congenital anomalies, as this period has passed. Patients should be seen in a multidisciplinary diabetic antenatal clinic and advised to self-monitor with regular premeal and postmeal capillary blood glucose levels. They may respond to changes in diet (consider referral to a dietician) and exercise alone. If these measures are insufficient, oral hypoglycaemic agents with or without insulin may be required. They should have serial growth scans to look for macrosomia with or without polyhydramnios.

Delivery and postnatal care

The planning of delivery is not always as rigid as in those with preexisting diabetes as the risk to the foetus may be less. Each case should be assessed individually taking into account any complications that may have developed.

Postnatally patients can discontinue their hypoglycaemic agents and should have a fasting plasma glucose test between

> **BOX 22.3 RISK FACTORS FOR GESTATIONAL DIABETES**
>
> - Body mass index >30 kg/m^2
> - Previous macrosomic baby weighing >4.5 kg
> - Previous gestational diabetes
> - First-degree relative with diabetes
> - Country of family origin:
>   - South Asian
>   - Black Caribbean
>   - Middle Eastern

6 and 13 weeks after delivery. If the postnatal fasting glucose is normal, then they should be offered an annual HbA1c due to their increased risk of developing type 2 diabetes. The foetus will still be at risk of hypoglycaemia in the immediate period post delivery, and therefore early feeds and close monitoring are advised. Patients with GDM should also be advised regarding weight loss and maintenance of a healthy diet with exercise and told of the high possibility of recurrence in future pregnancies.

Thyroid disease

Hypothyroidism

Hypothyroidism affects around 1% of pregnancies and is more common in those patients with a family history. Symptoms in pregnancy are similar to the nonpregnant patients:

- lethargy
- tiredness
- weight gain
- dry skin
- hair loss

These may be confused with normal pregnancy symptoms (cold intolerance, slow pulse rate and slow relaxing tendon reflexes are said to be discriminatory features in pregnancy). A goitre may also be present and should be carefully assessed when examining the patient.

In cases of known hypothyroidism preconceptual optimization of thyroid hormone levels with replacement therapy is very important as hypothyroidism itself can lead to subfertility. Up until 12 weeks, the foetus is entirely dependent upon maternal thyroid hormones. In severe cases of hypothyroidism, there is an association with miscarriage, reduced intelligence, neurodevelopmental delay and brain damage.

Most cases of hypothyroidism encountered in pregnancy are due to either autoimmune (Hashimoto/atrophic) thyroiditis or treated Graves disease, but it can also be due to drugs or following treatment for hyperthyroidism.

Table 22.2 Pregnancy-specific thyroid hormone values

Hormone	Nonpregnant	First trimester	Second trimester	Third trimester
Thyroid-stimulating hormone	0–4	0–1.6	0.1–1.8	0.7–7.3
Free T$_4$	11–23	11–22	11–19	7–15
Free T$_3$	4–9	4–8	4–7	3–5

In patients who are adequately treated, it is usual to continue the current dose of thyroxine and check levels in each trimester (see Table 22.2 for pregnancy-specific values). Those who require modifications of their dosing will need more frequent thyroid function tests (TFTs). The importance of compliance with medication to minimize the impact on the foetus should be emphasized to all patients.

Subclinical hypothyroidism is a term used to describe those with a high TSH and normal thyroxine concentration, but with no specific symptoms or signs of thyroid dysfunction. It affects 5% of the general population and is more common in women. There is no evidence that treatment with thyroxine improves pregnancy outcomes.

Postpartum thyroiditis is caused by a destructive autoimmune lymphocytic process. Patients usually present 3 to 4 months after delivery with hyper- or hypothyroidism. Most of the women recover without any treatment.

HINTS AND TIPS

Maternal thyroxin replacement is safe as very little amount of thyroxine crosses the placenta.

Hyperthyroidism

Hyperthyroidism, although less common than hypothyroidism, still affects around 1 in 800 pregnancies. Approximately 50% of those suffering from the disease have a family history of thyroid disease.

Symptoms of hyperthyroidism are the same as in the non-pregnant population and again can mimic normal pregnancy symptoms. These include sweating, palpitations, heat intolerance and vomiting. When examining the patient, look for the following signs:

- tachycardia
- tremor
- eye signs (exophthalmos)
- goitre
- palmar erythema

The presence of the first three signs is said to help distinguish hyperthyroidism from normal pregnancy symptoms.

About 95% of hyperthyroidism encountered in pregnancy is due to Graves disease, a condition where thyroid receptor antibodies stimulate thyroid hormone production. It can also be due to:

- drugs
- multinodular goitre
- thyroiditis

Again, if untreated patients may have difficulty conceiving, preconceptual counselling and optimization are vital, as untreated hyperthyroidism is associated with miscarriage, preterm labour and growth restriction.

TFTs should be measured in each trimester and assessed using pregnancy-specific values (Table 22.2). Antithyroid drugs such as propylthiouracil should be continued and carbimazole can be used from the second trimester onwards. β-Blockers may be required to improve symptoms of sweating, tachycardia and palpitations, and rarely surgery may be required, especially if obstructive symptoms from the goitre are present.

HINTS AND TIPS

Carbimazole is not preferred in the first trimester due to the risk of teratogenicity. Its use is associated with:

- aplasia cutis congenita (absence of a portion of skin, often localized on the head)
- craniofacial malformations (choanal atresia; facial dysmorphism)
- gastrointestinal tract and abdominal wall defects (exomphalos, oesophageal atresia, omphalo-mesenteric duct anomaly)
- cardiovascular system defects (ventricular septal defect)

About 1% of foetuses or neonates can suffer from neonatal thyrotoxicosis due to transplacental passage of thyroid-simulating antibodies. The condition should also be considered in foetuses or neonates of patients who are now hypothyroid as a result of thyroid treatment for Graves disease. Foetuses will exhibit signs of tachycardia, growth restriction and possibly a goitre, while neonates may present with jaundice, failure to gain weight, irritability or in severe cases heart failure.

Obesity

Obesity is one of the most commonly seen risk factors in obstetric practice affecting 21.3% of the antenatal population. Women with a body mass index (BMI) of 30 kg/m^2 or over have increased risk for:

- GDM
- Preeclampsia
- Fetal macrosomia
- Caesarean birth
- Vitamin D deficiency

Women with a booking BMI of 30 kg/m^2 or greater should be provided with information regarding the risks associated with obesity in pregnancy. There is conflicting evidence on optimal weight gain in this group of patients, therefore a healthy diet should be targeted rather than recommended weight targets.

During the antenatal period they should be offered:

- High-dose folic acid supplementation (5 mg).
- 150 mg aspirin daily, if they have another moderate risk factor for preeclampsia (see Chapter 21).
- GDM screening.
- Antenatal screening for choromosomal anomalies and 20-week screening ultrasound scan. Patients should be informed that ultrasound views may be limited due to raised BMI.
- Regular growth scans, as the SFH measurements will be inaccurate.
- Shared care between obstetricians and midwives.

Management of labour and delivery should involve a discussion with a senior obstetrician on an individual basis and women should be given the option of elective induction of labour at term. This may increase the chances of a vaginal delivery without changing the risks of adverse outcomes. To reduce the risk of excessive bleeding following birth, active management of the third stage of labour should be recommended.

CARDIOLOGY

Cardiovascular disorders and psychiatric disorders are leading causes and responsible for the same number of maternal deaths in the UK according to 2020 MBRACE report, together representing 30% of maternal deaths. Some cardiac conditions are related to extremely high risk of mortality and morbidity during pregnancy (see Box 22.4).

Congenital heart disease

Congenital heart disease includes patent ductus arteriosus, atrial septal defects and ventricular septal defects. The incidence

> **BOX 22.4 CARDIAC CONDITIONS ASSOCIATED WITH AN EXTREMELY HIGH RISK OF MORTALITY AND MORBIDITY**
>
> - Fontan circulation with any condition
> - Pulmonary artery hypertension
> - Severe ventricular dysfunction (with left ventricular ejection fraction less than 30%)
> - Severe mitral stenosis/symptomatic aortic stenosis
> - Severe aortic coarctation or recoarctation
> - Vascular Ehlers–Danlos syndrome
> - Aortic root >4.5 cm in Marfan syndrome
> - Ascending aorta >5 cm with bicuspid aortic valve
> - Tetralogy of Fallot >50 mm
> - Systemic right ventricular dysfunction
> - Turner syndrome with aortic size index >25 mm/m^2

of these in pregnancy is increasing as these women have undergone corrective surgery, and therefore can go on to have children themselves.

Following corrective surgery these heart defects cause little problem in pregnancy. These women should have consultant-led care and have an examination of the cardiovascular system at their first antenatal visit. If new symptoms arise during the pregnancy, such as tachycardia, chest pain or palpitations, they should be investigated with an echocardiogram and/or 24-hour ECG monitoring. Referral to a cardiologist may be necessary.

Acquired heart disease

The most common acquired heart disease in pregnancy is rheumatic fever, which is contracted in childhood and causes damage to one or more of the heart valves. It is more common in the migrant population and very rare in British-born women. First presentation of rheumatic heart disease could be in pregnancy, especially in migrants who have never been examined by a doctor.

Mitral stenosis

Mitral stenosis is the most common presentation of rheumatic heart disease seen in pregnancy. These women require an echocardiogram in pregnancy to assess severity of their disease. They may require treatment with β-blockers in pregnancy. The physiological changes in pregnancy can cause a deterioration in their condition. If there are any new signs or symptoms in pregnancy such as tachycardia, they will require reassessment.

Acute coronary syndrome

As women delay having children until their late 30s and early 40s, it is becoming increasingly more common to see myocardial infarctions and coronary artery disease in pregnancy. Coronary artery dissection and embolus are the more common causes in pregnancy than atherosclerosis. Box 22.5 presents the risk factors for ischaemic heart disease.

Acute coronary syndrome (ACS) is more common in the third trimester, intrapartum or postpartum and may not present with the usual symptoms of chest pain, but more atypical symptoms such as epigastric pain and nausea.

The management of ACS is the same in pregnancy as it is out of pregnancy. β-Blockers, aspirin, nitrates and heparin should be commenced. Thrombolysis and coronary angiography with stenting if required can be performed in pregnancy.

Aortic dissection

The risk of aortic dissection is increased in pregnancy and it is associated with a high mortality rate. It commonly presents with chest pain radiating between the scapulae and jaw pain (see Table 22.3 for the differential diagnosis of chest pain in pregnancy). There may be a difference in the blood pressure readings from the left and right arm.

Diagnosis involves various imaging modalities including a CXR looking for mediastinal widening or confirmation of dissection on echocardiography.

Once the diagnosis of aortic dissection has been made, the blood pressure needs to be controlled and plans to deliver the baby by caesarean section need to be made, before cardiac surgery to replace the aortic root can take place.

BOX 22.5 RISK FACTORS FOR ISCHAEMIC HEART DISEASE

- Obesity.
- Diabetes.
- Hypertension.
- Smoking.
- Hypercholesterolaemia.
- Multiparity.
- Age >35 years.
- Family history of ischaemic heart disease.

NEUROLOGY

Headache is a common presentation in pregnancy. See Table 22.4 for details.

Epilepsy

Epilepsy affects around 1 in 200 women of childbearing age and is one of the most common neurological conditions in

---

Table 22.3 Differential diagnosis of chest pain in pregnancy

Condition	Key characteristics	Investigations
Gastroesophageal reflux	Pain is usually retrosternal and could be related to eating. Resolves with antacid medication	-
Musculoskeletal	Pain could be positional or related to arm movements.	-
Pulmonary embolism	Sudden onset pleuritic or central chest pain. Look for tachycardia and VTE risk factors such as obesity, smoking (see risk factors for VTE).	Electrocardiogram (ECG) Chest X-ray Arterial blood gases V/Q* lung scan or CTPA**
Respiratory causes	Pneumothorax, pneumomediastinum – sudden onset pleuritic pain, associated with breathlessness Pneumonia- pleuritic pain, could be associated with fever, cough, sputum and breathlessness.	Chest X-ray Sputum culture Swab for viral culture Full blood count Blood culture CRP
Cardiac causes	Ischemic causes – pain is usually associated with nausea, sweating and dizziness. This group of conditions are seen more common in diabetics and smokers. Aortic dissection – pain severe, can radiate to interscapular area. Most common in late third trimester and first week postpartum.	ECG Troponin Chest X-ray Chest CT Echocardiogram Chest MRI

*Ventilation (V) Perfusion (Q) scan.
**CT pulmonary angiogram.

pregnancy. Similar to diabetes, the management of epilepsy should, ideally, begin preconceptually with the counselling of patients about the risks to the mother and foetus. It is very important that epileptic women who are of childbearing age should be offered effective contraception if not planning to conceive.

Preconception and antenatal care

Antiepileptic drugs (AEDs) should be reviewed to reduce exposure to teratogenic agents, such as sodium valproate. It is recommended that all epileptic women take folic acid 5 mg daily preconceptionally and continue later on in pregnancy.

As AEDs are known to be teratogenic, many patients are often concerned about the foetus, opting to discontinue therapy. However, patients should be carefully counselled against doing so and warned about the risk of status epilepticus and sudden unexpected death in epilepsy.

The aim of epilepsy treatment in pregnancy is to maintain a seizure-free status with monotherapy at the lowest possible AED dose. The approximate risk of congenital malformation for one AED appears to be around 6%, which is double the background rate. In addition, data on sodium valproate appear to show a significantly increased risk of congenital malformations, whereas lamotrigine and carbamazepine monotherapy have the least risk. Box 22.6 lists the known complications of AED use in pregnancy.

Due to the risk of congenital abnormalities, patients should undergo a detailed ultrasound scan with particular attention to:

- cardiac function
- neural tube status
- skeletal condition
- orofacial structures

The course of epilepsy is variable; as seizure frequency can improve or worsen, approximately two-thirds of women will not have any seizure deterioration. Levels of antiepileptic drugs can decrease during pregnancy due to increased hepatic metabolism and renal clearance. Seizures may therefore be difficult to control and dose increases may be required.

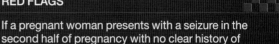

RED FLAGS

If a pregnant woman presents with a seizure in the second half of pregnancy with no clear history of epilepsy, then she should be treated for eclampsia until a diagnosis can be made (see Chapter 21).

Delivery and postnatal care

There is an increase in the risk of seizures around the time of delivery and the following first 24 hours. Therefore, women should be advised to continue their AED medication. This risk is sufficient enough to recommend that patients deliver in a hospital setting. Women with well-controlled epilepsy and no other risk factors can go on to have uncomplicated labour and vaginal

BOX 22.6 FETAL AND NEONATAL COMPLICATIONS OF ANTIEPILEPTIC DRUG USE IN PREGNANCY

- Orofacial clefts.
- Neural tube defects.
- Congenital heart disease.
- Haemorrhagic disease of the newborn.

Table 22.4 New differential diagnosis of headache in pregnancy

Condition	Key characteristics	Investigations
Hypertension/preeclampsia	Look for blurry and hyperreflexia (see Chapter 20)	Urinalysis Full blood count Coagulation
Epidural-related headache	Pain is often frontal and postural and associated with dural tap	-
Cerebral venous thrombosis (CVT)	Seen more often in postnatal period. Associated with signs of raised intracranial pressure.	Computed tomography (CT) venogram Venous angiography MRI
Idiopathic intracranial hypertension	Retro-orbital headache, common in patients with high BMI	CT/MRI of the brain Lumbar puncture
Migraines/tension headache	Migraines could be associated with prodromal symptoms. Tension headache, usually seen following periods of stress.	-

*Other causes of headache, such as meningitis, space-occupying lesions and subarachnoid haemorrhage, need to be considered when assessing a patient with headache.

delivery. However, triggers for seizures, that is, insomnia, stress, and pain, should be minimized during labour.

The neonates of women taking enzyme-inducing AEDs should receive 1 mg of vitamin K intramuscularly to prevent haemorrhagic disease of the newborn.

Breastfeeding is generally regarded as safe and should be encouraged. Postnatal education about safety measures should be given to all epileptic mothers such as the avoidance of excessive tiredness, changing the baby on the floor to prevent falls if a seizure occurs and also bathing the baby with another adult present, again in case of seizures.

> **ETHICS**
>
> The general driving restrictions that apply to epileptics also apply to pregnant women with epilepsy. Therefore, they should be informed that if they were to stop or reduce their antiepileptic drugs, they may experience a deterioration in their seizure control and this can affect their driving privileges.

GASTROINTESTINAL DISORDERS

Intrahepatic cholestasis of pregnancy

Intrahepatic cholestasis of pregnancy (ICP), previously called as obstetric cholestasis (OC) is a multifactorial condition characterized by itching especially of the palms and soles without a skin condition. It is associated with deranged liver function tests (LFTs) and occurs in the second half of pregnancy.

ICP affects around 0.7% of pregnancies in the UK and is more common in certain ethnic groups (1.2%–1.5% Indian or Pakistani origin).

The cause is not clearly understood, but a susceptibility to the cholestatic effects of oestrogen and progesterone is thought to be key. Given that a family history of the condition is often found (35%) genetic factors are thought to play a role.

Diagnosis

ICP should be considered in pregnant patients who have itching without any skin lesions and raised peak random total bile acid of 19 mmol/L. The diagnosis is more likely if itching and raised bile acid levels are resolved following the delivery of the foetus. Structured history and examination of the patient are essential to rule out other abnormalities of the liver. Women should be offered liver function and bile acid level measurements. Further laboratory tests or imaging are not routine in every woman with suspicion of ICP. However, additional tests could be considered if atypical clinical symptoms or severe early-onset ICP are present.

Maternal and perinatal risks

The risk of developing preeclampsia or GDM could be higher in patients with ICP. Therefore, blood pressure and urine monitoring should be carried out regularly, and testing for GDM should take place according to national guidance.

Risks to foetus:

- Stillbirth (risk is higher if bile acids more than 39 mmol/L and greatest where the levels exceed 100 mmol/L)
- Meconium-stained amniotic fluid
- A higher chance of both spontaneous and iatrogenic preterm birth

> **HINTS AND TIPS**
>
> Performing regular fetal ultrasound and cardiotocography do not predict or prevent stillbirth in women with ICP.

Antenatal care

Women with ICP need to be reviewed in a consultant-led maternity unit. LFTs and bile acids levels initially could be repeated after 1 week, and then frequency needs to be determined on an individual basis.

Treatment

There are no treatments available that improve pregnancy outcome (or raised bile acid concentrations) and treatments to improve maternal itching are of limited benefit. Chlorphenamine (Piriton), aqueous creams and ursodeoxycholic acid (UCDA) could be used for symptom control.

Delivery and postnatal care

Discussion about induction of labour depends on the levels of bile acids. Women should be advised that ICP itself does not impact their choice of mode of delivery. In uncomplicated ICP, follow-up needs to be arranged at least 4 weeks after delivery to confirm the resolution. Patients should be warned of the likelihood of recurrence in a future pregnancy. The choice of contraception or hormone replacement therapy is not influenced by ICP itself. However, if ICP occurred secondary to combined hormonal (oestrogen-containing) contraception, progestogen-only or nonhormonal methods should be preferred.

Acute fatty liver of pregnancy

Acute fatty liver of pregnancy (AFLP) is a rare (1 in 20,000), potentially fatal condition, which needs prompt recognition and management. Although the aetiology is poorly understood, a disorder of mitochondrial fatty acid oxidation may play a role. Risk factors include:

- First pregnancy
- Those carrying male foetuses
- Multiple pregnancy

The condition may be the same spectrum as preeclampsia and it may be difficult to distinguish from HELLP (*h*aemolysis, *el*evated liver enzymes (raised ALT), *l*ow *p*latelet count) syndrome. It is a reversible condition, which affects both the liver and the kidneys.

Patients may present with nausea, vomiting, anorexia, malaise, abdominal pain or polyuria. Jaundice, ascites, encephalopathy and mild proteinuric hypertension may also be present. The haematological and biochemical derangements are shown in Box 22.7.

Confirmation of the diagnosis with imaging is not always possible as changes may not be seen on ultrasound, computed tomography or MRI. Liver biopsy may be considered, but in practice is not usually done due to impaired coagulopathy.

Patients diagnosed with AFLP need multidisciplinary input and urgent delivery. Supportive measures with fluids, correction of hypoglycaemia and correction of coagulopathy are important and patients may need intensive care and dialysis. In severe cases, liver transplant may be necessary.

INFECTIOUS DISEASES

Human immunodeficiency virus (HIV)

Screening
In the UK all women are advised to have screening for human immunodeficiency virus (HIV) at the booking appointment. Identification of HIV-infected individuals then allows appropriate care to improve maternal health and reduce the risk of transmission to the foetus from approximately 25% to

---

BOX 22.7 ACUTE FATTY LIVER OF PREGNANCY BLOOD RESULTS

- ↑ Alanine transaminase
- ↑ Alkaline phosphatase
- ↑ Bilirubin
- ↑ White cell count
- Hypoglycaemia (severe)
- ↑ Uric acid
- Coagulopathy

---

less than 1%. The implementation of routine antenatal HIV screening has made mother-to-child transmission a rare occurrence in the UK.

Additional interventions for HIV-positive women include screening for hepatitis C, offering vaccinations against hepatitis B and screening for genital infection in the first trimester and at 28 weeks.

Testing for the patient's partner and any other children should be offered.

ETHICS

A major barrier to compliance with testing and treatment is the fear of stigmatization and patients should be reassured regarding confidentiality. It is good practice to ensure the patient's partner is aware of the diagnosis, as there may be health implications to them that need to be addressed. Patients with a new diagnosis should be encouraged to inform their partners.

Antenatal care
Patients with HIV should be followed up by a multidisciplinary team involving HIV specialists, obstetricians, specialist midwives and paediatricians. The use of combined antiretroviral therapy (cART) has been shown to dramatically reduce the risk of vertical transmission. Therefore,

- Patients who conceive whilst taking cART, should continue to do so.
- Patients who are not on cART but require it (following assessment) should commence treatment as soon as possible.
- All pregnant patients should be on cART irrespective of viral load by 24 weeks of gestation.

HINTS AND TIPS

Patients on certain antiretroviral treatments, such as tenofovir, should be screened for gestational diabetes due to their association with impaired glucose tolerance.

Delivery and postnatal care
A plan for the mode of delivery is usually determined at 36 weeks of gestation. Patients will have their viral load measured and if <50 copies/mL, a vaginal delivery will be offered.

Patients who have a high viral load will be offered a planned caesarean section with zidovudine cover (an antiretroviral) commenced 4 hours prior to delivery and continued until cord clamping).

In resource-rich countries, the avoidance of breastfeeding is recommended (to prevent transmission) and formula milk is used as an alternative. It is, however, not always possible in developing countries.

Once delivered all neonates are treated with antiretrovirals as soon as possible (ideally within 4 hours). The neonate will be tested at regular intervals and, if not breastfed, a negative test at 18 months ensures the child is not affected.

HINTS AND TIPS

Three steps are known to reduce rates of vertical transmission of HIV:

- antiretroviral medication
- elective caesarean section
- avoidance of breastfeeding

Varicella zoster virus (VZV)

In pregnancy, primary infection with VZV can cause maternal mortality/morbidity and may affect the foetus as well. Mothers have the risk of having severe pneumonia, hepatitis and encephalitis, and foetuses are at risk of congenital varicella syndrome (CVS) and neonatal varicella.

Screening

In the UK it is not routine to perform universal serological antenatal testing for VZV. Women should be asked about a previous infection and advised to inform healthcare workers if they come into contact with chicken pox/shingles during pregnancy. When seronegative women are identified, they could be offered immunization out of the pregnancy.

Management

If a woman nonimmune to VZV pregnant has had significant exposure to chicken pox, she should be offered varicella

zoster immunoglobulin (VZIG) as soon as possible. VZIG will still be effective when given up to 10 days after contact. The reason for the administration of VZIG is that it may prevent or at least attenuate chickenpox in nonimmune pregnant women and it may also reduce the risk of the development of fetal varicella syndrome (FVS).

HINTS AND TIPS

VZIG should not be given once the pregnant woman has developed chickenpox rash as there is no therapeutic benefit at this point.

For pregnant women with chickenpox infection, symptomatic treatment and hygiene are advised to prevent secondary bacterial infection of the lesions. If they present within 24 hours of the onset of the rash oral aciclovir should be given especially after 20 weeks of gestation. Intravenous aciclovir should be given to patients with severe infection.

The timing of the varicella infection is important in determining the risk to the foetus:

- In the first trimester, the risk of miscarriage does not appear to be increased if chickenpox occurs in the first trimester.
- If the patient develops varicella in the first 28 weeks of pregnancy – a small risk of FVS.
- Maternal infection in the last 4 weeks of a woman's pregnancy – a significant risk of varicella infection of the newborn.

Patients should be referred to fetal medicine at 16 to 20 weeks or 5 weeks following the infection for a detailed ultrasound examination to look for signs of FVS. FVS is characterized by one or more of the following findings:

- skin scarring (usually in a dermatomal distribution)
- eye abnormalities (microphthalmia, chorioretinitis or cataracts)
- limb abnormalities (hypoplasia)
- neurological abnormalities (microcephaly, cortical atrophy, mental retardation or dysfunction of bowel and bladder sphincters)

Defects do not occur at the time of initial infection immediately, most of the time develop later due to subsequent in utero viral reactivation.

A planned delivery should be postponed for at least 7 days after the onset of the maternal rash if there are no other contraindications. This will allow the passive transfer of antibodies from mother to foetus.

PSYCHIATRIC ILLNESS

Psychiatric disorders are one of the two main causes of maternal death in the UK according to the 2020 MBRACE report, responsible for 15% of maternal deaths.

Depression

Depression is one of the most common mental health problems that occurs during pregnancy and in the postnatal period. Around 10% of pregnant women will experience clinically significant depressive symptoms during pregnancy. It is important to identify risk factors and provide support for these women as depression can be associated with suicide. Antenatal depression can be challenging to diagnose as some symptoms of depression such as sleep deprivation, and lack of energy are commonly observed in normal pregnancies. However, symptoms of low mood, anxiety, loss of appetite, insomnia, low self-esteem, lack of energy, failure to find enjoyment and suicidal ideation should be actively enquired about. Risk factors for depression are shown in Box 22.8.

Any patient with a history of depression or who is currently suffering from depression should be referred for specialist counselling, usually in the form of a perinatal mental health team. Both pharmacological and nonpharmacological (cognitive behavioural therapy) treatments may be required.

Following the delivery of a child, it is normal for mothers to have some emotional and behavioural changes. Initially, they feel excited and high called 'pinks'. Between days 3 and 5 tearfulness, labile mood and irritability are common symptoms and called 'baby blues'. This is usually self-limiting and lasts around 48 hours. Healthcare professionals should make sure that blues is resolving, to be able to pick up postnatal depression in cases where symptoms persist/worsen.

Puerperal psychosis

Puerperal psychosis is an acute-onset condition which develops in a previously well woman after childbirth and affects women around 1 to 2 in 1000 births. It usually starts abruptly around 2 weeks postnatally and presents with mania, delusions and hallucinations (both auditory and visual). Patients appear agitated and may exhibit disinhibited behaviour.

> **BOX 22.8 RISK FACTORS FOR DEPRESSION DURING AND AFTER PREGNANCY**
>
> - History of postnatal depression
> - History of depression unrelated to pregnancy
> - In vitro fertilization pregnancy
> - History of abuse
> - Multiple pregnancy
> - Drug misuse
> - Poor social support
> - Low socioeconomic status
> - Low educational achievement
> - Poor pregnancy outcome (e.g., illness in pregnancy, premature or difficult delivery, neonatal illness or death, diagnosis of congenital anomaly antenatally or neonatally)

Puerperal psychosis is more common in patients with bipolar disorder (BD) or if they have had previous puerperal psychosis. Treatment invariably involves admission to hospital for both the safety of the mother and baby, ideally to a specialist mother and baby unit to prevent separation. Antipsychotic medications such as haloperidol may be required. Organic causes of psychosis (infection, drug withdrawals, etc.) must be excluded.

Schizophrenia

Schizophrenia affects around 1 in 100 women of childbearing age. Patients are followed up by multidisciplinary teams specialized in mental health disorders.

Hallucinations, delusions or an abnormal affect may be encountered. For the patients on antipsychotic medication, the lowest dose is used with a reduction in the dose towards term to prevent toxicity in the neonate. Breastfeeding on antipsychotics is not advised.

Bipolar disorder

BD is a condition characterized by episodes of acute illness mixed with periods of relative normality. Many of the drugs used to treat BD are teratogenic, and therefore careful assessment must be made to balance the risk of harm from a relapse in pregnancy against the risk of damage to the foetus. Lithium use is associated with cardiac defects. Again, management by specialist perinatal mental health teams is advised and particular attention needs to be paid to the puerperium when acute episodes are common.

Substance abuse

Substance abuse in pregnancy poses a risk to the health of the mother and the foetus. This risk is both direct (i.e., from the abused substance itself) and indirect (i.e., from risk allied to drug use like the transmission of infection from injecting drug use).

Booking assessments are an opportunity to screen for substance abuse. This particular group may represent a challenge even if they are identified, as their attendance for antenatal care may be poor. Therefore, care from specialist midwives may improve engagement as continuity of care is provided.

Cocaine abuse is associated with growth restriction, placental abruption, stillbirth and neonatal death. Opiates are associated with growth restriction, preterm labour and neonate dependence.

Alcohol abuse is known to cause fetal anomalies and fetal alcohol syndrome. Safe amounts of alcohol intake are the subject of much continuing debate and most people would recommend no alcohol at all, especially in the first trimester. Patients who wish to continue drinking alcohol should not exceed 1 to 2 units once or twice a week and binge drinking should be strongly discouraged.

Referral to drug and alcohol treatment services is important and patients should be offered a detoxification programme where appropriate.

Smoking cessation advice should be offered at every visit and when accepted, an appropriate referral made. Smoking is associated with growth restriction, placental abruption, cot death and childhood asthma, and therefore educating patients about the risks posed by both active and passive smoking is very important. It is important to arrange serial growth scans for these women as the risk of intrauterine growth restriction is high.

● Chapter Summary

- As women are delaying their pregnancies until a later age, we are encountering more pregnancies complicated by medical disorders.
- In ideal circumstances, the medical disorder should be managed prior to conception so that treatment can be optimized in terms of using nonteratogenic agents as well as maintaining good maternal health.
- A multidisciplinary approach should be used when managing women with complex medical disorders.
- Pregnancies complicated by medical disorders require more frequent consultant-led antenatal visits and monitoring often with additional ultrasound scans.

UKMLA Conditions
Anaemia
Depression
Diabetes in pregnancy
Epilepsy
Obesity and pregnancy
Substance use disorder
Varicella zoster
VTE in pregnancy

UKMLA Presentations
Breathlessness (shortness of breath)
Chest pain
Headache
Mental health problems in pregnancy

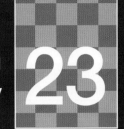
ABDOMINAL PAIN IN PREGNANCY

When assessing abdominal pain in pregnancy it is important to find out whether or not the cause is obstetric as the management options will alter accordingly. Table 23.1 shows the systems that may be involved.

History

With diverse differential diagnoses, the history is very important to identify the cause of the pain. Table 23.2 gives a summary of the points elicited from the history and examination findings that help to make the diagnosis.

Presenting symptoms

As with any history of pain, its characteristics are important. The acronym SOCRATES can be used for assessing pain:

Site – generalized or specific
Onset – sudden or gradual
Character – continuous or intermittent, stabbing or burning
Radiation – to the pelvis, back or thighs
Associations – gastrointestinal or genitourinary
Time course – duration
Exacerbating/relieving factors
Severity

Examination

Examination of the patient should be performed as described in Chapter 1. A vaginal examination may be considered. A speculum examination is appropriate to exclude bleeding, for example, in the presence of placental abruption (see Chapter 20). A digital examination may be indicated if the history and abdominal palpation suggest that the patient is in labour, to determine if there is cervical change.

COMMON PITFALLS

When examining a nonpregnant patient who has an ovarian cyst torsion is likely to elicit tenderness and guarding in the iliac fossa. Depending on the gestation, this might not be so specific in a pregnant patient because the gravid uterus interferes with the usual anatomical landmarks. Similarly, tenderness at McBurney point, which is typical of appendicitis, may be difficult to elicit in a patient who is late in the second or in the third trimester of pregnancy for a similar reason.

HINTS AND TIPS

When examining an obstetric patient, remember that they might feel faint when lying flat on their back for too long, secondary to pressure on the large vessels reducing venous return to the heart and causing supine hypotension. Pregnant patients should be examined with a left lateral tilt where possible.

Table 23.1 Differential diagnoses of abdominal pain in pregnancy

System involved	Pathology
Obstetric	Labour Placental abruption Symphysis pubis dysfunction Ligament pain Preeclampsia/HELLP syndrome Acute fatty liver of pregnancy
Gynaecological	Ovarian cyst rupture/torsion/haemorrhage Uterine fibroid degeneration
Gastrointestinal	Constipation Appendicitis Gallstones/cholecystitis Pancreatitis Peptic ulcer disease
Genitourinary	Cystitis Pyelonephritis Renal stones/renal colic

HELLP, *Haemolysis, elevated liver enzymes, low platelets.*

Investigations

Box 23.1 gives a summary of the investigations that should be considered and Fig. 23.1 provides an algorithm for the investigation of abdominal pain.

Table 23.2 Making a diagnosis from the history and examination

Differential diagnosis	Clinical features
Labour (see Chapter 26)	Intermittent pain, usually regular in frequency, associated with uterine tightening. The presenting part of the foetus is usually engaged. Vaginal examination shows cervical change.
Placental abruption (see Chapter 20)	Mild or severe pain, more commonly associated with vaginal bleeding. The uterus is usually tender on palpation and can be irritable or tense. There might be symptoms and signs of preeclampsia.
Symphysis pubis dysfunction	Pain is usually low and central in the abdomen just above the symphysis pubis, which is tender on palpation. Symptoms are worse with movement.
Ligament pain	Commonly described as sharp pain, which is bilateral and often associated with movement.
Preeclampsia/HELLP (see Chapter 21)	Epigastric or right upper quadrant pain, associated with nausea and vomiting, headache and visual disturbances. On examination there is hypertension and proteinuria.
Acute fatty liver of pregnancy	Epigastric pain or right upper quadrant pain, associated with nausea, vomiting, anorexia and malaise.
Ovarian cyst (see Chapter 11)	Unilateral pain, which is intermittent and might be associated with vomiting.
Uterine fibroids (see Chapter 5)	Pain is localized and constant. Fibroid may be noted on palpation and is tender.
Constipation	Usually suggested by the history, can cause lower abdominal discomfort and bloating.
Appendicitis	Pain associated with nausea and vomiting. Tenderness with guarding and rebound might be localized to the right iliac fossa depending on gestation. Patient may be pyrexial and have raised inflammatory markers.
Gallstones/cholecystitis	Right upper quadrant or epigastric pain which might radiate to the back or to the shoulder tip. Tenderness in the right hypochondrium, pyrexia present with cholecystitis.
Pancreatitis	Epigastric pain radiating to the back, associated with nausea and vomiting. Occurs more commonly in the third trimester.
Peptic ulcer	Epigastric pain associated with food. There might be heartburn, nausea and even haematemesis.
Cystitis	Usually suggested by history of dysuria, with pain and tenderness in the lower abdomen or suprapubically.
Renal stones/renal colic/ pyelonephritis	Loin pain that might radiate to the abdomen and groin, possibly associated with vomiting and rigors. Pyrexia is present with pyelonephritis.

HELLP, *Haemolysis, elevated liver enzymes, low platelets.*

Management

This depends on the cause of the pain and the gestation of the pregnancy. With regard to the obstetric causes, caesarean section or induction of labour (IOL) might need to be considered. For example, in severe preeclampsia, the benefits of delivery to the mother's health can outweigh the risks to the foetus of preterm birth. Placental abruption might be severe enough to compromise the foetus, and then delivery should be expedited.

However, most conditions can be managed conservatively. This includes analgesia in the presence of renal stones or antibiotics for pyelonephritis.

HINTS AND TIPS

Multidisciplinary team management of patients with suspected medical or surgical complications in pregnancy is essential (e.g., renal stones or cholecystitis). In the case of preterm labour, management must be in conjunction with the paediatricians. Do not forget to liaise with the anaesthetists for analgesia if delivery is indicated or for assistance with fluid replacement and airway management.

LARGE FOR DATES OR SMALL FOR DATES

Differential diagnosis

The growth of a pregnancy is estimated by measuring the symphysis–fundal height (SFH) after 24 weeks' gestation (see Chapter 1). This takes into account the size of the foetus, the liquor volume and the maternal structures, including the uterus. Before deciding whether the SFH is abnormal or not, last menstrual period and the scan reports should be checked to confirm the gestation of the pregnancy, and also whether it is a singleton pregnancy.

The differential diagnoses of the large-for-dates (LFD) or small-for-dates (SFD) uterus can be considered in two categories:

1. fetal or placental
2. maternal

A foetus found to be SFD can be categorized according to its growth pattern diagnosed with serial ultrasound scans:

- Small for gestational age (SGA): the foetus is small for the expected size at a certain gestation, but continues to grow at a normal rate as the pregnancy progresses.
- Intrauterine growth restriction (IUGR): the foetus is small or normal-sized for the expected size at a certain gestation, but the growth rate slows down as the pregnancy progresses.

BOX 23.1 SUMMARY OF INVESTIGATIONS TO BE CONSIDERED IN A PATIENT WITH ABDOMINAL PAIN

- Full blood count.
- Clotting studies.
- Group-and-save sample.
- Urea and electrolytes.
- Liver function tests.
- C-reactive protein.
- Glucose.
- Urinalysis/midstream urine/24-hour urine collection for protein or protein-to-creatinine ratio.
- Ultrasound scan of the uterus, ovaries, kidneys, liver and gall bladder.

HINTS AND TIPS

The symphysis–fundal height (SFH) measurement should be ± 3 cm equal to the number of weeks of pregnancy after 24 weeks (i.e., at 32 weeks a normal SFH will be between 29 and 35 cm). A discrepancy of more than 3 cm indicates large for a dates, and less than 3 cm is suggestive of small for dates.

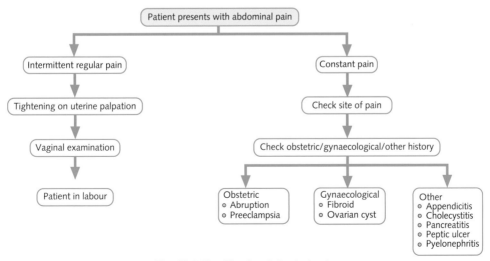

Fig. 23.1 Algorithm for abdominal pain.

History

- With respect to LFD uterus, a patient who had gestational diabetes in a previous pregnancy is at risk of developing the same condition again (see Chapter 22).
- A previous history of a baby that was SGA or IUGR, whether in relation to preeclampsia or not, increases the risk of a future pregnancy being similarly affected.
- A diagnosis of uterine fibroids or an ovarian cyst, either prior to pregnancy or in early pregnancy, can cause the SFH to palpate as LFD.
- Preexisting diabetes increases the chance of fetal macrosomia and polyhydramnios. The abdomen will palpate LFD, as in gestational diabetes.
- Fetal infection with cytomegalovirus or rubella may produce polyhydramnios, so the woman should be asked about recent flu-like illness or rash.

Current maternal disease increases the risk of IUGR, and therefore an SFD uterus (see Chapter 22):

- renal disease including renal transplantation
- hypertension
- congenital heart disease
- severe anaemia
- sickle-cell disease
- systemic lupus erythematosus
- cystic fibrosis
- human immunodeficiency virus (HIV) infection

HINTS AND TIPS

Social aspect of the history is important in this group of patients in view of the possible risk factors.

The ethnicity of the patient can be relevant in an small-for-dates patient. The growth charts used in most units were derived from Caucasian populations, in whom the average birthweight is greater than, for example, an Asian population. Hence some units have developed customized growth charts for each particular patient group.

Smoking in pregnancy is a major cause of a foetus being SGA, so that the abdomen palpates as SFD. It affects growth in the third trimester. Alcohol and illegal drug use are also causes of being small for gestational age, and so all these factors must be checked in the antenatal history.

Examination

See Chapter 1.

COMMON PITFALLS

Patients with a raised body mass index (BMI) can have undiagnosed small-for-gestational-age or intrauterine growth restriction babies as their symphysis–fundal height measurements are not accurate due to their body habitus. Serial growth scans should be arranged for women with a BMI >35 kg/m^2.

Investigations

Figs. 23.2 and 23.3 provide algorithms for the investigation of the LFD and SFD uterus.

Blood tests

- In the case of an LFD uterus where fetal macrosomia is suspected:
  - A glucose tolerance test should be arranged – for gestational diabetes.
  - Maternal antibodies [immunoglobulin M (IgM) and IgG] rubella and cytomegalovirus(CMV) – if polyhydramnios present – for fetal infection.
- SFD:
  - The blood investigations for PET – if patient is hypertensive.
  - Maternal antibodies (rubella/CMV) – for fetal infections.

HINTS AND TIPS

If there is no evidence of uteroplacental insufficiency, the other causes of the foetus being small for dates should be excluded. Look for fetal abnormalities and check for signs of in-utero infection with an ultrasound scan.

Ultrasound of the foetus

Plotting ultrasound measurements of head circumference, abdominal circumference and femur length on a growth chart is the main method of monitoring fetal growth, either LFD or SFD. In the case of SFD, serial measurements, at least 2 weeks apart, should be taken to distinguish between SGA and IUGR.

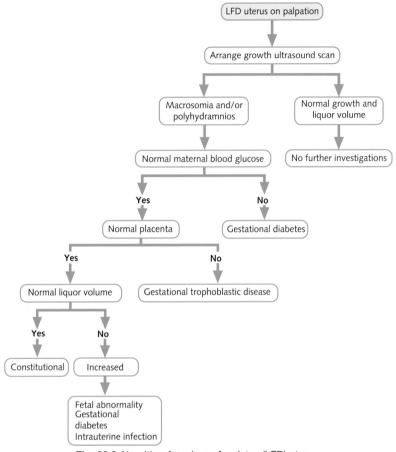

Fig. 23.2 Algorithm for a large-for-dates (LFD) uterus.

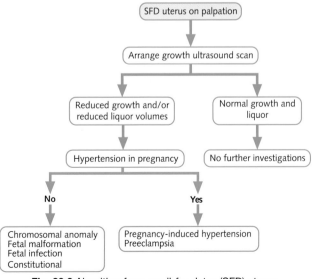

Fig. 23.3 Algorithm for a small-for-dates (SFD) uterus.

The latter is often secondary to uteroplacental insufficiency. With IUGR, the foetus preferentially diverts blood to the vital organs. There is less blood to the kidneys, and therefore reduced production of liquor (oligohydramnios), as well as less storage of glycogen in the fetal liver. The latter results in a tailing off of the abdominal circumference measurement.

HINTS AND TIPS

The fetal causes of oligohydramnios are related to its ability to produce urine and thus liquor (e.g., renal agenesis). The fetal causes of polyhydramnios are secondary to its inability to swallow liquor (e.g., oesophageal atresia or musculoskeletal disorders).

Ultrasound of the placenta and liquor volume

Trophoblastic disease is usually excluded at the 12-week dating scan by checking the structure of the placenta (see Chapter 18). This condition very rarely presents later in pregnancy with a uterus that palpates LFD.

A scan can also be used to measure the liquor volume objectively. The amniotic fluid index is the sum of the fluid pockets in the four quadrants of the abdomen. The amount varies with gestation, but the normal range is 5 to 25 cm. Liquor volume is also measured in terms of the deepest vertical pocket. During scan, the deepest pocket of fluid that is free of umbilical cord or fetal parts is measured vertically. A measurement of <2 cm indicates oligohydramnios, 2 to 8 cm is normal and >8 cm indicates polyhydramnios. Box 23.2 shows the causes of increased or decreased liquor.

Doppler studies

In conjunction with growth scans and measurement of the liquor volume, Doppler waveforms of the blood flow in the uteroplacental and fetal circulations can be used to assess the foetus. Increased placental vascular resistance, for example, in preeclampsia, changes the pattern of the flow in the umbilical artery. There is normally flow towards the placenta during fetal diastole. However, as the placental resistance increases, diastolic flow becomes absent and then reversed. Other vessels can also be examined within the foetus, including the middle cerebral artery and the ductus venosus, to look for patterns of flow redistribution or, in severe cases, heart failure which can occur if the placental blood flow is insufficient.

Maternal ultrasound

Ultrasound scan is useful to diagnose uterine fibroids or the presence of ovarian cysts which make the maternal abdomen palpate as large for dates.

BOX 23.2 CAUSES OF INCREASED OR DECREASED LIQUOR VOLUME

Increased liquor volume	Decreased liquor volume
Diabetes	Ruptured membranes
Fetal abnormality	Fetal abnormality
Multiple pregnancy	Aneuploidy
Fetal infection	Fetal infection
	Intrauterine growth restriction
	Maternal drugs (e.g., atenolol)

Cardiotocography

The cardiotocography (CTG) can be used to assess the IUGR foetus. When not in labour, the tracing might be abnormal if the uteroplacental insufficiency is severe. The presence of the following should be excluded:

- reduced variability
- bradycardia
- tachycardia
- decelerations

Management

Management of LGA (large for gestational age) will depend on gestation, underlying conditions (such as diabetes) and maternal preferences. There is conflicting evidence on IOL for LGA pregnancies. 'Big baby trial' is a UK-based ongoing large prospective study which aims to find out if IOL should be recommended in pregnancies with LGA.

A senior obstetrician should be involved in determining the timing and mode of delivery of SGA/IUGR pregnancies. Most of the time these pregnancies result in IOL or caesarean section before the due date.

REDUCED FETAL MOVEMENTS

Patients start feeling fetal movements between 18 and 20 weeks' gestation and it is recognized as a sign of fetal well-being. Fetal movements quickly develop a regular pattern and any reduction or change in this pattern may be an important clinical sign that may indicate the foetus is not thriving in utero. Women should be taught to monitor their baby's own pattern of movements and present to hospital if they have noticed a reduction or absent movements.

History

Normal fetal movements imply that the foetus' central nervous system and musculoskeletal systems are functioning. In the history, identify if this is the first episode of reduced fetal movement, and quantify the duration and nature of reduced fetal movements. Risk factors for stillbirth and growth restriction need to be identified. These include:

- hypertension
- IUGR
- diabetes
- smoking
- previous stillbirth
- primiparous
- multiple episodes of reduced fetal movements
- congenital malformation
- maternal obesity

Drug and social history are important as some sedating drugs such as alcohol, benzodiazepines, methadone or opioids can cross the placenta and cause reduced fetal movements.

A review of the anomaly ultrasound and placenta location should be undertaken as those women with an anterior placenta may have a reduced perception of fetal movements. Foetuses with major congenital malformations may move less due to abnormalities within their muscular, skeletal or central nervous systems.

Examination and investigations

- Routine examination as covered in Chapter 1.
- A CTG should be performed if patient is in the third trimester. A normal CTG (see Chapter 27) will indicate that the foetus is healthy with an intact autonomic nervous system.
- An ultrasound scan for growth and liquor volume assessment could be performed especially, if there are persistently reduced movements even with a normal CTG, or if there is an abnormal SFH measurement.

Management

Management will depend on gestation and maternal preferences. IOL may be considered especially if persistently reduced movements at term.

● Chapter Summary

- Taking a thorough history from a pregnant patient presenting with abdominal pain can identify treatable causes.
- You should perform an abdominal, speculum and vaginal examination for patients presenting with abdominal pain in the second and third trimesters of pregnancy.
- Perform an ultrasound to assess fetal growth in patients who present measuring large or small for dates and investigate further if the ultrasound scan is abnormal.
- When a woman presents with reduced fetal movements, she should be fully assessed and induction of labour should be considered if the pregnancy is at full-term gestation.

UKMLA Presentations
Reduced/change in fetal movements
Small for gestational age/large for gestational age

Multiple pregnancies account for 2% to 3% of all live births. The incidence has been rising due to increased maternal age and artificial reproductive techniques. The risk of pregnancy complications such as preterm birth and growth restriction is greater in multiple pregnancies compared to singleton pregnancies.

AETIOLOGY OF TWINS

Zygosity and chorionicity

The majority of twins (75%) are dizygotic, that is, they arise from the fertilization of two ova by two sperm. Each foetus has its own chorion, amnion and placenta – dichorionic diamniotic placentation. The placentae can appear fused if implantation occurs close together. These twins can be of the same or different sexes and will have different genetic constitutions (i.e., they have no more similarities than any siblings; Fig. 24.1).

Monozygotic twins (25%) arise following the fertilization of a single ovum by a single sperm, which then completely divides so that each twin has the same genetic makeup. Cell division may occur at different stages of embryonic development, giving rise to different structural arrangements of the membranes (Fig. 24.1). A third of monozygotic twins establish at the eight-cell stage, so that two separate blastocysts form and implant. These twins will thus have dichorionic diamniotic placentation. About two-thirds of monozygotic twins have monochorionic diamniotic placentation: that is, a single blastocyst implants, developing a single chorion; the inner cell mass divides into two so that each embryo has its own amnion. The least common type of monozygotic twins occurs by later splitting of the inner cell mass, before the appearance of the primitive streak, to produce a single amniotic cavity – monochorionic monoamniotic twins. Splitting even later than this results in conjoined twins. The incidence of monozygotic twins is constant around the world, at about 4 per 1000 births.

DIAGNOSIS OF CHORIONICITY

Diagnosis

Nowadays, multiple pregnancies are diagnosed by routine dating ultrasound scan at 11 to 14 weeks' gestation. Clinical situations in which the diagnosis should be suspected include a patient who presents with hyperemesis gravidarum, or if clinical examination reveals either a large-for-dates uterus or multiple fetal parts in later pregnancy.

Antenatally

The optimal way to determine chorionicity by ultrasound at 11 to 14 weeks' gestation is to assess the area between the interfetal membrane and placenta. This area involves a triangular placental tissue projection in DC twins, called lambda (λ) sign. Whereas in MC twins there is no placental tissue projection and this represents

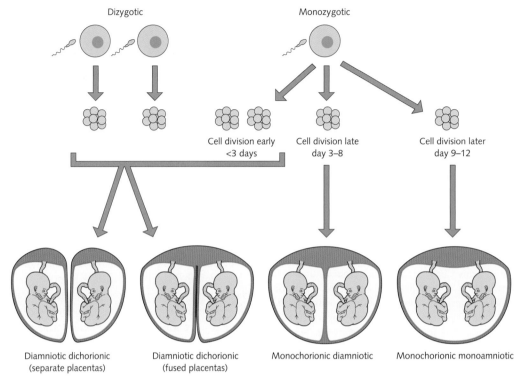

Diamniotic dichorionic
(separate placentas)

Diamniotic dichorionic
(fused placentas)

Monochorionic diamniotic

Monochorionic monoamniotic

Fig. 24.1 Aetiology of twinning.

the T sign. If there is no dividing membrane between the foetuses, they are monochorionic monoamniotic twins. The ideal time to identify chorionicity is the first trimester as with advancing gestation λ sign regresses in 15% of DC pregnancies.

Fetal sex can also be assessed by ultrasound. If they are discordant, then the pregnancy must be dichorionic (as the foetuses must come from two separate ova and sperm). Localization of the placental sites may also be helpful. If the placentae can be seen as being completely separate, then similarly, the pregnancy must be dichorionic.

Postnatally

At this stage, chorionicity can be determined by:

- macroscopic and microscopic examination of membranes
- analysis of red blood cell markers
- DNA probes

COMPLICATIONS

A multiple pregnancy must be treated as a high-risk pregnancy. The majority of pregnancy-related complications are more common in multiple pregnancies (e.g., gestational diabetes or preeclampsia). There are also certain problems that are specific to multiple pregnancies.

RED FLAGS

The mother with a multiple pregnancy is at risk of any complication associated with a singleton pregnancy but all the risks are increased.

Fetal malformations

The frequency of fetal malformations is thought to be almost double in a twin pregnancy compared with a singleton pregnancy, especially for monochorionic twins (4% cf. 2%). In terms of screening for chromosomal anomalies, parents can be offered nuchal translucency and combined blood test screening. They must be counselled about the possibility of a high-chance result in one baby, but a low-chance one in the other. With an invasive procedure, there is a greater risk of pregnancy loss than in a singleton pregnancy. Separate sampling must be performed with dichorionic twins.

Antenatal assessment of fetal well-being and growth

In a multiple pregnancy, antenatal care should be led by a consultant in a unit with facilities for regular ultrasound scans to check fetal growth. These patients are reviewed more frequently compared to singleton pregnancies as the pregnancy-related risks are higher.

Serial ultrasounds are usually performed every 4 weeks from 24 weeks in a dichorionic pregnancy, and every 2 weeks from 16 weeks in a monochorionic pregnancy, to monitor growth. In a monochorionic pregnancy, the scans also monitor the development of twin-to-twin transfusion syndrome (see Twin-to-twin transfusion syndrome (TTTS) below).

Preterm labour

Spontaneous preterm labour occurs in 30% of twin pregnancies. If preterm labour is diagnosed, tocolytics should be considered to allow in utero transfer to a hospital with neonatal intensive care facilities and to allow time for steroids administered to the mother to improve lung maturation. Cervical suture is NOT recommended in twin pregnancies to prevent preterm delivery as data show no benefit (see Chapter 25).

Pregnancy-induced hypertension and preeclampsia

Hypertension is about three times more common in multiple pregnancies than in singleton pregnancies because of the larger size of the placental bed (see Chapter 21). Hypertension and preeclampsia often develop earlier and can be more severe than in a singleton pregnancy. National guidelines recommend consideration for aspirin 75 mg daily from 12 weeks' gestation to reduce the risk of preeclampsia.

Antepartum haemorrhage

The incidence of placental abruption and placenta praevia is increased in multiple pregnancies (see Chapter 20).

Twin-to-twin transfusion syndrome

TTTS results from an imbalance in the blood flow across the placental vascular communications between twins and complicates 10% to 15% of MC pregnancies. The donor foetus becomes anaemic and growth restricted, with oligohydramnios, and the recipient foetus becomes fluid overloaded with polyhydramnios.

This syndrome usually occurs in the second trimester, and therefore scanning every 2 weeks is advised from 16 weeks. The condition results in fetal death in up to 80% of cases if left untreated and a 10% risk of handicap in the surviving twin. Depending on the stage of the disease at diagnosis, up to 26 weeks, laser treatment to the placental anastomoses is generally the advised option to reduce discordant blood flow between the foetuses (known as 'fetoscopic laser ablation of the placenta). Amniodrainage may be appropriate for symptom relief at later gestations.

In MC pregnancies, fetal death of a twin in utero puts the surviving twin at risk of neurological damage (15%–26%). In addition, it can also affect the mother, who is at risk of developing disseminated intravascular coagulation due to thromboplastins being released into the circulation. Magnetic resonance imaging of the surviving twin has been used in some units to assess neurological morbidity. The pregnancy can be managed conservatively until the surviving twin reaches a gestation with a better likelihood of survival.

INTRAPARTUM MANAGEMENT OF A TWIN PREGNANCY

Box 24.1 summarizes the management of vaginal delivery in a twin pregnancy.

Delivery of twin pregnancy

The mode of delivery depends on the presentation of the first twin (presenting twin); twin one is cephalic in more than 80% of pregnancies. If presentation of twin one is anything other than cephalic, caesarean section is advised. In the case of higher-order multiple pregnancies, delivery is almost always by caesarean section.

For a vaginal delivery, the onset of labour can be spontaneous or induced; induction is advised by 36 to 37 weeks for a monochorionic twin pregnancy and by 37 to 38 weeks for a dichorionic pregnancy. The woman needs intravenous access and a sample of serum saved in the blood transfusion laboratory because of the risk of postpartum haemorrhage (see below). An epidural block is often recommended to allow for possible manipulation of the second twin in the second stage of labour.

Both fetal heart rates should be monitored continuously, either per abdomen or with a fetal scalp electrode on the first twin. If there is an abnormality in the heart rate pattern of twin one, fetal blood sampling might be appropriate (see Chapter 27). Concerns with twin two should lead to immediate delivery by caesarean section. The reasons for augmentation of labour and for instrumental delivery are similar to those in a singleton pregnancy (see Chapter 28).

Once the first twin is delivered, the lie and presentation of the second twin must be determined by abdominal palpation and ultrasound. External cephalic version can be used to establish a longitudinal lie. Intravenous syntocinon may be necessary to maintain uterine contractions and the delivery of the second twin occurs either as a cephalic presentation or by internal podalic version and breech extraction. Again, the reasons for instrumental delivery or caesarean section are similar to those of a singleton pregnancy.

Complications

Postpartum haemorrhage
Postpartum haemorrhage (see Chapter 31) is more likely with a multiple pregnancy than a singleton because of the larger placental site. Uterine atony due to the increased volume of the uterine contents – two foetuses, placentae, etc. – is a contributing factor. Active management of the third stage of labour is, therefore, appropriate, including routine use of a postpartum syntocinon infusion.

Locked twins
This is a very rare complication of vaginal deliveries when the first twin is breech. As the delivery proceeds, the aftercoming head of the first twin is prevented from entering the pelvis by the head of the cephalic second twin. If this is diagnosed in the first stage of labour, a caesarean section should be performed; during the second stage, general anaesthesia is necessary to allow manipulation.

HIGHER-ORDER MULTIPLE PREGNANCIES (TRIPLETS OR MORE)

In comparison to twin pregnancies, higher-order multiples are associated with a higher perinatal mortality rate and an increased incidence of the aforementioned antenatal complications. Fertility treatments have increased the number of high-order pregnancies and, in the case of in vitro fertilization, guidelines in the UK now advise that a maximum of two embryos should be replaced in a woman under the age of 40 years (see Chapter 16). Pregnancies of higher-order multiples may be formed by separate embryos. Alternatively, one of the embryos may split to form a monochorionic pair of twins.

Selective fetocide (multifetal pregnancy reduction)

With triplets or more, it is appropriate to counsel the parents about selective fetal reduction, with the aim of reducing the risks of late miscarriage and preterm labour by keeping only one or two babies. Several methods, such as chemical, thermal, radiofrequency and laser could be used depending on chorionicity as well as other factors. For example intracardiac potassium chloride cannot be performed on a monochorionic twin because the injected foetus shares placental circulation with its co-twin and, therefore, the drugs would affect both foetuses. It is usually performed at 12 to 14 weeks' gestation, after results of screening for Down syndrome have been obtained if the parents wish this test. Despite the procedure-related risk of miscarriage of up to 7%, the incidence of complications is low.

ETHICS

Care must be taken to establish a couple's religious and moral views regarding abortion, when counselling about selective fetal reduction in high-order multiple pregnancies. It must be balanced against the chances of taking home babies who have not been compromised by premature birth.

● Chapter Summary

- Monozygotic twins arise following fertilization of a single ovum by a single sperm which then divides, so that each twin has the same genetic material (identical twins).
- Dizygotic twins arise following fertilization of two ova by two sperm.
- Chorionicity relates to placentation and is ideally diagnosed on the dating ultrasound scan performed before 14 weeks' gestation.
- Twin pregnancies are high risk and consultant-led antenatal care is required and screening for pregnancy-related conditions such as gestational diabetes and preeclampsia should be undertaken.

PRETERM LABOUR AND BIRTH

Preterm is defined as babies born alive before 37 weeks of pregnancy completed – according to the WHO (World Health Organization). Preterm labour (PTL) is when labour begins before 37 weeks gestation, which can lead to preterm birth (PTB). It is important to establish PTL for several reasons:

1. PTL has a higher risk of complications than term labour, for example, abnormal lie or malpresentation.
2. Prematurity is the leading cause of neonatal morbidity and mortality in the UK – liaison with the paediatric team is essential – preterm babies have a significantly increased mortality rate compared with term babies.
3. Up to 34 + 0 weeks' gestation attempts should be made – if clinically appropriate – to stop the labour only to allow time for the administration of corticosteroids to the mother. This will boost fetal lung surfactant production and, therefore, reduce neonatal respiratory distress.

INCIDENCE

The incidence of PTL is currently around 8% in England and Wales, but this varies in different populations and the incidence is increasing. Risk factors for premature labour are presented in Box 25.1. The main causes of preterm delivery are given in Box 25.2.

Infection is thought to play a part in at least 20% of cases (Box 25.3 lists common pathogens implicated in PTL).

Iatrogenic preterm delivery, accounting for one-third of preterm deliveries, occurs when obstetricians decide that delivery is necessary in the interests of fetal or maternal health, due, for example, to severe preeclampsia, or when scans have shown severe intrauterine growth restriction of the foetus.

HISTORY

PTL may be rapid in onset and progress and is almost always unexpected. Therefore, a comprehensive history taking is important which must include the onset, frequency and intensity of abdominal pain (see Chapter 23). Intermittent, but regular abdominal pain suggests uterine contractions. PTL may be

---

BOX 25.1 RISK FACTORS FOR PRETERM LABOUR

- Previous preterm birth or mid-trimester loss (16 to 34 weeks of pregnancy)
- Previous preterm premature rupture of membranes
- Previous delivery by caesarean section at full dilatation
- History of cervical cerclage in a previous pregnancy
- Smoking
- Low socioeconomic group
- Maternal age (<18 years)
- Domestic violence, lack of social support
- UTI or vaginal infections such as bacterial vaginosis
- Chronic medical conditions
- Multiple pregnancy
- Uterine variants such as unicornuate uterus
- Previous cone biopsy or large loop excision of the transformation zone or trachelectomy

---

BOX 25.2 CAUSES OF PRETERM LABOUR

- Infection (e.g., chorioamnionitis, maternal pyelonephritis).
- Uteroplacental ischaemia (e.g., abruption).
- Uterine overdistension (e.g., polyhydramnios, multiple pregnancy).
- Cervical incompetence.
- Fetal abnormality.
- Iatrogenic (e.g., delivery for severe intrauterine growth restriction caused by preeclampsia).

BOX 25.3 PATHOGENS IMPLICATED IN PRETERM LABOUR

- Sexually transmitted: *Chlamydia*, *Trichomonas*, syphilis, gonorrhoea.
- Enteric organisms: *Escherichia coli*, *Streptococcus faecalis*.
- Bacterial vaginosis: *Gardnerella*, *Mycoplasma* and anaerobes.
- Group B streptococcus (if a very heavy growth).

associated with clear watery vaginal discharge, suggesting possible rupture of the membranes, or bleeding, as with an antepartum haemorrhage (see Chapter 20). As infections are the leading cause for PTL, urinary and gastrointestinal symptoms should be elicited, as well as systemic symptoms such as fever. A past medical history and a social history should be taken to identify the risk factors shown in Box 25.1.

EXAMINATION

The examination must include baseline observations – pulse, blood pressure, respiratory rate and temperature – to look for signs of possible infection. The following needs to be checked when performing abdominal palpation:

- abdominal tenderness – site, guarding, rebound
- uterine tenderness – site
- uterine tone – soft or irritable (e.g., abruption)
- uterine contractions – frequency and strength
- fetal lie, presentation and engagement

A sterile speculum examination should be performed on a woman with abdominal pain and/or discharge. A vaginal swab should be taken if there is a clear watery loss suggesting ruptured membranes or if an abnormal vaginal discharge is present. If there is no obvious pooling of liquor but the patient provides a good history of ruptured membranes, then a test for the presence of amniotic fluid can be performed (e.g., AmniSure test). A fetal fibronectin test is appropriate between 24 + 0 and 33 + 6 weeks – the vaginal swab should be taken at this time (see below). A digital examination may be necessary to check the dilatation of the cervix. A closed cervix in the presence of palpable uterine contractions is called 'threatened preterm labour'.

INVESTIGATIONS

As abnormal lie and malpresentation are far more common in preterm pregnancy, an ultrasound scan should be performed to confirm the presentation of the foetus (see Chapter 29). Up to 25 + 6 weeks' gestation, the presence of the fetal heartbeat should be confirmed with a Sonicaid. After this gestation, a cardiotocograph should be performed, which will assess fetal well-being as well as indicate uterine activity.

Evidence of fetal fibronectin in the mother's cervical secretions can be checked using a specific kit and a vaginal swab; absence of fetal fibronectin, i.e., a negative test, suggests that

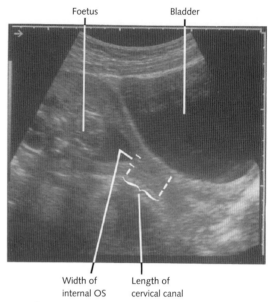

Foetus   Bladder

Width of   Length of
internal OS   cervical canal

Fig. 25.1 Transabdominal scan of cervical canal. *OS,* Obstetric ultrasound. (From Chudleigh T. *Obstetric Ultrasound: How, Why and When*. 3rd Edition. London: Churchill Livingstone; 2004. With permission from Elsevier.)

delivery is less likely and this may assist with management decisions such as the need for fetal steroids and tocolysis. Transvaginal scans may be used to examine the length of the cervix because cervical shortening is a predictor of preterm delivery (Fig. 25.1). Urinalysis must be performed to look for nitrites, which suggest a urinary tract infection.

MANAGEMENT

Box 25.4 summarizes the management plan for a woman who appears to be in PTL.

Liaison with the neonatal team and administration of steroids are vital. Some hospitals do not have facilities for treating babies born under certain gestations and in these cases transfer to the nearest appropriate unit is made, preferably prior to delivery known as an 'in utero transfer'. If the mother is unwell or if delivery is imminent, transfer of the baby can be arranged after delivery known as an 'ex utero transfer'. Ideally, the neonatologist will have an opportunity to counsel the woman and her partner about expectations when the baby is born and some of the problems that premature babies encounter.

BOX 25.4 MANAGEMENT CHECKLIST FOR A PATIENT PRESENTING IN THREATENED PRETERM LABOUR

- Assess for signs of a precipitant of preterm labour (e.g., sepsis, polyhydramnios, abruption, severe preeclampsia, obstetric cholestasis).
- Investigate with blood tests as appropriate, perform urine analysis and send midstream sample of urine.
- Determine the frequency and regularity of contractions.
- Ascertain fetal presentation and confirm with ultrasound.
- Monitor fetal heart with Sonicaid or cardiotocography if appropriate gestation.
- Perform a sterile speculum examination to examine the cervix and assess if membranes have ruptured. Take a high vaginal swab. A vaginal examination may be required to ascertain cervical dilatation.
- Consider corticosteroids.
- Give antibiotics if the membranes have ruptured or obvious signs of sepsis are present.
- Consider tocolysis (only to allow time for steroids or if it's required for intrauterine transfer).
- Contact neonatal team and arrange a transfer if necessary and appropriate.
- Discuss the mode of delivery with the patient.

COMMUNICATION

Parents need to be informed of problems encountered by children surviving extreme premature delivery, which include cerebral palsy, chronic lung disease, visual and hearing deficits and learning difficulties.

Tocolysis and steroids

Administration of drugs to reduce the uterine activity should be considered depending on:

- Cervical dilatation
- Need to administer steroids and allow time for them to be effective
- Need for in utero transfer

HINTS AND TIPS

Corticosteroids (betamethasone or dexamethasone) are given to the woman as two intramuscular injections 12 to 24 hours apart. They have been shown to significantly reduce neonatal respiratory distress by stimulating fetal surfactant production and are recommended for any woman in threatened preterm labour between 24 + 0 and 33 + 6 weeks' gestation. This can be extended up to 35 + 6 weeks if there are other risk factors such as intrauterine growth restriction. Repeated courses of steroid administration could be considered on an individual basis if the most recent course was given 7 days ago and the chances of delivery are high within the following 48 hours.

Table 25.1 Drugs used to treat preterm labour

Drug	Route of administration	Comments/side effects
Calcium-channel blockers (e.g., nifedipine)	Oral	Block calcium channels in the myometrium to reduce contractions. Not licenced in UK for this use. Side effects include headache, flushing and tremor.
Oxytocin receptor antagonists (e.g., atosiban)	Intravenous	Well tolerated but expensive. 8% experience headache.

The different drugs used to try to stop contractions are shown in Table 25.1. They have been shown to delay the number of women who deliver within 48 hours, but there is no clear evidence that they improve perinatal morbidity and mortality overall. They allow time for corticosteroids and, if necessary, transfer to another hospital able to offer neonatal care, as mentioned earlier. With all drugs, the side effects on mother and foetus must be balanced against the benefit of prolonging the pregnancy. Tocolysis should not be used in the following circumstances:

- Maternal illness that would be helped by delivery (e.g., preeclampsia)
- Evidence of fetal distress
- In the presence of chorioamnionitis

- When there has been significant vaginal bleeding, particularly if abruption is suspected
- Once the membranes have ruptured

Magnesium sulphate

In cases of established labour or planned preterm delivery where the gestation is below 30 weeks, a magnesium sulphate infusion should be commenced. This drug causes cerebral vasodilation and therefore provides the foetus with neuroprotection. It has been proven to reduce rates of cerebral palsy in preterm infants. At gestations between 30 and 33 + 6 weeks, an infusion can be considered.

Antibiotic therapy

Intrapartum antibiotics are offered to women who are in PTL. Antibiotics (erythromycin) are given prophylactically if the membranes have ruptured and the women are not in labour before term (around one-third of cases) to protect the foetus from ascending vaginal infection.

Mode of delivery

In most cases of PTL, it is possible to plan for a normal vaginal birth. There is no firm evidence to show that caesarean section is safer for the baby than vaginal delivery, especially when the presentation is cephalic. However, the caesarean section rate is higher than for term pregnancies because of a higher incidence of low-lying placenta, fetal distress and abnormal lie in prematurity. Caesarean section might have higher morbidity for the mother, particularly at very early gestations because the lower segment is not formed, increasing the necessity of having to use a classical uterine incision.

RED FLAGS

The following procedures are contraindicated in preterm labour:
- application of fetal scalp electrode
- fetal blood sampling
- ventouse delivery

PRETERM PRELABOUR RUPTURE OF MEMBRANES

Preterm prelabour rupture of membranes (PPROM) occurs in only 2% of pregnancies but is associated with 40% of preterm

deliveries. The principal issue is the risk of sepsis, both maternal and fetal. Maternal sepsis with ascending uterine infection can rapidly become overwhelming if not monitored and may cause severe morbidity and mortality, as well as affect future fertility. Sepsis in the infant is one of the three leading causes of mortality in the preterm infant, along with prematurity and pulmonary hypoplasia.

History and examination

History and examination should be performed as described earlier. A digital examination should only be performed if there are obvious signs of labour, as it may introduce infection higher up into the genital tract. A high vaginal swab should be taken.

Management

Management involves monitoring for symptoms and signs of clinical chorioamnionitis. Unwell women will be delivered without waiting for fetal maturation. These symptoms include:

- Feeling unwell such as fever or shivering
- abdominal pain
- Change in colour of vaginal loss from clear to green or brown
- Foul-smelling vaginal loss
- Raised maternal temperature, pulse or respiratory rate
- Tender uterus on palpation

Investigations include a cardiotocograph to exclude fetal tachycardia. Maternal blood tests can suggest infection including a raised C-reactive protein and white blood cell count. However, chorioamnionitis should not be discounted if these tests are normal in the presence of obvious clinical signs.

Expectant management (i.e., with no symptoms or signs of infection) involves:

- Administration of erythromycin (250 mg) four times a day for 10 days to reduce chorioamnionitis.
- Administration of corticosteroids to improve fetal lung maturity.

Some women will start to labour within 72 hours, but for those who do not, the general principle is to aim to deliver from 34 weeks of gestation. This will be either by induction of labour if the presentation is cephalic or by caesarean section with an abnormal lie. Tocolytics are not used in PPROM.

Management of future pregnancies

Prophylactic vaginal progesterone or cervical cerclage should be offered to reduce the risk of preterm delivery in future pregnancies if a patient has both:

- A history of spontaneous PTB – before 34 weeks or pregnancy loss from 16 weeks.

- A cervical length less than 25 mm between 16 and 24 weeks of gestation in the ongoing pregnancy – (transvaginal ultrasound).

There is no evidence to determine which of these options (progesterone vs. cervical cerclage) is superior in preventing PTB. Therefore, vaginal progesterone should be offered as an equal option with cervical suture. If a woman has only one of the risk factors mentioned earlier, then vaginal progesterone can still be considered. Also, patients who have a cervical length less than 25 mm (measured with transvaginal US between 16 and 24 weeks) cervical cerclage can be considered if there is a history of PPROM or cervical trauma.

Cervical cerclage

There are different types of cervical sutures classified based on the anatomical area in which the cerclage is inserted.

- Transvaginal cerclage (McDonald): A transvaginal purse-string suture placed at the cervical isthmus junction. The bladder is not mobilized and this is the most commonly used cerclage in clinical practice (see Fig. 25.2).
- High transvaginal cerclage requiring bladder mobilization (including Shirodkar): The purse-string suture is placed following bladder mobilization, to aim an insertion above the cardinal ligament level.
- Transabdominal cerclage: This type of suture is now usually inserted via a laparoscopy. The suture is placed at the cervicoisthmic junction.

Previous terminology (prophylactic, as a planned procedure, emergency, urgent, rescue) of cervical sutures has been recently changed as this could be ambiguous. The new terminology is based on the indication of the suture.

- History-indicated cerclage: Cerclage inserted in view of the previous history, performed as a prophylactic measure in asymptomatic women between 11 and 14 weeks of gestation. **Women with three or more previous PTBs should be offered a history-indicated cervical cerclage if the pregnancy is singleton.**
- Ultrasound-indicated cerclage: Cerclage inserted as a therapeutic measure in cases of cervical length shortening

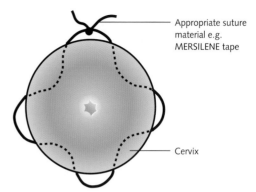

Fig. 25.2 The McDonald suture.

seen on serial transvaginal ultrasound. It is performed on asymptomatic women who do not have exposed fetal membranes in the vagina. Cervical length measurement is performed between 14 and 24 weeks of pregnancy by transvaginal scan, if measuring less than 25 mm and the patient has a history of PTB/PPROM/cervical trauma – cerclage can be offered.

- Emergency cerclage: Inserted in the case of premature cervical dilatation with exposed fetal membranes in the vagina. However, insertion of any suture can introduce infection and result in rupture of the membranes during the procedure or within a couple of weeks. This may lead to miscarriage or PTL depending on the gestation. Therefore prior to the procedure patients need to be informed about the risks and the benefits and the decision should be individualized.

RED FLAGS

Contraindications to cervical cerclage include:
- signs of infection
- vaginal bleeding
- uterine contractions
- ruptured membranes

Chapter Summary

- Preterm labour is defined as labour occurring before 37 weeks of gestation.
- Prematurity is the single largest cause of neonatal mortality and long-term handicap in otherwise normal babies.
- Cervical cerclage or vaginal progesterone pessaries could be offered as preventative measures.
- A course of corticosteroids should be considered for women in suspected preterm labour especially before 34 weeks of gestation, as this has been shown to significantly reduce neonatal respiratory distress.
- Magnesium sulphate infusion is neuroprotective for foetuses below 30 weeks and can be considered up to 33 + 6 weeks' gestation.
- Antibiotic treatment should be commenced once the membranes have ruptured in threatened preterm labour.
- The neonatal team should be informed at the earliest opportunity as they need to counsel the parents and prepare for the preterm delivery.

UKMLA Presentations

Labour

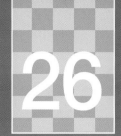
OBSTETRIC PELVIC EXAMINATION

Indications for performing this examination include assessment in labour, assessment of membrane rupture and vaginal bleeding. The examination involves:

- external inspection of the vulva
- internal inspection of the vagina and cervix
- vaginal examination if indicated

External examination

The blood flow through the vulva and vagina increases dramatically in pregnancy. The vulva might look swollen and oedematous secondary to engorgement. Vaginal discharge, leaking amniotic fluid or any bleeding and signs of female genital mutilation should be noted.

Internal inspection of the vagina and cervix

Examination of the vagina and cervix with a sterile speculum should be performed using an aseptic technique. Increased vaginal and cervical secretions are normal in pregnancy. Inspection of the cervix might reveal amniotic fluid draining through the cervical os. Digital examination in the presence of ruptured membranes is likely to increase the risk of ascending infection and is, therefore, usually avoided unless there are regular uterine contractions. Exclusion of cervical pathology is important in the presence of bleeding, such as a cervical polyp or ectropion.

Vaginal examination

This should be performed under aseptic conditions in the presence of intact membranes. Once the cervix has been identified, the following characteristics should be determined:

- dilatation
- length
- position of cervix
- consistency
- station of presenting part
- position of presenting part

Cervical dilatation is assessed in centimetres using the examining fingers. One finger's breadth is roughly 1 to 1.5 cm. Full dilatation of the cervix is equivalent to 10-cm dilatation.

When not in established labour, the normal length of the cervix is about 3 cm. Shortening occurs as the cervix effaces, becoming part of the lower segment of the uterus, in the presence of regular uterine contractions (Fig. 26.1). Softening of the cervix occurs as pregnancy progresses, aiding cervical effacement and dilatation. The consistency of the cervix can be described as firm, mid-consistency or soft. The position describes where the cervix is situated in the anteroposterior plane of the pelvis. As the cervix becomes effaced and dilated, it tends to become more anterior in position.

The 'station' of the presenting part is determined by how much the presenting part has descended into the pelvis. The station is defined as the number of centimetres above or below a fixed point in the maternal pelvis, the ischial spines. This should equate to the engagement found on abdominal palpation (Fig. 26.2).

Using the aforementioned characteristics, Bishop devised a scoring system (the Bishop score) to evaluate the 'ripeness' or favourability of the cervix (Table 26.1). This system is used as an objective tool when inducing labour to assess the cervix. The higher the score, the more favourable the cervix is and the more likely that induction of labour (IOL) will be successful.

CLINICAL NOTES

The routine examination for the process and progress of labour is cervical assessment.

When assessing progress in labour one must always comment on engagement of head, cervical dilatation, cervical effacement, station of head in relation to ischial spines, position of head, moulding, caput and liquor colour (e.g., meconium staining).

The Bishop score is used in the assessment of cervical favourability prior to induction of labour.

Defining the position of the presenting part

With a cephalic presentation, the anterior and posterior fontanelles and the sagittal sutures should be identified. The posterior fontanelle is Y-shaped and is formed when the three sutures between the occipital and parietal bones meet. The anterior fontanelle is larger, diamond-shaped and formed by the four

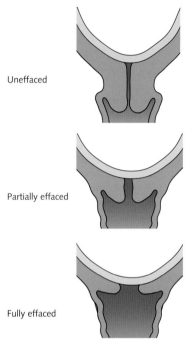

Fig. 26.1 Effacement of uterine cervix.

Uneffaced

Partially effaced

Fully effaced

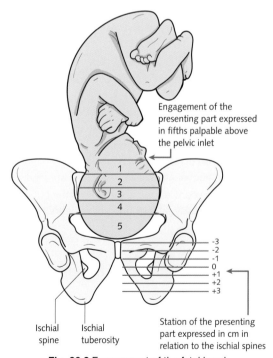

Engagement of the presenting part expressed in fifths palpable above the pelvic inlet

1
2
3
4
5

-3
-2
-1
0
+1
+2
+3

Ischial spine

Ischial tuberosity

Station of the presenting part expressed in cm in relation to the ischial spines

Fig. 26.2 Engagement of the fetal head.

Table 26.1	The Bishop score system			
Cervical characteristic	**Score**			
	0	**1**	**2**	**3**
Dilatation (cm)	0	1–2	3–4	> 4
Length (cm)	3	2	1	< 1
Station (cm)	3	2	1 or 0	+1 or +2
Consistency	Firm	Medium	Soft	
Position	Posterior	Mid	Anterior	

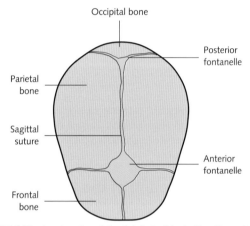

Occipital bone

Posterior fontanelle

Parietal bone

Sagittal suture

Anterior fontanelle

Frontal bone

Fig. 26.3 The landmarks of the fetal skull including the anterior and posterior fontanelles.

sutures between the meeting of the parietal and temporal bones (Fig. 26.3). The position of the presenting part can be defined as shown in Fig. 26.4. The presence of caput and moulding should also be checked as it is important to assess the progress of labour. Caput is the subcutaneous swelling on the fetal scalp that can be felt during labour and this increases if the labour is prolonged with failure of the cervix to dilate. 'Moulding' is the term used to describe the overlapping of the skull bones that occurs as labour progresses.

INTRODUCTION – LABOUR

Labour has three stages:

- First stage: from the onset of established labour until the cervix is fully dilated.
- Second stage: from full dilatation until the foetus is born.
- Third stage: from the birth of the foetus until delivery of the placenta and membranes.

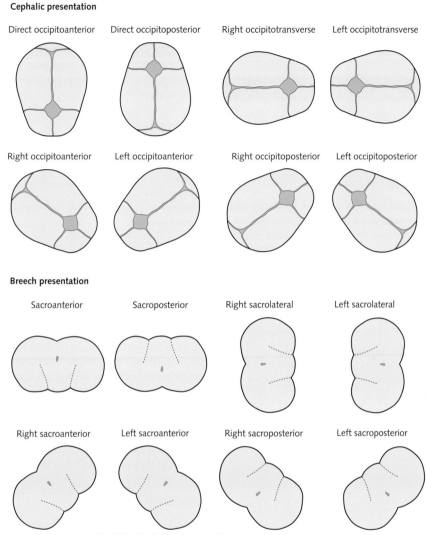

Cephalic presentation

Direct occipitoanterior   Direct occipitoposterior   Right occipitotransverse   Left occipitotransverse

Right occipitoanterior   Left occipitoanterior   Right occipitoposterior   Left occipitoposterior

Breech presentation

Sacroanterior   Sacroposterior   Right sacrolateral   Left sacrolateral

Right sacroanterior   Left sacroanterior   Right sacroposterior   Left sacroposterior

Fig. 26.4 Defining the position of the presenting part.

ONSET OF LABOUR

Prior to the onset of labour, painless irregular uterine tightenings, known as 'Braxton Hicks' contractions, become increasingly frequent. The presence of painful contractions can signal the onset of labour and women's perception of being 'in labour', however, professional cervical assessment is required. The actual onset of established labour is determined by:

• Painful regular contractions.
• Progressive cervical dilatation of ≥4 cm and effacement (Fig. 26.1).

These factors diagnose labour, with or without a 'show' (passage of a mucoid plug from the cervix, often blood-stained)] or ruptured membranes. Irregular contractions prior to cervical dilatation and effacement are part of the latent phase of labour, which may be very variable in duration.

The factors which are responsible for the onset of labour at term are not well understood. To some degree, it is thought to be mechanical, as preterm labour is seen more commonly in circumstances in which the uterus is overstretched, such as multiple pregnancies and polyhydramnios. Inflammatory markers such as cytokines and prostaglandins also play a role. The latter is thought to be present in the decidua and membranes in late pregnancy and is released if the cervix is digitally stretched at term to separate the membranes and help to initiate labour (a cervical sweep).

NORMAL PROGRESS IN LABOUR

Once the diagnosis of established labour has been made, progress is assessed by monitoring:

- uterine contractions
- dilatation of the cervix
- descent of the presenting part

The rate of cervical dilatation is expected to be approximately 0.5–1 cm/h in a nulliparous woman and 1–2 cm/h in a multiparous woman. A partogram is commonly used to chart the observations made in labour (Fig. 26.5) and to highlight slow progress, particularly a delay in cervical dilatation or failure of the presenting part to descend (see Chapter 29).

HINTS AND TIPS

Accurate diagnosis of the onset of labour is important when managing a labouring patient. Starting a partograph too early may lead to misdiagnosis of prolonged labour and can result in unnecessary interventions.

Progress of labour is determined by three factors:

- passages
- passenger
- power

Passages

Bony pelvis

The pelvis is made up of four bones:

- two innominate bones
- sacrum
- coccyx

The passage that these bones make can be divided into inlet and outlet, with the cavity between them (Fig. 26.6). The pelvic inlet is bounded by the pubic crest, the iliopectineal line and the sacral promontory. It is oval in shape, with its wider diameter being transverse. The cavity of the pelvis is round. The pelvic outlet is bounded by the lower border of the pubic symphysis, the ischial spines and the tip of the sacrum. Again, the shape is oval, but the wider diameter is anteroposterior.

When a woman stands upright, the pelvis tilts forwards. The inlet makes an angle of about 55 degrees with the horizontal; this angle varies between individuals and different ethnic groups. The presenting part of the foetus must negotiate the axis of the birth canal with the change of direction occurring by rotation at the level of the pelvic floor muscles (see the 'Soft tissues' section).

Soft tissues

The soft passages consist of:

- uterus (upper and lower segments)
- cervix
- pelvic floor
- vagina
- perineum

The upper uterine segment is responsible for the propulsive contractions that deliver the foetus. The lower segment is the part of the uterus that lies behind the uterovesical fold of the peritoneum and above the cervix. It develops gradually during the third trimester, and then more rapidly during labour. It incorporates the cervix as the cervix effaces, to allow the presenting part to descend.

The pelvic floor consists of the levator ani group of muscles, including pubococcygeus and iliococcygeus arising from the bony pelvis to form a muscular diaphragm along with the internal obturator muscle and piriformis muscle. As the presenting part of the foetus is pushed out of the uterus it passes into the vagina, which has become hypertrophied during pregnancy. It reaches the pelvic floor, which acts like a gutter to direct it forwards and allow rotation. The perineum is distal to this and stretches as the head passes below the pubic arch and delivers.

Passenger

The fetal skull consists of the face and the cranium. The cranium is made up of two parietal bones, two frontal bones and the occipital bone (see Figs. 26.7 and 26.3), held together by a membrane that allows movement. Up until early childhood, these bones are not fused and can overlap to allow the head to pass through the pelvis during labour; this overlapping of the bones is known as 'moulding'.

Fig. 26.7 shows the anatomy of the fetal skull, including the sutures between the bones, and the spaces known as 'fontanelles'. These are important landmarks that can be felt on vaginal examination in established labour and enable the position of the foetus to be assessed (see Fig. 26.4). The position is described in terms of the occiput in a cephalic presentation, and the sacrum in a breech presentation.

The degree of flexion and the position of the fetal skull determine the ease with which the foetus passes through

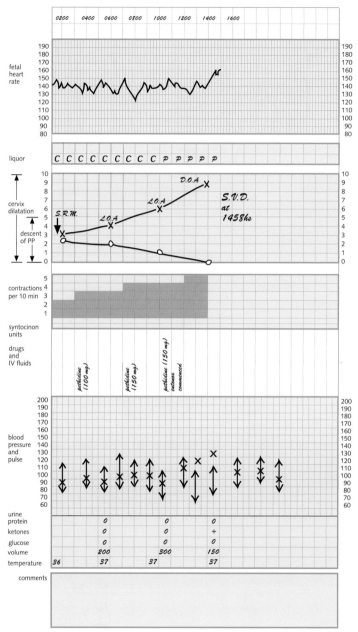

Fig. 26.5 A partogram showing progress and observations in labour. *C*, Clear liquor; *DOA*, direct occipito-anterior; *IV*, intravenous; *LOA*, left occipito-anterior; *P*, pink liquor; *PP*, presenting part; *SRM*, spontaneous rupture of membranes; *SVD*, spontaneous vaginal delivery.

the birth canal. Fig. 26.8 shows the diameters of the fetal skull. The diameter that presents during labour depends on the degree of flexion of the head. The head usually becomes more flexed with the increasing strength of the uterine contractions. Thus, the smallest diameters for delivery are the suboccipitobregmatic diameter, which represents a flexed vertex presentation, and the submentobregmatic diameter, which corresponds to a face presentation. The widest diameter is mentovertical, a brow presentation, which usually precludes vaginal delivery.

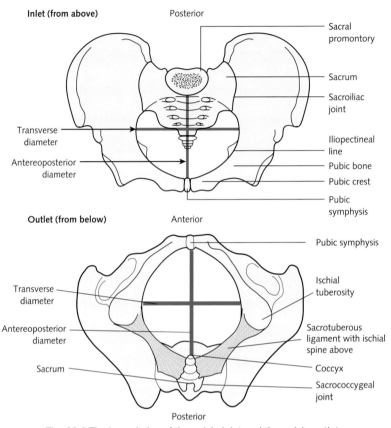

Fig. 26.6 The boundaries of the pelvic inlet and the pelvic outlet.

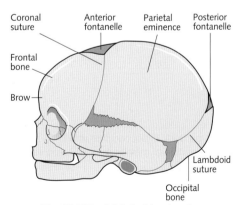

Fig. 26.7 The fetal skull landmarks.

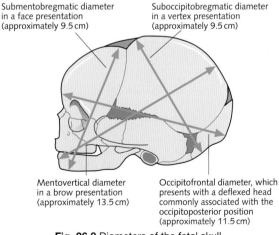

Fig. 26.8 Diameters of the fetal skull.

Power

The myometrial component of the uterus acts as the power to deliver the foetus. It consists of three layers:

- thin outer longitudinal layer
- thin inner circular layer
- thick middle spiral layer

From early pregnancy, the uterus contracts painlessly and irregularly (Braxton Hicks contractions). These contractions increase after the 36th week until the onset of labour. In labour, a contraction starts from the junction of the fallopian tube and the uterus on each side, spreading down and across the uterus with its greatest intensity in the upper uterine segment. Like any other muscle, the myometrium contracts and relaxes, but it also has the ability to retract so that the fibres become progressively shorter. This effect is seen in the lower segment: progressive retraction causes the lower segment to stretch and thin out, resulting in effacement and dilatation of the cervix (see Fig. 26.1).

During labour, the contractions are monitored for:

- strength
- frequency
- duration

The resting tone of the uterus is about 6 to 12 mmHg; to be effective in labour this increases to an intensity of 40 to 60 mmHg. There are usually three or four coordinated strong contractions every 10 minutes, each lasting approximately 60 seconds, to progress in labour.

In the second stage of labour, additional power comes from voluntary contraction of the diaphragm and the abdominal muscles as the mother pushes to assist delivery.

HINTS AND TIPS

The mechanism of delivery can be more easily remembered in four stages, thinking about how the head and shoulders must negotiate the transverse and anteroposterior diameters of the maternal pelvis inlet and outlet:

- flexion of the head
- internal rotation
- extension
- external rotation (restitution)

DELIVERY OF THE FOETUS

Active contractions of the uterus of increasing strength, frequency and duration cause passive movement of the foetus down the birth canal. At the beginning of labour, the foetus usually engages in the occiput transverse or occiput anterior position (i.e., in a position appropriate to the wider transverse diameter of the pelvic inlet). As labour progresses (Fig. 26.9A), the head becomes fully flexed so that the suboccipitobregmatic diameter is presenting.

As descent occurs through the pelvic cavity, internal rotation brings the occiput into the anterior position as it reaches the pelvic floor. This means that the head is now in the appropriate position to negotiate the wider diameter of the pelvic outlet, which is anteroposterior. In the second stage of labour, the occiput descends below the symphysis pubis (Fig. 26.9B) and delivers by extension. Increasing extension around the pubic bone delivers the face (Fig. 26.9C).

Delivery of the head brings the widest diameter of the shoulders (the bisacromial diameter) through the transverse diameter of the pelvic inlet into the pelvic cavity. External rotation or restitution occurs where the head rotates to a transverse position in relation to the shoulders (Fig. 26.10). This progresses with continuing descent and rotation of the shoulders to bring the bisacromial diameter into the anteroposterior diameter of the pelvic outlet. Further contractions and maternal effort enable the anterior shoulder to pass under the pubis, usually assisted by gentle downward traction on the head. Lateral flexion of the foetus delivers the posterior shoulder and the rest of the body follows (Fig. 26.11).

HINTS AND TIPS

Descent of the presenting part is assessed by both abdominal palpation (amount of head felt above the pelvic brim expressed in fifths = engagement) and vaginal examination (descent in relation to level of ischial spines = station).

MANAGEMENT OF LABOUR

The first stage of labour

When a patient presents in the first stage of labour, routine assessment of the mother and foetus is performed.

Maternal monitoring

Regular examination of the mother should include:

- pulse, blood pressure, respiratory rate, temperature
- urinalysis
- analgesia requirements
- abdominal palpation: symphysis fundal height, lie, presentation, engagement

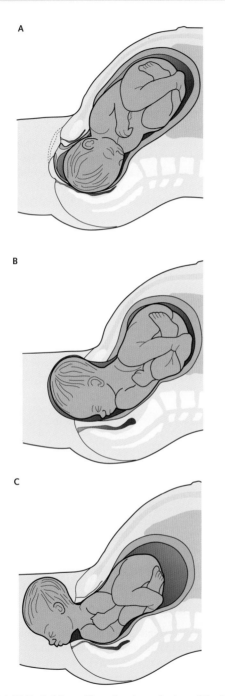

Fig. 26.9 (A) Early labour. There has been flexion of the fetal head. The cervix is effacing and has begun to dilate. (B) The second stage of labour. The head has undergone internal rotation to bring the occiput into the anterior position. The cervix is fully dilated. (C) Delivery of the head. Extension of the fetal neck occurs as the head passes under the pubic symphysis for its delivery.

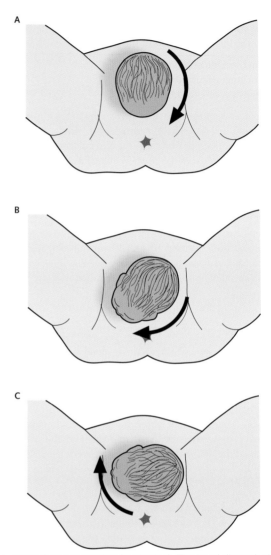

Fig. 26.10 External rotation (restitution). The head distends the perineum as it delivers in the occipitoanterior position and the external rotation occurs to allow delivery of the shoulders.

- contractions: strength, frequency, duration
- vaginal examination: degree of cervical effacement, cervical dilatation, station of presenting part in relation to ischial spines, position of presenting part, presence of caput or moulding (see Chapter 29)

There is delayed gastric emptying during pregnancy and labour. If an emergency general anaesthetic is needed, there is an increased risk of inhalation of regurgitated acidic stomach contents, causing Mendelson syndrome. Therefore, some

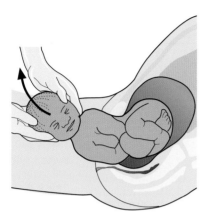

Fig. 26.11 Delivery of the shoulders. The anterior shoulder passes below the pubic symphysis, aided by axial traction of the head by the midwife or doctor. The posterior shoulder delivers as the head is gently guided upwards.

women may be advised to remain nil by mouth and take antacid therapy depending on their risk of needing an operative procedure.

If the membranes are ruptured, then the colour of the liquor must be documented, usually clear, blood-stained or having meconium present.

The need for analgesia during labour varies markedly between different women. Nonpharmacological techniques include the use of psychoprophylaxis, hypnosis, massage and transcutaneous electrical nerve stimulation. The pharmacological methods are summarized in Table 26.2.

Fetal monitoring

Intermittent auscultation or continuous fetal heart rate monitoring is appropriate, depending on the risk assessment. In a low-risk pregnancy, intermittent monitoring with a Sonicaid or with a Pinard stethoscope is sufficient, every 15 minutes during and after a contraction for 60 seconds in the first stage of labour, and every 5 minutes in the second stage.

If there are any risk factors during the pregnancy that have been present antenatally or are identified in labour, then continuous electronic monitoring with cardiotocography (CTG) should be performed. See Box 27.1 for indications for continuous monitoring.

In some patients, abdominal monitoring of the heart rate can be difficult, for example, if the patient is obese, and so a fetal scalp electrode can be applied directly to the head once the cervix is dilated and the membranes are ruptured. If monitoring suggests that the fetal heart rate pattern is pathological, a fetal pH by taking a blood sample from the fetal scalp known as 'fetal blood sampling' can be considered (see Chapter 27).

The second stage of labour

Once the cervix is fully dilated, the patient is encouraged to use voluntary effort to push with the contractions. If she has an epidural anaesthetic in situ, she might be less aware of an urge to push, and so a further hour can be allowed for the presenting part to descend with the contractions alone. Without an epidural, the mother may adopt various positions for the delivery of the foetus. As the head descends, the perineum distends and the anus dilates. Finally, the head crowns: the biparietal diameter has passed through the pelvis and there is no recession between contractions. The attendant can apply pressure on the perineum for support during delivery of the head and give consideration of an episiotomy. Once delivered, the neck is felt to exclude the presence of the umbilical cord which should be looped over the fetal head to prevent excessive tension in the cord as the body delivers.

After external rotation, lateral flexion of the head towards the anus (also known as 'axial traction') dislodges the anterior shoulder from behind the pubic symphysis with the next contraction. Lifting the head gently in the opposite direction delivers the posterior shoulder (Fig. 26.11). Holding the shoulders, the rest of the body is delivered either onto the bed or onto the mother's abdomen. Finally, the umbilical cord is secured with clamps and cut.

The third stage of labour

Management of the third stage of labour can be:

- physiological
- active

Women who have had an uncomplicated pregnancy and labour may choose to have a physiological third stage. This means that they do not receive any oxytocic drugs, the attendant waits for the umbilical cord to stop pulsating before it is cut and delivery of the placenta occurs passively. In situations where there is an increased risk of postpartum haemorrhage (PPH) or depending on parental choice, active management is advised.

Active management of the third stage has been shown to reduce the incidence of PPH (see Chapter 31). Management involves:

- using an oxytocic drug
- clamping and cutting the cord
- controlled cord traction

In most units, syntocinon (five units of oxytocin) or syntometrine (five units of oxytocin with 0.5 mg ergometrine) is given intramuscularly with the delivery of the anterior shoulder; it takes about 2 to 3 minutes to act. As the placenta detaches from the uterine wall, the cut cord will appear

Table 26.2 Pharmacological methods of analgesia in labour

	Technique	Indication	Effectiveness	Duration of effect	Side effects
Oxygen/nitrous oxide (Entonox)	Inhalation of 50:50 mixture with onset of contraction	First stage	<50% Takes 20–30 seconds for peak effect	Time of inhalation only	Does not relieve pain
Pethidine	Intramuscular injection 100–150 mg	First stage	<50% Takes 15–20 minutes for peak effect	Approximately 3 hours	Nausea and vomiting – give with an antiemetic Respiratory depression in the neonate (this is easily reversed with intramuscular naloxone)
Pudendal block	Infiltration of right and left pudendal nerves (S2, S3 and S4)	Second stage for operative delivery	Within 5 minutes	45–90 minutes	–
Perineal infiltration	Infiltration of perineum at posterior fourchette	Second stage prior to episiotomy Third stage for suturing of perineal lacerations	Within 5 minutes	45–90 minutes	–
Epidural anaesthesia	Injection via a catheter into the epidural space (L3–4)	First- or second-stage Caesarean section	Complete pain relief in approximately 95% of women within 20–30 minutes	Bolus injection every 3–4 hours or continuous infusion or patient-controlled administration	Transient hypotension – give intravenous fluid load Dural tap Risk of haemorrhage if abnormal maternal clotting Increased length of second stage because of reduced pelvic floor tone and loss of bearing-down reflex
Spinal anaesthesia	Injection into the subarachnoid space	Any operative delivery; manual removal of the placenta	Immediate effect	Single injection lasting 3–4 hours	Respiratory depression

to lengthen. There is usually some bleeding and the fundus becomes hard. Brandt-Andrews method of controlled cord traction is commonly used to deliver the placenta once it has separated to reduce the incidence of uterine inversion (Fig. 26.12). The placenta and membranes must be checked to ensure they are complete.

Finally, the vagina, labia and perineum are examined for tears that may require suturing (see Chapter 28). The uterine fundus is palpated to check that it is well contracted, approximately at the level of the umbilicus. The estimated blood loss should be recorded.

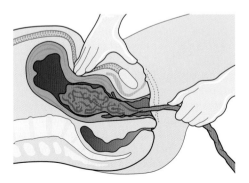

Fig. 26.12 Controlled cord traction to deliver the placenta.

INDUCTION OF LABOUR

Definition

IOL is defined as the artificial initiation of labour. In the UK, over 30% of labours are induced each year.

Indications

The rate of induction varies widely between different units. Table 26.3 summarizes possible reasons for IOL. In the UK, the most common indication is prolonged pregnancy, which is when a pregnancy continues beyond 41 weeks of gestation.

METHODS

> **HINTS AND TIPS**
>
> Prior to induction of labour, the favourability of the cervix should be assessed. This is usually done by using the Bishop score (Table 26.1).
> - unfavourable cervix = hard, long, closed, not effaced (low Bishop score)
> - favourable cervix = soft, beginning to dilate and efface (high Bishop score)

Membrane sweeping

During the examination of the uterine cervix, the examining finger passes through the cervical canal and rotates against the uterus to separate the membranes. If the cervix

Table 26.3 Indications for the induction of labour

Maternal	Severe preeclampsia
	Advanced maternal age
	Recurrent antepartum haemorrhage
	Preexisting disease (e.g., diabetes, essential hypertension)
	Gestational diabetes
	Social
Fetal	Prolonged pregnancy
	Intrauterine growth restriction
	Prelabour rupture of membranes
	Preterm premature rupture of membranes
	Intrauterine fetal death
	Suspected macrosomia

is closed, then massaging around the cervix achieves the same effect. This may trigger the onset of labour without the need for medical or mechanical methods. Patients should be informed that procedure could be painful and can cause vaginal bleeding.

Pharmacological and mechanical methods

Mechanical dilatators

Insertion of a double balloon catheter or osmotic cervical dilatators (dilates the cervix by absorbing fluid from surrounding tissues) are alternatives to pharmacological methods such as dinoprostone and misoprostol. These methods are preferred especially in women with a higher risk of hyperstimulation or who have had a previous caesarean scar.

Prostaglandins

Local application of a prostaglandin, usually prostaglandin E2, given as a vaginal gel, tablet or pessary, has been shown to ripen the cervix as part of the induction process and reduce the incidence of operative delivery when compared with the use of oxytocin alone. Used locally instead of systemically, the gastrointestinal side effects are minimized. Patients who have IOL with prostaglandins should have uterine activity and fetal monitoring in view of the risk of uterine hyperstimulation.

> **HINTS AND TIPS**
>
> **TACHYSYSTOLE VERSUS HYPERSTIMULATION**
>
> Tachysystole – more than five contractions in a 10-minute period associated with a normal fetal heart trace and the absence of fetal distress.
>
> Hyperstimulation – more than five contractions in a 10-minute period associated with an abnormal fetal heart rate pattern indicating the presence of fetal distress.

Amniotomy

Artificial rupture of the membranes is thought to cause local release of endogenous prostaglandins. It is done using an amnihook and may be part of the induction process or performed to accelerate slow progress in labour. It can also be done with an abnormal CTG to exclude meconium staining of the liquor,

Table 26.4 Complications associated with the use of amniotomy and oxytocin

Treatment	Complication
Amniotomy	Cord prolapse
	Infection
	Bleeding from a vasa praevia
	Placental separation
	Failure to induce efficient contractions
	Amniotic fluid embolism
Oxytocin	Abnormal fetal heart rate pattern
	Hyperstimulation of the uterus
	Rupture of the uterus
	Fluid overload

or to allow the application of a fetal scalp electrode. Table 26.4 shows the complications associated with amniotomy.

Oxytocin

An intravenous infusion of synthetic oxytocin (syntocinon) is commonly used to induce labour, and to stimulate contractions after amniotomy or spontaneous rupture of membranes. The dose must be carefully titrated according to the strength and frequency of the uterine contractions, and continuous fetal monitoring is necessary. Table 26.4 shows the complications associated with oxytocin.

● Chapter Summary

- Labour is defined as the onset of regular painful contractions associated with cervical change (dilatation and effacement).
- Progress in labour is determined by three factors: passage, passenger and power.
- Delivery of the foetus involves flexion of the head, internal rotation, extension and external rotation (restitution).
- Analgesia in labour is dependent on patient choice and includes Entonox, intramuscular opioids, local anaesthetic and regional anaesthetic.
- Induction of labour is the artificial initiation of uterine contractions to deliver the foetus. This can be done with the use of prostaglandin agents and/or artificial rupture of the membranes followed by the use of syntocinon or mechanical dilatators.

FETAL HEART RATE MONITORING IN LABOUR

Fetal heart rate (FHR) can be monitored by intermittent auscultation (IA) or cardiotocography (CTG) in labour depending on the initial risk assessment for fetal compromise at the onset of labour. IA now typically involves the use of a hand-held Doppler ultrasound device or historically, a Pinard stethoscope which is preferred in low-risk pregnancies. CTG is a form of continuous electronic FHR monitoring used to evaluate fetal wellbeing antenatally and during labour. As well as the FHR, the uterine activity is recorded while performing CTG. It has been used increasingly in the UK since the 1970s, with the aim of detecting fetal hypoxia before it causes perinatal morbidity or mortality, in particular cerebral palsy. However, the expected reduction in hypoxia-induced intrapartum perinatal mortality has not occurred and the role of CTG monitoring has been questioned as the rate of caesarean section increases. The need to constantly educate staff about the appropriate use of the CTG and its interpretation by fetal physiology and pattern recognition, and to audit standards in relation to patient care is essential. There are several guidelines to interpret FHR during labour that are present such as National Institute for Health and Care Excellence (NICE), International Federation of Gynaecology and Obstetrics (FIGO) and American College of Obstetrics and Gynecology (ACOG). This chapter is based on the NICE guidelines in fetal monitoring as in the UK; the majority of the obstetric units prefer NICE.

Monitoring in an uncomplicated pregnancy in labour

IA of the FHR may be appropriate for a healthy woman in labour who has had an uncomplicated pregnancy. This involves documenting the heart rate for a minimum of 60 seconds at least:

- every 15 minutes including after a contraction in the first stage of labour
- every 5 minutes including after a contraction in the second stage of labour

Continuous monitoring is recommended if IA is abnormal or any risk factors develop during the course of the labour, such as meconium-stained liquor.

Table 27.1 Indications for recommending continuous fetal monitoring

Categories	Indication for continuous monitoring
Maternal	Induced labour Previous uterine scar (caesarean section/ myomectomy) Preeclampsia Diabetes Antepartum haemorrhage Other maternal medical disease Maternal request
Fetal	Intrauterine growth restriction Prematurity Oligohydramnios Abnormal Doppler artery studies Multiple pregnancy Breech presentation
Intrapartum	Raise in baseline fetal heart rate (FHR) on intermittent auscultation (IA) Decelerations on IA Meconium-stained liquor Vaginal bleeding in labour Use of oxytocin for augmentation Epidural analgesia Maternal pyrexia Maternal tachycardia >120 bpm Postterm pregnancy Prolonged rupture of membranes >24 hours

Who should have continuous cardiotocography (CTG) monitoring?

Table 27.1 shows the maternal and fetal indications for recommending continuous monitoring.

FEATURES OF CARDIOTOCOGRAPHY (CTG)

Classify four features of CTG trace (contractions, baseline FHR, variability and decelerations) as white, amber or red (based on the level of concern) and use the presence of the accelerations alongside these four features when categorizing the overall trace.

- **Uterine contractions:** As well as monitoring the FHR, the CTG also monitors the frequency of uterine contractions. This is important, for example, if the patient is having intravenous oxytocin to stimulate/initiate contractions. Contractions more than five in 10 minutes will reduce the time of return to resting tone between contractions and this may lead to fetal hypoxia if occurring over a prolonged period.

    A tocodynamometer should be used to record contraction frequency and length on the CTG trace. This needs to be confirmed with palpation of the uterus, because the size of the peaks shown on the tracing may be related to the positioning of the monitor on the maternal abdomen or the thickness of the maternal abdominal wall.

- **Baseline FHR**: This is the mean level of FHR over a period of 5 to 10 minutes when FHR is stable. It is expressed as beats per minute (bpm) and is determined by the fetal sympathetic and parasympathetic nervous systems. The normal range is 110 to 160 bpm. In the preterm foetus, the baseline tends to be at the higher end of the normal range.

- **Baseline variability**: Minor fluctuations occur in the baseline FHR at 3 to 5 cycles/min. It is measured by estimating the difference in bpm between the highest peak and the lowest trough of change in a 1-minute segment of the trace. Normal baseline variability is 5 to 25 bpm.

- **Accelerations**: These are increases in the FHR of 15 bpm or more above the baseline rate, lasting 15 seconds or more. The presence of accelerations is usually a sign of a healthy foetus. Isolated absence of the accelerations on a CTG trace does not indicate fetal acidosis therefore this feature is not included in the categorization of the CTG by the recent NICE guidance.

- **Decelerations**: These are falls in the FHR of more than 15 bpm below the baseline, lasting 15 seconds or more. Different types of decelerations can be seen, depending on their timing with the uterine contractions:
    1. Early decelerations: the FHR slows at the same time as the onset of the contraction and returns to the baseline at the end of the contraction in an identical pattern with every contraction. These are usually benign.
    2. Variable decelerations: the timing of the slowing of the FHR in relation to the uterine contraction varies within the time frame of the contraction. The deceleration is of rapid onset and recovery, with a particular shape on the recording, known as 'shouldering'. It represents a normal physiological response by the foetus to the stress of a contraction in association with the compression of the umbilical cord. However, other features might make this type of deceleration more suspicious, such as loss of the normal baseline variability or loss of the shouldering.
    3. Late decelerations: the FHR begins to fall during the contraction, with its trough more than 20 seconds after the peak of the contraction and returning to baseline after the contraction.

The CTG has been categorized by NICE guidelines, as shown in Table 27.2:

- Normal: no amber or red features (all four features are white) (Fig. 27.1)
- Suspicious: one feature is amber
- Pathological: two or more features are amber or one is red (Fig. 27.2)

PHYSIOLOGY

The principle of monitoring during labour is to detect fetal hypoxia and, therefore, prevent fetal acidaemia and cell damage.

Acute fetal hypoxia

In a previously well foetus, this can occur secondary to:

- uterine hyperstimulation
- placental abruption
- umbilical cord compression
- sudden maternal hypotension (e.g., insertion of regional anaesthesia)
- uterine rupture

These conditions can result in an increase in the FHR baseline, with decelerations, produced by a baroreceptor-mediated response, as the fetal blood pressure is affected. If the FHR baseline falls, and this is prolonged to more than 3 minutes (i.e., a fetal bradycardia), the ongoing fetal hypoxia may result in myocardial ischaemia.

Table 27.2 Categorization of the features of the fetal heart rate according to National Institute for Health and Care Excellence (NICE) guidelines

Feature	White	Amber	Red
Contractions	<5 in 10 minutes	≥5 in 10 minutes*	-
Baseline (bpm)	Stable baseline of 110–160	Increase ≥ 20 bpm from the start of labour or since the last review 100–109 bpm** Unable to determine	<100 >180
Variability (bpm)	5–25	<5 for between 30 and 50 minutes >25 for up to 10 minutes	<5 more than 50 minutes >25 more than 10 minutes Sinusoidal
Decelerations	No decelerations Early decelerations Variable decelerations that are not evolving to have concerning characteristics***	Repetitive variable decelerations with any concerning characteristics for less than 30 minutes Variable decelerations with any concerning characteristics for more than 30 minutes Repetitive late decelerations for less than 30 minutes	Repetitive variable decelerations with any concerning characteristics for more than 30 minutes Repetitive late decelerations for more than 30 minutes Acute bradycardia, or a single prolonged deceleration lasting 3 minutes or more

*Contractions leading to reduced resting time/hypertonus.
**Continue usual care if stable throughout labour if there is normal variability and no decelerations.
***Such as lasting more than 60 seconds, reduced variability within the deceleration, failure or slow return to baseline, loss of previously present shouldering.

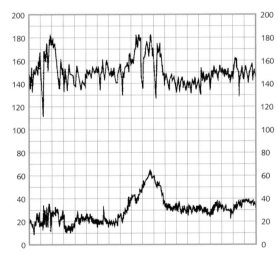

Fig. 27.1 Fetal heart acceleration during a uterine contraction with normal baseline variability.

Chronic fetal hypoxia

If there has been chronic uteroplacental insufficiency during the pregnancy, for example, secondary to preeclampsia, then the foetus is at increased risk of hypoxia during labour. Reduced intervillous perfusion during uterine contractions or maternal hypotension can exacerbate underlying reduced placental perfusion. This can result in FHR decelerations persisting after the uterine contraction has stopped (late decelerations), and

an increase in the fetal cardiac output with an increase in the baseline heart rate. This may be followed by reduced heart rate variability as the fetal chemoreceptors respond to ongoing fetal hypoxia. Prolonged hypoxia eventually produces cerebral and myocardial damage.

CLINICAL NOTES

Remember to look at the changes in the cardiotocograph over time. For example, after 8 hours in labour in a term baby, the baseline rate may be 155 bpm (i.e., within the normal range) but if it was 120 bpm at the start of labour, then this rise is significant and pathology such as fetal infection should be excluded.

ASSESSMENT OF THE PATIENT IN LABOUR

Baseline maternal observations

Temperature
A raised maternal temperature might explain fetal tachycardia, for example, if there are ruptured membranes for >24 hours increasing the risk of fetal and maternal infection.

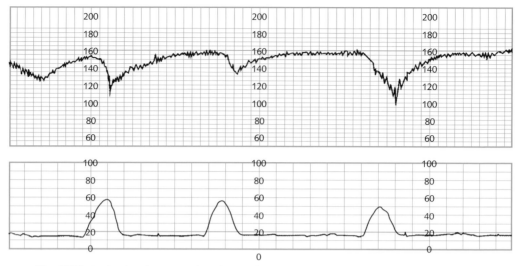

Fig. 27.2 Late decelerations occurring after uterine contractions with reduced baseline variability.

Pulse

This might be raised in conjunction with maternal pyrexia. In the presence of fetal bradycardia, the maternal pulse should be checked to ensure the monitoring is recording FHR and not the mother's heart rate. This can be excluded by checking with an ultrasound scan. To aid differentiation between FHR and maternal heart rate, a fetal scalp electrode (FSE) can be applied, provided the cervix is at least 1 to 2 cm dilated and the membranes are ruptured.

Blood pressure

Administering epidural anaesthesia can be associated with maternal hypotension. This results in reduced blood flow to the uterus and can cause fetal bradycardia. Therefore, intravenous fluids are administered and blood pressure is regularly checked when the medication is given.

Abdominal palpation

- Uterine size
- Engagement of presenting part
- Scar tenderness in a patient with a previous caesarean section
- Uterine tone

The size of the maternal abdomen should be assessed to check if it is large or small for dates (see Chapter 23). The engagement of the presenting part is important to assess progress in labour (see Chapter 26). In a patient who has previously had a caesarean section, the presence of scar tenderness should be elicited; scar rupture is commonly associated with an abnormal CTG and vaginal bleeding. Another cause of vaginal bleeding with an abnormal CTG is placental abruption (see Chapter 20). If this is suspected, the uterus will typically feel hard and tender.

The uterine contractions should be palpated, especially if the patient's labour is being stimulated by intravenous oxytocic agents. Hyperstimulation can cause an abnormal FHR. There should be a resting tone between contractions.

Vaginal examination

As well as assessing the dilatation of the cervix to determine the progress in labour the presence of the fetal cord must also be excluded. A cord prolapse, as it is known, is associated with fetal bradycardia as the blood vessels in the cord spasm. This is an emergency situation requiring immediate delivery by caesarean section if the cervix is not fully dilated.

A vaginal examination may also be indicated to apply an FSE to aid distinguishing between maternal heart rate and FHR. If the membranes are broken liquor should be checked to see if there is meconium or blood stain as part of the risk assessment.

MANAGEMENT OF THE PATIENTS BASED ON THE CARDIOTOCOGRAPHY (CTG) TRACE

The management based on the categorization of the CTG is shown in Fig. 27.3. When there is a concern about the foetus' wellbeing the following possible underlying causes need to be looked for and conservative measures should be taken:

- Cord compression – can affect the blood flow to the foetus and can cause CTG changes. Recommended measure: change maternal position.

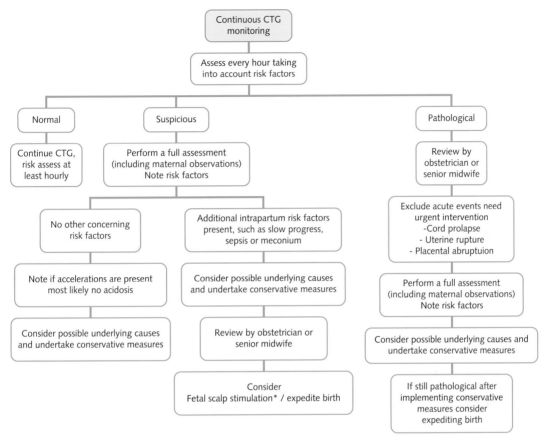

*Absence of an acceleration in response to fetal scalp stimulation is an alarming sign that foetus is affected by hypoxemic stress and expedited birth may be needed.

Fig. 27.3 Algorithm for cardiotocograph (CTG) monitoring.

- Maternal hypotension – can cause CTG changes by altering the blood flow to the uterus – usually seen following the epidural top-up.

  Recommended measure: intravenous fluids/call anaesthetist for review.

- Excessive uterine contractions – can result in hypoxic stress to the foetus.

  Recommended measure: stop oxytocin / consider tocolytics (terbutaline).

  Fetal scalp is no longer routinely performed for pathological CTG traces because of the limited evidence available.

HINTS AND TIPS

Do not offer intravenous fluids to treat fetal heart rate (FHR) changes unless the patient is hypotensive or septic. Maternal facial oxygen therapy also is not recommended as a conservative measure as there is no benefit and can cause harm to foetus.

Chapter Summary

- Fetal monitoring in labour can be intermittent or continuous depending on the risk factors associated with the pregnancy.
- The five features of a cardiotocograph (CTG) are contractions, baseline rate, variability, acceleration and decelerations.
- The principle of monitoring during labour is to detect fetal hypoxia and, therefore, prevent fetal acidaemia and cell damage.

MLA Presentations
Complications of labour

28

INTRODUCTION

For all interventions in obstetrics, the following general principles apply:

- Make sure all documentation includes the time and date, a legible signature and a printed name.
- Clearly record the indication for the intervention, the abdominal and vaginal examination findings as appropriate and the operative findings including any complications.
- Obtain informed consent from the patient, either verbal or written, depending on the procedure.

ASSISTED VAGINAL DELIVERY

Choosing the most appropriate instrument depends on the clinical circumstances and operator's choice and their level of skill. Forceps and vacuum extraction are linked with different advantages and disadvantages. Failure rates, maternal anxiety, cephalo/subgaleal haematoma and retinal haemorrhage are more common with vacuum delivery; while significant vulvo-vaginal tears, skull fracture, facial nerve palsy are more likely with forceps delivery. There is no significant difference between both types of instruments in birth by caesarean section, low Apgar scores at 5 minutes and the need for phototherapy.

Rotational births should be performed/supervised by expert clinicians. The instrument options for rotational delivery are Kielland's rotational forceps, manual rotation followed by direct traction forceps or vacuum and rotational vacuum extraction.

Please see Table 28.1 for indications of instrumental delivery.

Table 28.1 Indications for assisted vaginal birth

Type of indication	Description
Maternal	Lack of progress Maternal exhaustion or distress Medical conditions to avoid Valsalva (e.g., cardiovascular disease)
Fetal	Suspected fetal compromise (pathological cardiotocograph (CTG) trace, thick meconium)
Combined	Both maternal and fetal indications often coexist

VENTOUSE DELIVERY

Since the 1950s, when the vacuum extractor was invented in Sweden, it has increasingly been seen as the instrument of choice for assisted vaginal delivery. Metal cups (Fig. 28.1C) were used initially, either anterior cups or posterior cups. Subsequently, silicone rubber ones (Fig. 28.1A) were developed and more recently, the disposable handheld KIWI® cup (Fig. 28.1B). Metal and standard ventouse are rarely used in modern-day obstetrics. The metal cups are more likely to be associated with trauma to the vagina or the fetal scalp, but may be more appropriate for delivery in certain situations, such as the presence of excessive caput on the fetal head. Along with the KIWI® cups, they are useful in the presence of a fetal malposition. Both the metal and silicone cups are available in different diameters depending on the gestation of the foetus. It is not an appropriate instrument at less than 34 weeks' gestation and should be used with caution between 34 and 36 weeks' gestation. Table 28.2 presents the complications of instrumental delivery.

Technique for ventouse

All types of cup rely on the same technique. The cup is applied in the midline over or just anterior to the occiput, avoiding the

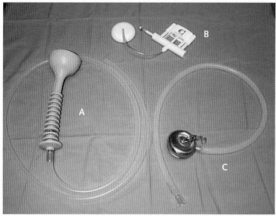

Fig. 28.1 Ventouse cups. (From Simms R, Hayman R. Instrumental vaginal delivery. *Obstet Gynaecol Reprod Med* 23:270–78, 2013. Elsevier.)

Table 28.2 Complications of instrumental delivery

Type of complication	Description
Maternal	Genital tract trauma (cervical/vaginal/vulval) with risk of haemorrhage and/or infection
Fetal	Ventouse delivery is likely to cause a chignon (scalp oedema) or, less commonly, a cephalohaematoma (subperiosteal bleed) Forceps can cause bruising if not appropriately applied, or rarely facial nerve palsy or depression skull fracture

surrounding vaginal mucosa. The suction pressure in the cup is raised to 0.6–0.8 kg/cm² or equivalent, either by connection to a separate machine or with the handheld mechanism found within the KIWI®cup.

Traction with the maternal contractions and with maternal effort should be along the pelvic curve, that is, initially in a downwards direction and then changing the angle upwards as the head crowns. This action basically mimics the passage of the fetal head during a normal delivery, but uses the vacuum pump to increase traction and flexion.

The operator should judge whether an episiotomy is needed and the procedure should be complete within approximately 15 minutes of cup application. The cardiotocograph (CTG) should monitor the fetal heart rate throughout and, in most units, it is standard practice for a paediatrician to be present.

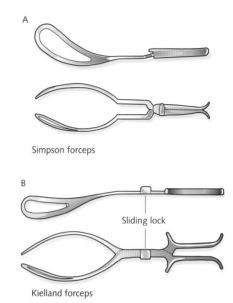

Fig. 28.2 Types of forceps.

FORCEPS DELIVERY

Over the last three to four centuries, forceps have been used for delivery. There are two main types of forceps (Fig. 28.2):

- nonrotational or traction forceps (Simpson, Anderson, Neville Barnes or Wrigley)
- rotational forceps (Kielland)

Technique for forceps

The blades of nonrotational forceps are applied to the head, avoiding trauma to the vaginal walls. The direction of traction is similar to that of the ventouse, with episiotomy performed when the head crowns to give more space (Fig. 28.3).

Use of the rotational forceps involves a slightly different technique: the knobs on the blades must always point towards the occiput; asynclitism can be corrected using the sliding mechanism of the handles and then rotation achieved prior to traction in the manner described earlier.

> **RED FLAGS**
>
> Instrumental delivery should not be attempted if the head is above the ischial spines because of the risks of excessive traction to the foetus – a caesarean section is indicated.

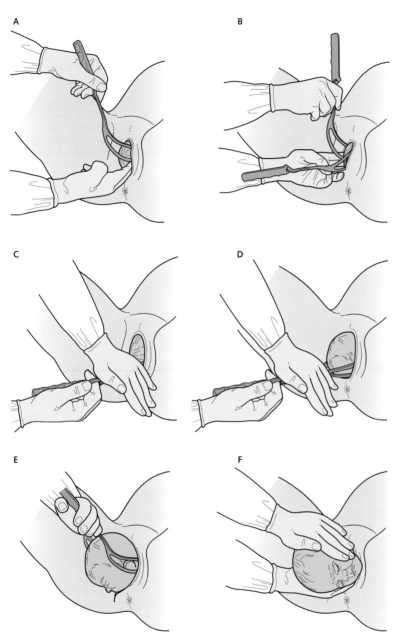

A

B

C

D

E

F

Fig. 28.3 Forceps delivery: change the application of blades.

EPISIOTOMY

The purpose of an episiotomy is to increase the diameter of the vulval outlet by making an incision in the perineal body. Since the 1980s, the routine episiotomy rate has been reduced dramatically because studies have demonstrated its association with increased blood loss, as well as long-term morbidities such as pain and dyspareunia. However, there are still indications for its use (Table 28.3).

HINTS AND TIPS

To make them easier to remember, the indications or complications for any intervention can be divided into maternal and fetal.

Table 28.3 Indications for episiotomy

Type of indication	Description
Maternal	Female circumcision (consider if previous perineal reconstructive surgery)
Fetal	Instrumental delivery
	Breech delivery
	Shoulder dystocia
	Abnormal cardiotocograph

Right mediolateral episiotomy
Midline episiotomy

Fig. 28.4 Types of incision for episiotomy.

Two techniques are used for episiotomy (Fig. 28.4). Both should be performed with adequate analgesia, either an epidural, pudendal or perineal infiltration with local anaesthetic, and should start in the midline at the posterior fourchette:

1. Mediolateral: widely used in the UK, this type of incision is more likely to protect the anal sphincter if the incision extends during delivery.
2. Midline: this technique is widely used in the USA and, although it is easier to repair and likely to result in less postpartum pain, it is more likely to involve the anal sphincter if it extends.

Repair of an episiotomy should be performed by an experienced operator. There should be adequate light and appropriate analgesia. A three-layer technique is normally practiced, with absorbable sutures (Fig. 28.5):

- First layer – vaginal skin: identify the apex of the incision and suture in a continuous layer to the hymen to oppose the cut edges of the posterior fourchette.
- Second layer – perineal body: deep sutures to realign the muscles of the perineal body.
- Third layer – perineal skin: continuous subcuticular or interrupted sutures to close the skin.

An examination of the vagina should be performed to ensure that the apex of the episiotomy is secure. Rectal examination should ensure the rectal mucosa has not been broached by any deep sutures because this can result in fistula formation.

> **RED FLAGS**
>
> At the end of the procedure, all needles and swabs should be accounted for as a retained swab or instrument is classified by NHS Improvement as a 'Never event'.

PERINEAL REPAIR

Approximately 70% of mothers who deliver vaginally will sustain some degree of perineal trauma. This can be classified as:

- First degree: involves skin only.
- Second degree: involves skin and perineal muscle.
- Third degree: includes partial or complete rupture of the anal sphincter (see Table 28.4).
- Fourth degree: as for third degree, but also involves the anal mucosa.

The principles for repair are the same as for episiotomy. Some first-degree tears can be allowed to heal by primary or secondary intention if they are not actively bleeding. It is very important to recognize and repair appropriately any damage to the anal sphincter or mucosa; failure to do so can result in long-term morbidity, such as urgency of stool, or incontinence of flatus or faeces (this occurs in approximately 5% of women).

> **COMMUNICATION**
>
> Approximately 3% of patients sustain a third- or fourth-degree tear. These patients need to be debriefed postnatally regarding the extent of their tear. They should be advised to take antibiotics, analgesia and laxatives during their recovery. They may also require referral for physiotherapy depending on local policy. The discussion should involve mode of delivery and risks in a future pregnancy alongside a patient information leaflet.

CAESAREAN SECTION

Caesarean section was first described by the ancient Egyptians. It was used increasingly throughout the 20th century such that

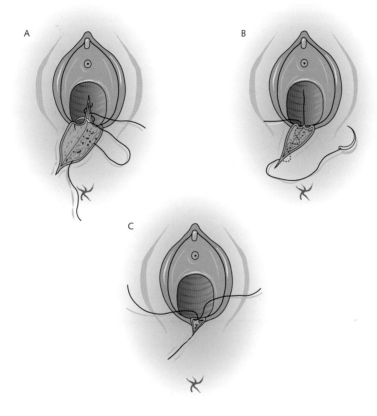

Fig. 28.5 Repair of an episiotomy. (A) Suturing the vaginal wall. (B) Suturing the perineal muscles. (C) Subcuticular sutures to the perineal skin. Tying the strands together – the knot disappears beneath the vaginal mucosa.

Table 28.4 Classification of third- and fourth-degree tears

Grade 3a tear	Less than 50% of external anal sphincter (EAS) thickness torn
Grade 3b tear	More than 50% of EAS thickness torn
Grade 3c tear	Both EAS and internal anal sphincter (IAS) torn
Fourth-degree tear	Injury to the perineum involving the anal sphincter complex (EAS and IAS) and anorectal mucosa

rates of 25% are now common in units in the UK. The lower segment procedure (lower segment caesarean section (LSCS)) was introduced in the 1920s and has largely replaced the 'classical' midline uterine incision. Although the latter is sometimes indicated for preterm delivery with a poorly formed lower segment or for a preterm abnormal lie, it is associated with higher rates of haemorrhage and rupture in future labours (up to 5% for midline operation, <1% for lower segment procedure).

Indications for lower segment caesarean section

Some of the indications for a caesarean section are listed in Table 28.5. The majority of the time decision is individual and based on women's risk factors and wishes.

Technique for lower segment caesarean section

An elective LSCS is usually performed at 39 or more weeks' gestation. Delivery at and after this gestation reduces the

Table 28.5 Indications for lower segment caesarean section

Type of indication	Description
Maternal	Previous caesarean section Placenta praevia Maternal disease (e.g., fulminating preeclampsia) Maternal request with no obstetric indication Active primary genital herpes simplex virus Human immunodeficiency virus disease depending on viral load
Fetal	Breech presentation Twin pregnancy if the presentation of first twin is not cephalic Abnormal cardiotocograph or abnormal fetal blood sample in first stage Cord prolapse Delay in first stage of labour (e.g., due to malpresentation or malposition)

respiratory morbidity in the infant – transient tachypnoea of the newborn. With regional analgesia more commonly used than general analgesia, a low transverse skin incision is made. The rectus sheath is cut and the rectus muscles divided. The utero-vesical peritoneum is incised to allow the bladder to be reflected inferiorly. The lower uterine segment is incised transversely and the foetus is delivered manually (instrumental delivery may be needed in selected cases).

Intravenous oxytocin is given by the anaesthetist and the placenta and membranes are removed. The angles of the uterine incision are secured to ensure haemostasis and then the uterus is closed with an absorbable suture, usually in two layers. The rectus sheath is closed to avoid incisional hernias and, finally, the skin is closed with either an absorbable or nonabsorbable suture.

ETHICS

You cannot proceed to caesarean section without consent from the mother even if there is acute fetal distress. This can be verbal or written consent.

Complications of lower segment caesarean section

Although LSCS has become an increasingly safe procedure, particularly with the introduction of regional anaesthesia, there is still significant morbidity associated with it:

- Haemorrhage – all patients should have a group-and-save sample sent; cross-match blood for certain patients (e.g., those with placenta praevia).
- Infection – reduced by routine use of prophylactic antibiotics.
- Thromboembolic disease – prophylaxis in all patients for up to 6 weeks depending on other risk factors.
- Visceral injury – damage to bladder or bowel, particularly with a history of previous abdominal surgery, most commonly a previous LSCS.
- Gastric aspiration – particularly with general anaesthetic (Mendelson syndrome), is reduced by routine use of antacids.
- Future pregnancy – may be suitable for vaginal birth after caesarean (VBAC; see the following section) or may be advised repeat LSCS. This carries an increased risk of complications such as morbidly adherent placenta.

Vaginal birth after caesarean

In patients who have had a pregnancy complicated by caesarean section, options for future deliveries should be discussed. For the majority of women who have had one previous LSCS, vaginal delivery can be offered if they go into spontaneous labour (VBAC). The main serious fetal and maternal risk is scar rupture, which occurs in 0.5% of pregnancies. In the case of a classical caesarean, the possibility of scar rupture in labour is high (up to 5%) and thus repeat LSCS would be recommended.

Patients who agree to VBAC need to be counselled regarding care in labour, as well as possible recourse to repeat LSCS:

- intravenous cannula
- full blood count and group-and-save sample available in laboratory
- continuous CTG monitoring
- monitor vaginal loss to exclude bleeding
- monitor abdominal pain: scar rupture can present with continuous pain, as opposed to intermittent contractions

With appropriate monitoring, vaginal delivery rates of approximately 70% can be expected.

Chapter Summary

- The aim of operative vaginal delivery is to replicate a vaginal delivery to expedite the delivery and reduce neonatal and maternal morbidity.
- Perineal trauma should be assessed by appropriately trained staff who can correctly identify a third-degree tear after all types of deliveries (spontaneous or assisted) and arrange an immediate repair to reduce maternal morbidity.
- A caesarean section is major abdominal surgery and is associated with an increased risk of bleeding, infection, thromboembolic disease and visceral injury.
- A vaginal birth after caesarean section is associated with a 0.5% risk of scar rupture and women should be counselled adequately.

FAILURE TO PROGRESS IN LABOUR

As described in Chapter 26, labour and delivery require the interaction of three components – the passages, the passenger and power – as part of a dynamic process:

- passages: the shape and size of the hard bony pelvis and soft tissues
- passenger: the size, presentation and position of the foetus
- power: this is mainly involuntary (strength and frequency of uterine contractions) but also voluntary (diaphragm and abdominal muscles)

Any of these factors can be involved in the failure of labour to progress normally, as summarized in Table 29.1. Once the diagnosis of labour has been made, a primiparous patient is expected to progress (by the cervix dilating), at approximately 0.5–1 cm/h and a multiparous patient by 1–2 cm/h.

Failure to progress related to the bony pelvis

Abnormal bony shape

Antenatal X-ray pelvimetry and routine pelvic assessment by vaginal examination are no longer performed (as they were unreliable indicators). However, certain points in a patient's history and examination can give clues to the likelihood of failure to progress in labour due to an abnormal pelvis (Table 29.2). Although still rare, one of the common problems is a previous pelvic fracture.

Cephalopelvic disproportion

With true cephalopelvic disproportion (CPD), the size of the pelvis is not in proportion to the foetus. It should be suspected antenatally if the head does not engage at term, particularly in a woman of short stature. Usually, a trial of labour is still appropriate, but in some cases an elective caesarean section is planned. During labour, CPD is diagnosed if the head remains unengaged on abdominal palpation. This is confirmed by assessing station on vaginal examination and by the presence of caput (swelling under the fetal scalp caused by reduction in venous return) and moulding. However, these signs are more commonly found simply with malposition rather than with true CPD.

Table 29.1 Differential diagnoses for failure to progress in labour

Bony passages	Abnormal-shaped pelvis Cephalopelvic disproportion
Soft passages	Uterine/cervical fibroids Cervical stenosis Circumcision
Passenger	Fetal size Fetal abnormality Fetal malpresentation Fetal malposition
Power	Lack of coordinated regular strong uterine contractions

Table 29.2 Causes of abnormalities of the bony pelvis

Congenital	Acquired
Osteogenesis imperfecta Ectopia vesicae Dislocation of the hip	Kyphosis of the thoracic or lumbar spine Scoliosis of the spine Spondylolisthesis Pelvic fractures Rickets/osteomalacia Poliomyelitis in childhood

Failure to progress related to the soft tissues of the pelvis

Uterus

A uterine malformation, such as the presence of a midline septum (a Müllerian or developmental abnormality), might prevent the foetus from lying longitudinally so that a malpresentation is responsible for failure to progress. This can also be rarely caused by uterine fibroids, which may increase the SFH (symphysis pubis fundal height) measurement during pregnancy and obstruct labour. The presence of a cervical fibroid might even necessitate a caesarean section.

Cervix

Failure of the cervix to dilate during labour despite adequate uterine contractions is rarely secondary to cervical scarring causing stenosis. This could be the result of cervical amputation or cone biopsy.

Vagina

Congenital anomalies of the vagina rarely cause problems with respect to labour and delivery, except in patients who have had reconstructive surgery. Other types of surgery, such as a colposuspension for urinary stress incontinence or repair of a vesicovaginal fistula, generally indicate the need for an elective caesarean section at term, but more to prevent recurrent symptoms rather than because of possible slow progress in labour.

Vulva

Previous perineal tears or episiotomy should not present difficulties during delivery. More problematic is a female circumcision (female genital mutilation (FGM)), which may necessitate an anterior episiotomy to prevent more severe tears and the risk of fistula formation. Ideally, this patient should have been assessed antenatally to make the appropriate plan of care including surgery for reversal of FGM before 20 weeks' gestation.

Ovary

Ovarian cysts in pregnancy are usually incidental findings at routine ultrasound. They can present with abdominal pain during pregnancy, secondary to torsion or haemorrhage (see Chapter 11). They do not cause slow progress in labour because they rise up out of the pelvis as the uterus increases in size.

Failure to progress related to the passenger

Fetal size

The possibility of a large foetus might be suggested by the patient's past medical history, for example, type 1 diabetes, or from the antenatal history, with development of gestational diabetes or hydrops fetalis from rhesus isoimmunization or parvovirus infection (see Chapter 23). In a multiparous patient, it is useful to check the weights of previous deliveries as an assessment of the ability to deliver the current infant.

Abdominal palpation is not always accurate as a method of diagnosing a large foetus, although this should be done to assess engagement of the presenting part in labour. Ultrasound is more accurate, provided that gestational age has been correctly estimated early in pregnancy.

During labour, on vaginal examination, the cervix may be felt to be increasingly oedematous. Signs of caput or moulding may be noted on the fetal head (Chapter 26). Caput is the boggy swelling on the fetal head as subcutaneous oedema of the scalp develops.

Fetal abnormality

Routine ultrasound scanning is likely to diagnose abnormalities such as a congenital goitre or a lymphangioma. These extend

the neck, so that the normal process of flexion cannot take place. This may result in a face or brow presentation (see earlier). Abdominal enlargement caused by the presence of ascites, multicystic kidneys or an umbilical hernia may make delivery difficult. Abnormalities of the fetal skull such as anencephaly should be suspected in labour if the head does not engage and the sutures feel widely spaced on vaginal examination. This condition is a type of spina bifida, again routinely diagnosed on ultrasound scan.

Fetal malposition

The fetal head normally engages with an occiput transverse position. With descent, the head rotates to an occipitoanterior position as described in Chapter 26. Any position other than occipitoanterior can be associated with failure to progress in labour, namely:

- occipitoposterior (OP) position
- occipitotransverse position

Approximately 20% of vertex presentations in early labour are occiput posterior. Diagnosis is determined by abdominal palpation:

- maternal lower abdomen that is flattened or concave
- fetal back cannot be palpated anteriorly
- fetal limbs that can be palpated anteriorly

On vaginal examination, the positions of the sutures and fontanelles are determined (see Chapter 26). If the anterior fontanelle is palpable vaginally, then the head is deflexed. If only the posterior fontanelle can be felt, then the head is flexed. This degree of flexion allows the smallest diameter of the head to present. It will, therefore, be more likely to rotate at the pelvic floor and proceed to normal vaginal delivery. The majority of OP positions will rotate during labour in the presence of adequate contractions. The minority will not rotate, but will deliver vaginally in the OP position (face to pubes) if the pelvis is large enough, while some will need rotation either manually or with an instrument (see Chapter 28).

Fetal malpresentation

Any presentation other than a vertex presentation is a malpresentation. The vertex is the area between the parietal eminences and the anterior and posterior fontanelles (Fig. 26.4). The most common malpresentation is the breech presentation, while others include shoulder, brow and face presentations.

Malpresentation can occur by chance, but it can also be caused by fetal or maternal conditions that prevent the vertex from presenting to the pelvis (Table 29.3).

Table 29.3 Causes of malpresentation

Maternal	Contraction of the pelvis
	Pelvic tumour (e.g., fibroid)
	Mullerian abnormality
	Multiparity
Foetoplacental	Prematurity
	Placenta praevia
	Polyhydramnios
	Multiple pregnancy
	Fetal anomaly
	• hydrocephalus
	• extension of the fetal head by neck tumours
	• anencephaly
	• decreased fetal tone

Breech presentation

The incidence of breech presentation increases with decreasing gestation with a prevalence of 3% at term. There are three types of breech presentation (Fig. 29.1):

- extended or frank breech (approximately 50%)
- flexed or complete breech (approximately 25%)
- footling breech (approximately 25%)

There is increased perinatal mortality and morbidity associated with vaginal breech delivery when compared with the cephalic presentation of comparable birthweight at term. This is usually associated with difficulty in delivering the aftercoming head. The fetal trunk is softer than the head and can pass through the pelvis easily, which may result in entrapment of the aftercoming head.

MANAGEMENT

There are three management options for a breech presentation:

- external cephalic version (ECV)
- elective caesarean section
- planned vaginal breech delivery

External cephalic version

An attempt is made to turn the foetus to a cephalic presentation by manual manipulation through the maternal anterior abdominal wall. This is usually performed at around 37 weeks' gestation, to allow time for spontaneous version, and to minimize the number of successful versions turning back to breech. Contraindications to ECV include:

- pelvic mass
- antepartum haemorrhage
- placenta praevia
- multiple pregnancy
- ruptured membranes

ECV is usually performed under ultrasound guidance on the labour ward because of the small risk of fetal distress requiring immediate caesarean section (1:300). Success rate is around 50%. Rhesus-negative women should be given anti-D immunoglobulin following the attempted version because of the possibility of foetomaternal transfusion.

Management of labour with a breech presentation

This is classified as high-risk delivery, therefore should be in an obstetric unit with an attendant neonatologist with continuous fetal heart rate monitoring. Epidural anaesthesia is encouraged because of the increased chances of manipulation during delivery.

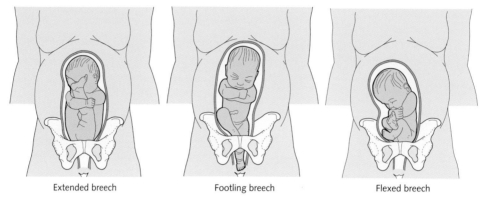

Extended breech   Footling breech   Flexed breech

Fig. 29.1 Classification of breech presentation.

During the second stage, the breech should be allowed to descend onto the pelvic floor before active pushing is commenced. If descent does not occur, this could indicate disproportion or an unexpectedly large foetus, and caesarean section is indicated.

RED FLAGS

Cord prolapse

Defined as the descent of the umbilical cord through the cervix before the presenting part when the membranes are ruptured. Cord prolapse is not common–overall incidence is up to 0.6%. However, in noncephalic presentations, it is more common, seen in 1% in patients with breech presentation.

It is associated with perinatal death mainly because of

- birth asphyxia – at home delivery settings
- prematurity and congenital malformations – at hospital settings

The risk of cord prolapse should be considered in the antenatal management of malpresentation due to higher risk of cord prolapse and admission to hospital after 37 weeks is common practice. Prolonged deceleration immediately after membrane rupture is a common presentation and healthcare professionals should assess for cord prolapse if fetal bradycardia occurs.

Once the diagnosis is made, immediate delivery should be planned. The mode of delivery depends on the cervical assessment. If delivery is imminent, a vaginal delivery could be considered. If diagnosis is made in community, then immediate transfer to hospital with a knee–chest position or left lateral (ideally head down and a pillow under the hip), to release the pressure on the cord, is essential.

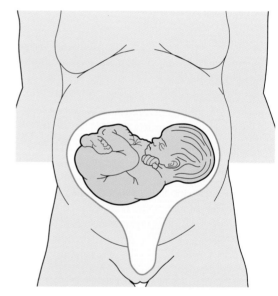

Fig. 29.2 Transverse lie.

Transverse lie and unstable lie

A transverse lie occurs when the long axis of the foetus is transverse to that of the mothers, usually with the shoulder presenting (Fig. 29.2). When the fetal lie is different at each palpation, the lie is said to be 'unstable'. The incidence of transverse lie diagnosed in labour with a single foetus is approximately 1 in 500 women. The most serious complication of a transverse lie is cord prolapse, and this is associated with spontaneous rupture of membranes, either antenatally or in labour. Admission to hospital from 37 weeks' gestation until delivery is indicated where immediate delivery is possible if the membranes spontaneously

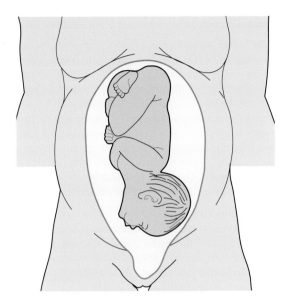

Fig. 29.3 Face presentation.

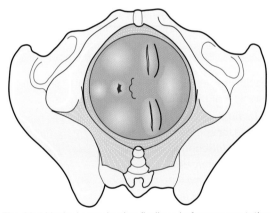

Fig. 29.4 Vaginal examination findings in face presentation.

rupture. If a transverse lie is diagnosed in early labour, ECV may be attempted only if the membranes are intact.

Face presentation

The incidence of face presentation in labour is 1 in 300 labours and occurs when the head is fully extended (Fig. 29.3). Diagnosis is usually made during vaginal examination in labour when the supraorbital ridges, the bridge of the nose and the alveolar margins in the mouth are palpable (Fig. 29.4). During labour, the face becomes oedematous and may be mistaken for a breech presentation. The chin (mentum) is the denominator and the submentobregmatic diameter is 9.5 cm (Fig. 26.4), i.e.,

the same as the suboccipitobregmatic diameter when the head is fully flexed, so vaginal delivery is possible. Flexion of the head to allow vaginal delivery is possible only in the mentoanterior position, which occurs in 75% of cases.

HINTS AND TIPS

Face presentation will deliver vaginally if it is mentoanterior but NOT if it is mentoposterior.

Management of a face presentation in labour is essentially the same as for a vertex presentation. Mentoposterior positions rotate spontaneously to mentoanterior in 50% of cases, usually in the second stage of labour, and in those that do not, a caesarean section is indicated.

COMMUNICATION

Patients with a face presentation need to be counselled that during labour the face becomes swollen and the baby can look very bruised when delivered and that this is not permanent and will settle.

Care must be taken during vaginal examination because fetal eyes can be damaged by trauma or antiseptic lotions.

Brow presentation

The incidence of brow presentation in labour is approximately 1 in 500. Vaginal examination reveals a high presenting part, a palpable forehead with orbital ridges in front and the anterior fontanelle behind. With a brow presentation, the mentovertical diameter of 13.5 cm presents (Fig. 26.4). An average-sized foetus will not engage with a normal-sized pelvis and this will result in obstructed labour. When the fetal head is small in relation to the maternal pelvis, descent might occur, allowing flexion of the head as it reaches the pelvic floor. Signs of disproportion will lead to a caesarean delivery.

Failure to progress related to the power

The frequency, duration and strength of the contractions are assessed with uterine palpation. The cardiotocograph reports the frequency and duration. However, the recording of the strength can be altered by position of the monitor on the abdomen and maternal obesity and so this must be assessed on palpation. Inefficient uterine activity can be diagnosed if labour is prolonged and the contractions are:

- uncoordinated
- fewer than 3 to 4 in 10 minutes
- lasting less than 60 seconds

After thorough abdominal and vaginal examinations, and with normal fetal monitoring, careful use of oxytocic drugs, usually intravenous syntocinon infusion, can improve the contractions. Caution must be taken to avoid too frequent contractions because this can reduce the oxygen exchange in the placental bed and lead to fetal hypoxia. Patients should be on continuous CTG (cardiotocography) monitoring.

Particular care is essential in a multiparous patient because the diagnosis of inefficient uterine action is much less common than in a primiparous patient. A fetal malposition, malpresentation or increased fetal size should be considered as the cause of the slow progress; inappropriate use of oxytocic drugs is associated with uterine rupture in this group.

MANAGEMENT OF FAILURE TO PROGRESS

This depends on the cause. Contractions may be improved with:

- artificial rupture of membranes (ARM)
- use of intravenous syntocinon

ARM is thought to release local prostaglandins and can increase the rate of labour progression. The strength and frequency of the uterine contractions can also be improved by administration of an infusion of intravenous syntocinon (synthetic oxytocin). However, caution must be exercised in a multiparous patient. In general, labour proceeds more rapidly in a second pregnancy. Therefore, if progress is slow, fetal size and position must be considered so that excessive contractions do not put the patient at risk of uterine rupture with syntocinon. Regular strong contractions will help to correct a fetal malposition by rotating the head against the pelvic floor muscles, as well as improving descent. Malpresentation may be managed as described earlier.

The presence of good contractions over several hours but without significant progress in terms of cervical dilatation and descent of the presenting part should alert the physician to consider delivery by caesarean section.

Failure to progress in the second stage of labour should be assessed in the manner already described and instrumental delivery considered (see Chapter 27). If the head is almost crowning, then an episiotomy might be all that is necessary to expedite vaginal delivery.

SHOULDER DYSTOCIA

Shoulder dystocia is a problem of the pelvic inlet preventing delivery of the shoulders once the head is out. This occurs because the shoulders fail to pass through the pelvic inlet; it is not a problem with the outlet or the perineum. The essential point is not to use excessive traction and nonaxial pull direction on the fetal head and to facilitate delivery of the shoulders because this risks damage to the brachial plexus nerve roots in the neck. Increasing hypoxia occurs while the foetus is lodged in the vagina, with pressure on the umbilical cord. The more common injury to the foetus is Erb palsy caused by damage to nerve roots C4, C5 and C6, which can have serious long-term neurological sequelae. Manoeuvres to aid delivery include:

- Lie the patient flat.
- McRoberts position – the hips are flexed in knee–chest position to widen the anteroposterior diameter of the pelvis.
- Suprapubic pressure to dislodge the anterior shoulder.
- Internal rotation techniques to try and rotate the anterior shoulder from under the pubic symphysis.
- Deliver the posterior arm.

This situation is an emergency and should therefore be practised as a regular drill by all the staff in the maternity unit. A senior neonatologist should be called to attend urgently to assess the baby at delivery.

HINTS AND TIPS

A useful pneumonic for the management of shoulder dystocia – HELPERR:

call for **help**

evaluate for episiotomy

legs into McRoberts

suprapubic **p**ressure

enter manoeuvres (internal rotation)

remove posterior arm

roll onto all fours

COMMUNICATION

Because of the high rate of litigation associated with shoulder dystocia due to the long-term sequelae of Erb palsy, meticulous documentation is important. Shoulder dystocia proformas should be used with careful documentation of the timing of each manoeuvre and who performed it. There must be clear documentation as to which shoulder was anterior during the delivery.

Chapter Summary

- The most common malpresentation is a breech presentation. Management options at term are external cephalic version, vaginal breech delivery or caesarean section depending on the history and the patient's wishes.
- Other malpresentations include transverse lie, oblique lie, face presentation and brow presentation.
- Failure to progress in labour can be due to an abnormality of the passage, passenger or powers.
- Management of failure to progress in labour due to inadequate contractions can be treated with ARM followed by the use of a syntocinon infusion.
- Cord prolapse is an obstetric emergency where the umbilical cord descends through the cervix before the presenting part, following the rupture of membranes.
- Following the diagnosis of cord prolapse an immediate delivery should be planned. The mode of delivery will depend on the cervical assessment. If delivery is imminent, vaginal delivery could be considered.
- Shoulder dystocia occurs when the anterior shoulder of the baby fails to pass under the symphysis pubis following the delivery of the fetal head. There are various manoeuvres to aid delivery.

UKMLA Conditions
Cord prolapse

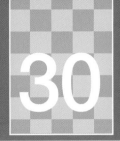

INTRODUCTION

Despite advances in prenatal and antenatal care, stillbirth is still a common occurrence with 1 in 200 births in the UK.

Investigations into the cause of stillbirth by means of maternal investigations and a postmortem are aimed at reducing the risk of this devastating situation recurring in a future pregnancy. However, more than 50% of stillbirths were found to be unexplained (Table 30.1).

DEFINITIONS

- Stillbirth: A baby that is born with no signs of life at or after 24 completed weeks of pregnancy.
- Intrauterine death: A foetus in utero greater than 24 completed weeks of pregnancy is found to have no cardiac activity.

Table 30.1 Causes of stillbirth

Type of condition	Causes of stillbirth
Maternal condition	Diabetes (preexisting and gestational) Preeclampsia Sepsis Obstetric cholestasis Acute fatty liver Thrombophilias (e.g., protein C and protein S resistance, factor V Leiden mutation, antithrombin III deficiency)
Fetal condition	Infection: *Toxoplasma*, *Listeria*, syphilis, parvovirus Chromosomal abnormality Structural abnormality Rhesus disease leading to severe anaemia Twin-to-twin transfusion syndrome (affects monochorionic twins only) Intrauterine growth restriction Alloimmune thrombocytopaenia
Placental condition	Postmaturity Abruption Placenta praevia: significant bleed Cord prolapse

DIAGNOSIS

Most commonly a diagnosis of an intrauterine death is made when the patient presents with a history of reduced fetal movements. Occasionally it will be made during a routine antenatal visit when the clinician is unable to auscultate the fetal heart. It can also present with symptoms of the event that caused the baby to die, for example, antepartum haemorrhage and abdominal pain associated with placental abruption (see Chapter 20).

When a patient presents with reduced fetal movements and there are difficulties in auscultating the fetal heart using a cardiotocography machine or handheld Doppler, this should prompt rapid referral to a trained clinician to perform an ultrasound scan. If there is no fetal heart activity, then the diagnosis of an intrauterine death can be made. Ideally, this should be verified by a second appropriately trained individual.

BREAKING BAD NEWS

Conveying the diagnosis of an intrauterine death to the parents can be one of the most challenging entities a clinician ever has to do. It is imperative that the parents are told straight away in a sensitive and empathetic manner using clear unambiguous terms. Occasionally, if a mother presents on her own, one should offer to call her partner or a relative to come and join her.

COMMUNICATION

Breaking bad news is an important skill for all clinicians. Think about the environment in which you are going to do this and ensure the patient has the appropriate support. Also, try to give the patient the time she needs, so if possible, hand over bleeps to colleagues as these could be a distraction.

HISTORY

Taking a history from a patient diagnosed with an intrauterine death is aimed at:

- assessing maternal wellbeing
- identifying potential causes

Using the handheld obstetric notes to review their past obstetric and medical history or by direct questioning of the patient, the following points should be identified:

- Maternal rhesus group: Mothers that are rhesus negative should be investigated to rule out the possibility of rhesus disease as a cause of the stillbirth (see Chapter 19).
- Trisomy screening: If patients are found to have a high-chance result, it is likely that a chromosomal abnormality may be the cause. Note that screening tests are not diagnostic, therefore chromosomal abnormalities still could be the cause.
- Ultrasound: The anomaly ultrasound scan and any subsequent growth scans should be reviewed, as any abnormality (either structural or growth related) may indicate a potential cause.
- Antepartum haemorrhage: Recurrent bleeds or, indeed, a large bleed may indicate a placental abruption or vasa praevia (a situation where unprotected placental vessels course through the membranes and if ruptured can lead to rapid loss of fetal blood and fetal death; see Chapter 20).
- Ruptured membranes: Any history of vaginal fluid loss may indicate a breach in the fetal membranes exposing the foetus to ascending infection (chorioamnionitis).
- Itching: Itching mainly affecting the palms and soles may indicate intrahepatic cholestasis of pregnancy, which is associated with an increased risk of stillbirth (see Chapter 22).
- Signs of maternal illness: Fever, rash or vomiting may indicate an intercurrent illness as the cause of the fetal demise. Listeria, toxoplasmosis and parvovirus are all possible infections that can lead to intrauterine death.

EXAMINATION

A thorough general examination is important to identify any potential signs of maternal illness. Even in the absence of a preceding maternal illness, an intrauterine death can lead to maternal sepsis and/or coagulopathy. The examination should include:

- maternal pulse
- blood pressure
- respiratory rate
- temperature
- looking for rashes (may indicate maternal infection)

The uterus should also be palpated to assess its size, tone and contour. A uterus that is larger than one would expect for the gestation may indicate polyhydramnios, which can be secondary to maternal diabetes (see Chapter 22). A uterus that is smaller than expected may indicate intrauterine growth restriction. A tender firm uterus may indicate placental abruption, whereas a tender but soft uterus may indicate chorioamnionitis.

INVESTIGATIONS

Investigations in the setting of an intrauterine death are aimed at:

1. Assessing the current state of maternal wellbeing.
2. Identifying a potential cause of the stillbirth.
3. Possibly identifying any prognostic factors for future pregnancy.

It is important that parents are told that in around 50% of all cases, no cause will be found. However, investigations are still essential – if a cause is found, this may be vital in preventing recurrence.

Haematology and biochemistry

- Full blood count: Assess maternal haemoglobin levels in the context of a haemorrhage, maternal white cells for infection; platelets for coagulopathy
- C-reactive protein: Useful in infection, although nonspecific as to the site.
- Urea and electrolytes: Assess renal function in preeclampsia, haemorrhage and sepsis, also useful as a baseline.
- Liver function tests: Assess in preeclampsia, obstetric cholestasis, haemorrhage and sepsis, also useful as a baseline.
- Coagulation screen: Assess the possibility of coagulopathy.
- Kleihauer: Essential for ALL women (not just those who are rhesus negative) to estimate a foetomaternal haemorrhage. This will also allow dose calculation of anti-D in rhesus-negative patients.
- Maternal thrombophilia screen with or without antibody screen: Indicated if intrauterine growth restriction or hydrops is identified, respectively.
- Random blood sugar and HbA1c: May indicate gestational diabetes or indeed previously undiagnosed type 1 or type 2 diabetes.
- Maternal thyroid function: May indicate occult thyroid disease.
- Parental karyotyping: Indicated if fetal karyotype indicates an unbalanced translocation or if fetal karyotyping is not possible and features indicate a chromosomal cause.

Microbiology

- Urinalysis and midstream urine: Assess the possibility of urinary tract infection; proteinuria may indicate preeclampsia and ketonuria in a diabetic patient would prompt assessment to rule out ketoacidosis.
- Blood cultures, vaginal swabs and cervical swabs: Should be performed if sepsis is suspected as they will allow accurate identification of a pathogen and appropriate antibiotic therapy.
- Placental and fetal swabs should be taken to rule out chorioamnionitis.
- Maternal infection serology: Parvovirus B19, toxoplasmosis, rubella, cytomegalovirus, syphilis (TORCH screen).

Pathology

A postmortem examination should be offered to all parents when an intrauterine death has been diagnosed. It is carried out by a specialist perinatal pathologist. A full postmortem involves an examination of the placenta and fetal karyotype, as well as the foetus. A limited postmortem allows the parents to specify the organs or body compartments they wish to be examined. This can be of relevance when a specific organ abnormality was suspected antenatally, for example, on the anomaly scan. An external postmortem examination can be performed using imaging modalities, but this is likely to give only limited information. It is important to inform parents that agreeing to a postmortem may affect the timing of funeral arrangements.

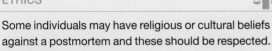

ETHICS

Some individuals may have religious or cultural beliefs against a postmortem and these should be respected. An external postmortem examination with imaging or placental examination only may be acceptable. Informed consent involves explaining that such tests will give less information.

MANAGEMENT

Once an intrauterine death has been confirmed and the parents have been informed, it is important to allow them the time to absorb the information, as well as start to grieve. Subsequently, a plan of care needs to be made detailing the method of delivery.

In most cases a vaginal delivery will be the most suitable way to deliver the foetus, having less impact on mode of delivery for a subsequent pregnancy. An antiprogesterone (mifepristone) is given orally and then after 36 to 48 hours, a course of prostaglandins (e.g., misoprostol) is administered, either orally or vaginally. For gestations nearer term, an oxytocin infusion may be used as an alternative to prostaglandin.

Rarely, labour is contraindicated (e.g., multiple previous caesarean sections or extensive uterine surgery), and a caesarean section may be required.

COMMUNICATION

Following delivery, the parents are encouraged to hold the baby (if they wish to do so) and mementoes such as pictures and foot/hand prints are taken. Religious ceremonies can also take place if the parents wish.

AFTER DELIVERY

Most units have a specialist midwife who acts as a direct contact for the patient and ensures appropriate follow-up counselling and investigations take place. They will report all stillbirths to MBRRACE-UK who are responsible for confidential enquiries. In the UK, support should include details about the Stillbirth & Neonatal Death charity (SANDS), which offers support to parents. The immediate period following a stillbirth is a very vulnerable time for the mother and she is at significant risk of postnatal depression (see Chapter 31). Mothers should be offered cabergoline to suppress lactation if they wish to do so.

It is very important to arrange a follow-up appointment with the consultant in charge of their care to ensure all investigations that were performed are reviewed and a plan made for future pregnancies. If no particular cause for the stillbirth was identified, then the couple can be offered consultant-led antenatal care with regular growth scans in the following pregnancy and induction of labour at an appropriate gestation can be considered. As always, cases need to be handled with great sensitivity and care.

Chapter Summary

- A stillbirth occurs when a baby is born with no signs of life at or after 24 completed weeks of pregnancy.
- An intrauterine death occurs when a foetus in utero greater than 24 completed weeks of pregnancy is found to have no cardiac activity.
- More than 50% of stillbirths have no cause identified.
- Diagnosis of an intrauterine death is by detecting no fetal heart activity on ultrasound scan. A second clinician should confirm this.
- Investigations to identify a cause for the stillbirth should be undertaken and include haematology, biochemistry, microbiology and a postmortem.
- Vaginal delivery is the most suitable mode of delivery in the majority of cases unless there are contraindications.
- A follow-up appointment should be offered to these couples to discuss results from investigations performed, plans for future pregnancies and concerns or questions that the couple may have.

UKMLA Presentations
Intrauterine death

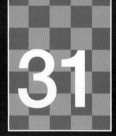

POSTPARTUM HAEMORRHAGE

Definitions

Postpartum haemorrhage (PPH) refers to excessive bleeding from the genital tract following delivery of the infant. Blood loss of around 200 to 300 mL is usually expected with a vaginal birth. PPH is classified as either primary or secondary:

- **Primary PPH**: Blood loss of >500 mL within 24 hours of delivery. This is often described as 'minor' if between 500 and 1000 mL and 'major' if >1000 mL or associated with hypovolaemic shock.
- **Secondary PPH**: Abnormal or excessive bleeding from the genital tract between 24 hours and 12 weeks after delivery.

INCIDENCE AND RISK FACTORS

Obstetric haemorrhage remains one of the major contributors to maternal mortality worldwide. Primary PPH occurs in about 5% of deliveries in developed countries, but this incidence rises to 28% in the developing world. Risk factors for PPH are shown in Table 31.1.

Aetiology of primary postpartum haemorrhage (PPH)

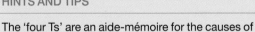

HINTS AND TIPS

The 'four Ts' are an aide-mémoire for the causes of primary postpartum haemorrhage (PPH):

- Tone (90% of cases)
- Trauma
- Tissue
- Thrombin

Note that PPH is often multifactorial. For example, uterine atony in the presence of a retained placenta.

Tone

Uterine atony refers to poor uterine contractility and is the commonest cause of primary PPH, accounting for 75% to 90%

Table 31.1 Risk factors for postpartum haemorrhage (PPH)

Maternal factors	Pregnancy factors
Grand multiparity	Multiple pregnancy
Uterine fibroids	Fetal macrosomia
Maternal age >35 years	Polyhydramnios
High BMI	Prolonged 2nd and 3rd stage
Coagulation disorders	of labour
Antenatal anaemia	Previous postpartum
	haemorrhage (PPH)
	Antepartum haemorrhage in
	current pregnancy
	Placenta accreta or praevia
	Instrumental delivery
	General anaesthesia
	Retained placental tissue/
	products of conception
	Genital tract trauma
	Infection: endometritis
	Uterine rupture

of cases. Bleeding postdelivery most commonly arises from the placental site. In normal physiology, the uterus contracts following delivery, causing intramyometrial blood vessels at the placental bed to constrict, thus arresting bleeding. Factors affecting uterine contractility will predispose to PPH. Examples include uterine fibroids, prolonged labour and previous PPH. Over-distension of the uterus, such as in fetal macrosomia, multiple pregnancy and polyhydramnios, also increases the risk of uterine atony and PPH.

Trauma

Genital tract trauma can occur with a normal vaginal delivery, either from an episiotomy or from a vaginal, cervical or perineal tear. Trauma is more common with an instrumental delivery, especially with the use of forceps, in particular, Kielland forceps. Therefore, the genital tract, including a rectal examination, should always be checked for signs of trauma once the placenta has been delivered. As the genital tract is extremely vascular during pregnancy, even a small laceration can result in profuse bleeding very quickly!

The average blood loss at caesarean section is 500 mL. Placenta praevia, accreta or prolonged labour may increase this. In prolonged labour, the presenting part may become impacted in the pelvis, making delivery more difficult. This can cause the incision on the uterus to tear, which may increase blood loss.

Uterine rupture is rare and is an uncommon cause of PPH in the UK. It is associated with high rates of maternal and fetal morbidity and mortality. Incidence has fallen dramatically with the introduction of the lower segment procedure (<1%), as opposed to the classical vertical incision of the uterus (up to 5%). Uterine rupture is usually seen in patients who undergo labour having previously had a caesarean section. These patients should be counselled preoperatively on the risks of vaginal birth after caesarean section (VBAC) and monitored closely on labour ward. Spontaneous rupture is much less common, usually seen in grandmultiparous women and associated with the use of syntocinon to augment labour. Uterine rupture can present with an abnormal cardiotocograph in labour, or with continuous abdominal pain and vaginal bleeding. Diagnosis is made at laparotomy and the treatment is surgical – either repair of the rupture or hysterectomy.

Tissue

The presence of retained products of conception (RPOC) or placental tissue prevents the uterus from contracting effectively, resulting in bleeding from the placental bed. The placenta should be delivered within 30 minutes in the case of active management of the third stage, and within 60 minutes with physiological management.

The placenta may be abnormally invasive, increasing the risk of retained placental tissue. This occurs on a spectrum, from superficial attachment to the myometrium (placenta accreta), to invasion into the myometrium (placenta increta), and finally invasion through the entire wall of the uterus and through the uterine serosa (placenta percreta). The latter may even invade surrounding pelvic organs including the bladder and bowel. Risk factors for placenta accreta spectrum include previous caesarean section and placenta praevia.

Thrombin

Coagulation disorders can be acute or chronic (preexisting). Preexisting conditions such as inherited vascular disorders (e.g., von Willebrand's) are usually known about antenatally. HELLP syndrome in association with preeclampsia can be acquired in pregnancy. Disseminated intravascular coagulation (DIC) can present acutely, secondary to placental abruption or maternal sepsis. PPH may also lead to DIC, which itself exacerbates blood loss.

Assessment

Primary PPH is a common but important obstetric emergency. Acute haemorrhage may occur suddenly and rapidly become life-threatening. Awareness of risk factors, familiarity with interventions and a multidisciplinary team approach is essential in the management of PPH.

Always begin with ABC – Airway, Breathing, Circulation. Note the patient's appearance (is she pale or unresponsive?). Check the heart rate, respiratory rate and blood pressure. Blood loss should be estimated as accurately as possible, for example, by weighing pads. It is common to underestimate the loss.

Intravenous access should be established with two wide-bore cannulae. Blood should be sent for a full blood count (to determine haemoglobin and platelet count), coagulation screen (including fibrinogen), renal and liver function tests (to establish baseline) and group-and-save. Depending on the degree of haemorrhage, cross-matching blood in preparation for transfusion may be necessary.

Careful clinical examination is required to determine the cause of the bleeding so that appropriate management can be instigated. Carry out a focused abdominal examination and assess the size and tone of the uterus (whether the uterus is contracted or not). The uterine fundus should be at or below the level of the umbilicus. If it is above, there might be retained placental tissue, or the uterus could be filling with clots. Check that the placenta and membranes have been delivered and are complete. Ensure that the cotyledons appear complete and that there is no suggestion of a succenturiate lobe. Consider that the bleeding might be coming from trauma to the genital tract. The patient should be examined in sufficient light and with adequate analgesia (either local or regional) to exclude lacerations to the cervix, vagina and perineum.

CLINICAL SKILLS: ASSESSMENT OF THE PATIENT WITH PRIMARY POSTPARTUM HAEMORRHAGE (PPH)

- Resuscitation: ABC (airways, breathing, circulation)
- Quantify the blood loss
- General appearance
- Observations: heart rate, blood pressure, respiratory rate
- Establish intravenous access
- Send bloods for full blood count (FBC), Urea and electrolytes (U&Es), coagulation screen, group-and-save or crossmatch
- Abdominal examination: assess size and tone of the uterus
- Check that the placenta and membranes have been delivered and are complete

ASSESS FOR GENITAL TRACT TRAUMA

Management

A multidisciplinary approach to management is very important, involving liaison between the obstetrician, the anaesthetist and the haematologist. Fig. 31.1 provides an algorithm for the management of primary PPH. As the cause of PPH may be multifactorial, interventions are usually undertaken simultaneously until the bleeding is under control.

Tone

Uterine atony is the commonest cause of PPH and initial management therefore involves stimulating myometrial contractions and improving uterine tone. The following measures are usually instituted in turn:

- Palpate the fundus of the uterus and 'rub up' a contraction by massaging it abdominally.
- Perform bimanual compression.
- Empty the bladder – an indwelling catheter should be left in place to monitor urine output.

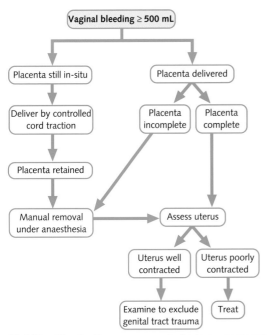

Fig. 31.1 Algorithm for the management of primary postpartum haemorrhage. (Source: Kay SE, Sandhu CJ. *Crash Course Obstetrics and Gynaecology*. Elsevier; 2019: 219–226. © 2019.)

- Administer uterotonic drugs, commonly five units of IV oxytocin (may be repeated) followed by an oxytocin infusion of 40 units in 500 mL of isotonic crystalloids at 125 mL/hour. IV or IM ergometrine 0.5 mg may also be administered in patients without a history of hypertension in pregnancy or cardiac disease.
- Consider the use of prostaglandins, either IM carboprost (also known as haemabate) 0.25 mg or sublingual/rectal misoprostol 800 mcg. These should be used with caution in women with asthma.
- IV tranexamic acid (an antifibrinolytic agent) 1 g has been shown to improve outcomes.

Should the bleeding continue despite pharmacological measures, surgical interventions should be initiated sooner rather than later. An intrauterine balloon can be inserted either vaginally or abdominally if inserted during caesarean section. The balloon is filled with water and works by applying pressure directly to the placental bed, tamponading the bleeding. Uterine compression sutures (e.g., B-Lynch or modified compression sutures) are a form of haemostatic brace suture that require a laparotomy for its insertion but can also be performed at the time of caesarean section. Sutures are placed around the body of the uterus to maintain compression. Stepwise uterine devascularization and internal iliac artery ligation may be performed but the latter requires a high degree of surgical skill and training, and is associated with a risk of ureteric injury. Depending on local facilities, interventional radiology procedures such as arterial embolization can be considered. These measures all have the benefit of controlling bleeding without resorting to hysterectomy, hence preserving fertility. However, prompt recourse to hysterectomy may be essential to reduce maternal morbidity and mortality, especially in cases of uterine rupture or placenta accreta spectrum.

Trauma

Bleeding while the uterus is firmly contracted is strong evidence of genital tract trauma. Lacerations should be repaired as soon as possible with appropriate analgesia. There should be good light and an aseptic technique should be applied to minimize infection. Suturing may need to take place in theatre, for example, cervical lacerations bleed profusely and may need to be repaired under general anaesthesia.

Tissue

If the placenta is still in situ, delivery should be attempted by controlled cord traction. Once delivered, the placenta must be examined to ensure the cotyledons and membranes are complete. If delivery of the placenta fails or is incomplete, manual removal will be necessary under regional or general analgesia. This is usually performed with antibiotic cover to reduce the risk of postpartum endometritis.

In cases of placenta accreta spectrum, it may be appropriate to leave the placenta in situ to be absorbed over time, especially if the patient is not bleeding. This is associated with a high risk of infection and secondary PPH, and the patient will require close monitoring following discharge. More commonly, however, the patient has significant bleeding and surgery is necessary, including hysterectomy.

Thrombin

Blood should be cross-matched and transfused and any coagulation defects corrected with fresh frozen plasma and cryoprecipitate to avoid going into DIC. A plasma fibrinogen level of greater than 2 g/L should be maintained during ongoing PPH. Platelets should be transfused when the platelet count reaches 75×10^9/L.

Complications of postpartum haemorrhage (PPH)

Sheehan syndrome

Rarely, PPH can lead to infarction of the pituitary gland, resulting in hypopituitarism. The size and oxygen demand of the pituitary gland increases during pregnancy, making it vulnerable to injury in severe blood loss. This can lead to failure of lactation, secondary amenorrhoea, hypothyroidism and adrenal crises.

Prevention of postpartum haemorrhage (PPH)

During the antenatal period, this should begin with identifying patients with preexisting anaemia as well as those with risk factors. Careful history taking would identify women with a known inherited coagulation factor deficiency or those who have had a previous PPH. Antenatal anaemia, defined as a haemoglobin level of <110 g/L at booking and <105 g/L at 28 weeks should be investigated and treated appropriately. This has been shown to reduce morbidity associated with PPH. Haematinic supplements such as folate and B12 may be used. Oral iron supplementation is commonly prescribed for iron-deficiency anaemia, although intravenous iron should be considered in those who do not respond to oral therapy.

During labour, PPH may also be anticipated, for example, in a patient who has a prolonged labour ending with a difficult instrumental delivery of a large baby. Active management of the third stage of labour is routine in most obstetric units, and is associated with an up to 50% reduction in the incidence of PPH. This involves:

- Administration of a uterotonic, typically IM oxytocin 10 units
- Controlled cord traction to deliver the placenta
- Clamping and cutting of the umbilical cord

Secondary postpartum haemorrhage (PPH)

Aetiology

Causes of secondary PPH include:

- RPOC or placental tissue
- Infection of the uterine cavity (endometritis)
- Rarely, gestational trophoblastic disease (molar pregnancy)

Clinical presentation

The patient may present with a persistent and offensive-smelling vaginal discharge, or prolonged and heavy vaginal bleeding in the presence of RPOC. Fever and lower abdominal pain are more likely to be associated with postpartum endometritis.

Assessment

Basic observations should include heart rate, blood pressure, respiratory rate and temperature. Tachycardia and pyrexia may be present with endometritis. Perform an abdominal examination. The height of the uterine fundus should be checked because the uterus will usually remain poorly contracted if there is retained placenta tissue. Tenderness is usually suggestive of endometritis. Speculum examination may also reveal offensive-smelling vaginal discharge. A bulky, tender uterus with an open cervical os may point to a diagnosis of RPOC (Fig. 31.2).

Bloods should be sent for a full blood count (to determine haemoglobin, white blood cell and platelet count), blood

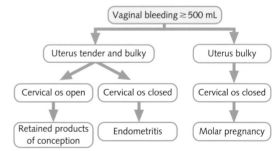

Fig. 31.2 Algorithm for the differential diagnoses of secondary postpartum haemorrhage (Source: Kay SE, Sandhu CJ. *Crash Course Obstetrics and Gynaecology*. Elsevier; 2019: 219–226. © 2019.)

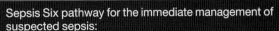

cultures, coagulation screen and group-and-save. A raised white blood cell count is an indication of infection. Depending on the estimated blood loss and haemoglobin level, cross-matching blood might be necessary. High vaginal and endocervical swabs should be sent for culture. A transvaginal ultrasound scan is helpful in excluding the presence of RPOC. Surgical evacuation of the uterus performed under ultrasound guidance will yield tissue for histological analysis to confirm the diagnosis.

Management

Definitive management of secondary PPH depends on the cause and clinical situation. If bleeding is light and there are no other signs of infection, a conservative approach with antibiotic treatment is sometimes taken but this requires clinical judgement and clear safety-netting. Endometritis requires treatment with broad-spectrum antibiotics (to cover aerobic and anaerobic organisms), either oral or intravenous, depending on clinical severity. RPOC usually requires removal of retained tissue, either by manual vacuum aspiration (MVA) or evacuation of retained products (ERPC) under general anaesthesia. The postpartum uterus is soft and susceptible to perforation. As a result, ERPC should ideally be performed under ultrasound guidance.

POSTNATAL INFECTION

Also known as 'puerperal infection', postnatal infection is defined as a maternal temperature of >38°C on any occasion in the first 14 days after delivery. The causative agent is commonly Group A streptococcus, found on the skin and in the respiratory tract, although other bacterial, viral or fungal pathogens may also be responsible. Localized infection may quickly lead to septic shock, rapid deterioration, multisystem organ failure and ultimately death.

Worldwide, sepsis remains a leading cause of maternal morbidity and mortality. Pregnant and postpartum women are highly susceptible to infection due to their immunocompromised state, and early recognition of the signs and symptoms of sepsis followed by prompt commencement of antibiotics is important. The 'Sepsis Six Care Bundle' was developed by the UK Sepsis Trust in 2013. It provides a quick reference guide to the urgent measures that should be completed within an hour of diagnosis of sepsis. Use of such care pathways has been shown to reduce the morbidity and mortality from sepsis if undertaken promptly. With improved hygiene and the use of antibiotics, the incidence of postnatal infection has fallen over the last 50 years.

> **RED FLAGS**
>
> Sepsis Six pathway for the immediate management of suspected sepsis:
> - Administer high-flow oxygen: Maintain oxygen saturations >94%.
> - Take blood cultures: Also consider sending urine cultures, high vaginal and endocervical swabs, wound swabs and sputum cultures if appropriate.
> - Administer broad-spectrum antibiotics according to local microbiology guidelines.
> - Administer intravenous fluids.
> - Check serial serum lactate levels: If >4 mmol/L, escalate to intensive care.
> - Monitor hourly urine output: Insert a urinary catheter if required in order to monitor fluid balance.

Sites of infection

- Uterus
- Caesarean section wound
- Perineal wound
- Chest
- Urinary tract
- Breast

History

The site of infection is usually obvious from the patient's history. Dysuria and urinary frequency would indicate a urinary tract infection. The presence of loin pain, rigors and fever may suggest an ascending infection to the kidneys causing pyelonephritis. Cough, coryzal symptoms and shortness of breath point towards a chest infection. This is typically a postoperative complication, seen after caesarean section.

Endometritis is more common following an operative intervention (such as caesarean section, instrumental delivery or manual removal of placenta). It typically presents with lower abdominal pain, fever, offensive-smelling vaginal discharge and heavy/prolonged bleeding. RPOC must be excluded. Caesarean section wound infections often present with purulent discharge, bleeding, erythema and pain. It is now routine practice to administer prophylactic antibiotics at the time of a caesarean section to decrease the incidence of wound and uterine infection.

Infection in the perineum can present with pain, redness, purulent vaginal discharge and wound breakdown. There is usually a history of a vaginal tear or episiotomy. Acute mastitis, or infection of the breast, typically presents at the end of the first week after delivery, as organisms that colonize the baby affect the breast. Patients can present with breast pain, erythema and fever.

Examination

A thorough examination of all body systems should be conducted as shown in Fig. 31.3.

It is important to note that patients may deteriorate rapidly with sepsis. Plotting the patient's observations on a Modified Early Warning Score (MEWS) chart can help to detect such patients and allow early escalation for critical/intensive care support. Red flag symptoms include:

- Confusion
- Hypotension: Systolic blood pressure ≤90 mmHg (or steadily dropping)
- Heart rate >130 beats per minute
- Respiratory rate >25 breaths per minute
- Oxygen saturations <92%
- Nonblanching rash: mottled, ashen, cyanotic appearance
- Lactate ≥2 mmol/L
- Oliguria (not passed urine in 18 hours)

Investigations

White blood cell count and C-reactive protein levels may be raised. Blood cultures are indicated in the presence of a fever ≥38°C. Other relevant investigations may be appropriate depending on the suspected source of infection:

- High vaginal and endocervical swabs
- Perineal wound swabs
- Caesarean section wound swabs
- Urine culture
- Sputum sample

Management

The antimicrobial treatment of choice will usually depend on local microbiology guidelines, but usually involves a broad-spectrum antibiotic and anaerobic cover with metronidazole for 5 to 7 days. Flucloxacillin is more appropriate for mastitis or wound infections because the usual pathogen is *Staphylococcus*. Any abscess may require surgical incision and drainage. In the event of wound breakdown, resuturing is not usually performed and the wound is allowed to heal by secondary intention.

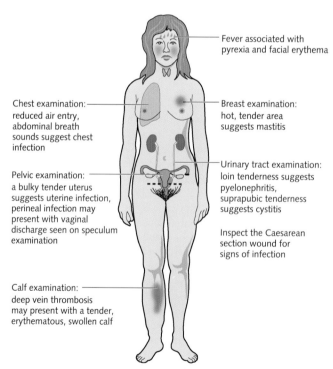

Fig. 31.3 Examination of the patient with postnatal pyrexia. (Source: Kay SE, Sandhu CJ. *Crash Course Obstetrics and Gynaecology*. Elsevier; 2019: 219–226. © 2019.)

POSTNATAL MENTAL HEALTH

Incidence

Mental health disorders are a major cause of maternal morbidity and mortality and left untreated, can have a detrimental impact on health in infancy and childhood. The United Kingdom's Confidential Enquiry into Maternal Deaths (MBR-RACE-UK) is an annual investigation looking into the deaths of women who died during pregnancy, childbirth and up to 1 year following delivery. The 2022 report found that deaths by suicide had risen three-fold since the previous report, and that maternal suicide was now the leading cause of direct maternal deaths occurring during pregnancy and within a year of delivery.

COMMUNICATION

Risk factors for postnatal mental illness include a previous history of mental health disorder either in or outside of pregnancy, as well as a family history of general and perinatal mental illness. Therefore, it is essential to enquire about these sensitively in the antenatal period to aid prediction and allow early detection and management of postnatal mental disorders. Early referral to perinatal mental health teams and multidisciplinary team management is essential.

Patients should be made aware that most psychotropic medications are relatively safe in pregnancy and breastfeeding. Many patients choose to discontinue medications during pregnancy, which increases the risk of relapse and deterioration of mental health disorders especially in the postpartum. The decision to continue or initiate any drug should be made together with the patient, in the context of a multidisciplinary team, weighing the risks and benefits. It is important to note that untreated mental illness carries the greatest risk to both maternal and infant outcomes.

Care should ideally take place in the community although in some cases, admission to a mother and baby unit may be necessary during an acute episode.

'Baby Blues'

Around 50% to 80% of women across all cultures and backgrounds will experience transient feelings of tearfulness, emotional lability, irritability and anxiety in the first few days after delivery. The predominant mood, however, is happiness. Peak incidence is between days 3 and 5, and symptoms usually settle within a week with reassurance and support from family and friends.

Postnatal depression

Depression is one of the most common mental health disorders among women during pregnancy and in the postpartum, affecting up to 25% of pregnant women and new mothers. Risk factors for postnatal depression have been listed previously in Chapter 22. Common symptoms are shown in Box 31.1. Symptoms of postnatal depression tend to have a gradual onset, with a peak incidence between 4 and 6 weeks postpartum.

Identification of risk factors during the antenatal period and early recognition of symptoms is important so that patients are referred promptly to the mental health team. Several screening tools have been developed and validated for use, including the Edinburgh Postnatal Depression Scale (EPDS) and 'Whooley' questionnaire.

Both pharmacological and nonpharmacological treatments may be necessary. Nonpharmacological modes of treatment include cognitive behavioural therapy (CBT), counselling and psychotherapy. As with any drug in pregnancy and breastfeeding, pharmacological treatment should be considered if the benefits outweigh the risks. Selective serotonin reuptake inhibitors (SSRIs), in particular sertraline, are the preferred antidepressants due to their relative safety profile in pregnancy and breastfeeding. Tricyclic antidepressants can be given safely both

---

BOX 31.1 SYMPTOMS OF POSTNATAL DEPRESSION

- Persistent low/depressed mood, sadness, tearfulness
- Lack of interest/pleasure in usual activities (anhedonia)
- Feeling worthless, guilty or inadequate
- Impaired concentration, poor memory, difficulty making decisions
- Insomnia and early morning awakening
- Diminished appetite or weight loss
- Fatigue, diminished energy
- Social withdrawal and poor self-care
- Ambivalence towards the baby
- Thoughts of self-harm or suicide

antenatally and postnatally, although they are generally not recommended in women at risk of self-harm due to the risk of overdose. Electroconvulsive therapy is safe.

Postpartum (puerperal) psychosis

Postpartum psychosis is rare although the most serious of the postnatal mental health disorders, affecting 2 in 1000 deliveries. Risk factors include:

- Personal history of bipolar affective disorder (35% risk)
- Previous postpartum psychosis or psychotic illness (50% risk of recurrence)
- Family history of bipolar affective disorder or postpartum psychosis (25% risk)

Postpartum psychosis tends to present with sudden onset within the first 2 weeks of delivery. Common symptoms are shown in Box 31.2. There is usually a combination of mania, depressive and psychotic symptoms, and the patient may rapidly deteriorate. During an acute episode, treatment usually involves admission to a mother and baby unit. This is due to the high risk of suicide and harm to self and others, as well as risk to both physical and mental health with the illness itself. A combination of antipsychotics, antidepressants and mood stabilizers is often initiated. Prognosis is generally good, although risk of relapse is high especially in the first few weeks. Due to the high rate of recurrence, these patients should be referred early in their next pregnancy to the perinatal mental health team, and a management plan put in place.

BOX 31.2 SYMPTOMS OF POSTNATAL PSYCHOSIS

- Delusions: persecutory beliefs, grandiosity, suspiciousness, fear
- Confusion and disorientation
- Hallucinations (auditory and visual)
- Insomnia and early morning awakening
- Irritation and agitation
- Lability of mood
- Often a combination of mania, depression and psychotic symptoms

---

THROMBOEMBOLIC DISEASE

Thromboembolic disease remains the leading cause of direct maternal deaths during and up to 6 weeks postdelivery. Chapter 22 describes the risk factors, diagnosis and management in detail. The postpartum period carries the highest risk of developing VTE and women should undergo a risk assessment postnatally as risk factors may have changed in the third trimester and depending on the mode of delivery. In the UK, LMWH is usually offered for 10 days postdelivery, although this may be extended to 6 weeks in women classified as high risk. Women should be safety-netted on the signs and symptoms of deep vein thrombosis (DVT) and PE, and encouraged to mobilize and avoid dehydration.

Chapter Summary

- Primary postpartum haemorrhage (PPH) is defined as bleeding more than 500 mL within 24 hours of delivery. The commonest causes of primary PPH are uterine atony and genital tract trauma.
- Secondary PPH is defined as bleeding more than 500 mL that starts 24 hours after delivery and occurs within 6 weeks. Common causes of secondary PPH are endometritis and retained products of conception (RPOC).
- Use the ABC (airways, breathing, circulation) approach when initially assessing a bleeding patient.
- Puerperal infection is defined as a maternal temperature of 38°C maintained for 4–6 hours in the first 14 days after delivery.
- Postnatal depression is one of the most common medical diseases of pregnancy, with 10% of women fulfilling the criteria for a depressive disorder; psychosis is much rarer, affecting 0.2% of births.
- Postdelivery, women should be risk assessed for thromboprophylaxis.

INTRODUCTION

Maternal collapse is a rare but serious event that requires prompt effective management. The Royal College of Obstetricians and Gynaecologists (RCOG) defines maternal collapse as 'an acute event involving the cardiorespiratory systems and/or brain, resulting in a reduced or absent conscious level (and potentially death), at any stage in pregnancy and up to six weeks after delivery'. The aim of this chapter is to give an overview of the main causes and initial management. The causes are summarized in Fig. 32.1.

Maternal deaths include any woman who dies from the time of conception up to 1 year postnatally. It is a rare but traumatic and distressing experience for all involved. It has wide-reaching implications not only for the family of the deceased but also for the medical team, with the lessons that can be learned from the tragedy being important both clinically and personally. This chapter discusses the National Confidential Enquiry that collates patient case details and publishes the lessons that need to be learnt across all units.

THE COLLAPSED PATIENT

The prospect of a collapsed pregnant patient can be very daunting for any clinician. The use of maternity or obstetric early warning charts can help recognize those patients at risk of collapse. As with any patient, the importance of summoning help and following the airway, breathing, circulation (ABC) guide of management is paramount. There are, however, important differences in management of the pregnant patient, compared with a nonpregnant patient:

- Maintenance of a left lateral tilt or utero displacement during resuscitation to prevent aortocaval compression and increase venous return to the heart.
- The mother always takes priority over the foetus and unless needed to aid maternal resuscitation, delivery of the foetus should be delayed until the mother is stable.

- Fig. 32.2 shows an algorithm for the initial management of the collapsed patient.

CAUSES OF MATERNAL COLLAPSE

HINTS AND TIPS

When investigating the causes of maternal collapse remember 4 Hs and 4 Ts, as for nonpregnant patients:

- hypovolaemia
- hypoxia
- hypo/hyperkalaemia (and other electrolyte disturbances)
- hypothermia
- thromboembolism
- toxicity
- tension pneumothorax
- tamponade

Fig. 32.3 outlines the significant physiological changes that the body undergoes during pregnancy.

Haemorrhage

Haemorrhage is the most common cause of collapse in obstetric patients. In many cases, the bleeding will be obvious, or revealed. However, in cases such as occult placental abruption, ruptured ectopic pregnancy or haemorrhagic cyst, it may be concealed and a high index of clinical suspicion is required. Sixteen mothers died from haemorrhage in the last confidential enquiry into causes of maternal death (*Mothers and Babies: Reducing Risk through Audit and Confidential Enquiries across the UK (MBRRACE) 2018–2020,* published in November 2022).

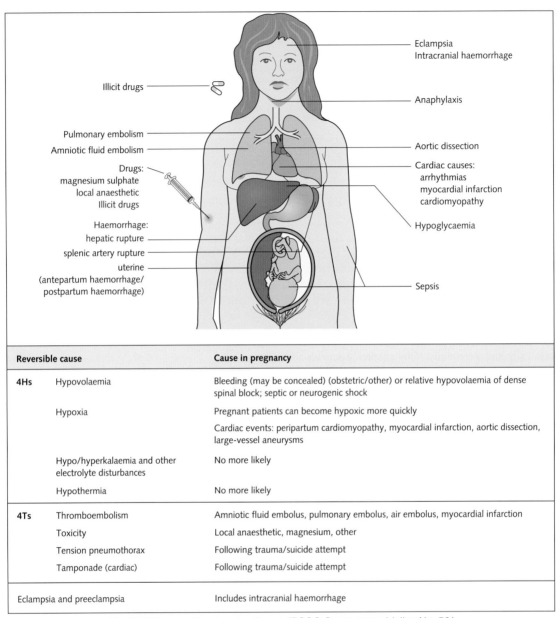

Illicit drugs

Pulmonary embolism
Amniotic fluid embolism

Drugs:
magnesium sulphate
local anaesthetic
Illicit drugs

Haemorrhage:
hepatic rupture
splenic artery rupture
uterine
(antepartum haemorrhage/
postpartum haemorrhage)

Eclampsia
Intracranial haemorrhage

Anaphylaxis

Aortic dissection
Cardiac causes:
arrhythmias
myocardial infarction
cardiomyopathy

Hypoglycaemia

Sepsis

Reversible cause		Cause in pregnancy
4Hs	Hypovolaemia	Bleeding (may be concealed) (obstetric/other) or relative hypovolaemia of dense spinal block; septic or neurogenic shock
	Hypoxia	Pregnant patients can become hypoxic more quickly
		Cardiac events: peripartum cardiomyopathy, myocardial infarction, aortic dissection, large-vessel aneurysms
	Hypo/hyperkalaemia and other electrolyte disturbances	No more likely
	Hypothermia	No more likely
4Ts	Thromboembolism	Amniotic fluid embolus, pulmonary embolus, air embolus, myocardial infarction
	Toxicity	Local anaesthetic, magnesium, other
	Tension pneumothorax	Following trauma/suicide attempt
	Tamponade (cardiac)	Following trauma/suicide attempt
Eclampsia and preeclampsia		Includes intracranial haemorrhage

Fig. 32.1 Causes of maternal collapse. (*RCOG Green-top guideline No. 56.*)

Major haemorrhage can be due to:

- placenta praevia/accreta
- placental abruption
- uterine rupture or a nonobstetric intraabdominal bleed (splenic rupture, etc.)
- postpartum haemorrhage (PPH)

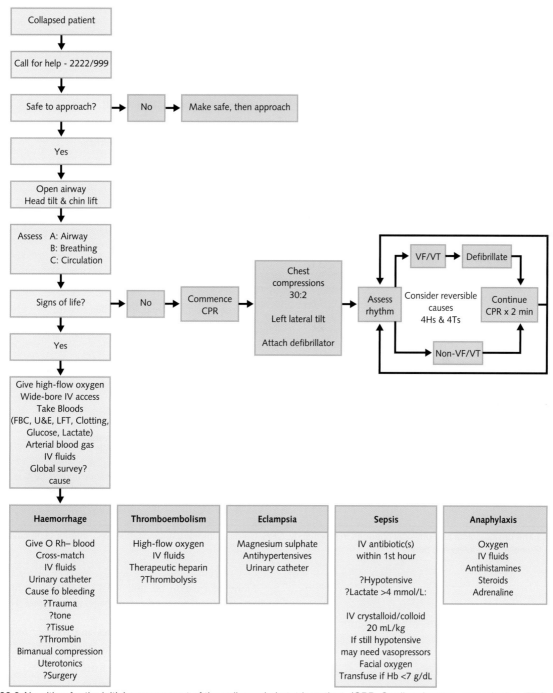

Fig. 32.2 Algorithm for the initial management of the collapsed obstetric patient. (*CPR,* Cardiopulmonary resuscitation; *FBC,* full blood count; *IV,* intravenous; *LFT,* liver function test; *U&E,* urea and electrolytes; *VF,* ventricular fibrillation; *VT,* ventricular tachycardia.)

System	Changes in pregnancy	Impact on resuscitation
Cardiovascular system		
Plasma volume	Increased by up to 50%	Dilutional anaemia Reduced oxygen carrying capacity
Heart rate	Increased by 15–20 bpm	Increased CPR circulation demands
Cardiac output	Increased by 40% Significantly reduced by pressure of gravid uterus on IVC	Increased CPR circulation demands
Uterine blood flow	I0% of cardiac output at term	Potential for rapid massive haemorrhage
Systemic vascular resistance	Decreased	Sequesters blood during CPR
Arterial blood pressure	Decreased by 10-15 mmHg	Decreased reserve
Venous return	Decreased by pressure of gravid uterus on IVC	Increased CPR circulation demands Decreased reserve
Respiratory system		
Respiratory rate	Increased	Decreased buffering capacity, acidosis more likely
Oxygen consumption	Increased by 20%	Hypoxia develops more quickly
Residual capacity	Decreased by 25%	Hypoxia develops more quickly when apnoeic
Arterial pCO$_2$	Decreased	Decreased buffering capacity, acidosis more likely
Laryngeal oedema	Increased	Difficult intubation
Other changes		
Gastric motility	Decreased	Increased risk of aspiration
Lower oesophageal sphincter	Relaxed	Increased risk of aspiration
Uterus	Enlarged	Diaphragmatic splinting reduces residual capacity and makes ventilation more difficult Aortocaval compression causes supine hypotension, reduces venous return and significantly impairs CPR
Weight	Increases	Large breasts may interfere with intubation, makes ventilation more difficult

Fig. 32.3 The physiological and physical changes in pregnancy. *CPR,* Cardiopulmonary resuscitation; *IVC,* inferior vena cava. (*RCOG Green-top guideline No. 56.*)

HINTS AND TIPS

Remember the 4 Ts for causes of postpartum haemorrhage (PPH):

1. **Tone:** uterine atony
2. **Trauma:** vaginal tears or uterine angle extensions at caesarean section
3. **Thrombin:** Underlying clotting disorders
4. **Tissue:** retained placenta or retained products of conception

More information on individual causes can be found in Chapter 20 (Antepartum haemorrhage) and Chapter 31 (Postnatal complications).

National management guidelines and training tools have helped the management of haemorrhage including:

- Use of maternity early warning charts.
- Prompt recognition and resuscitation.
- Involvement of a senior multidisciplinary team (i.e., haematologists, anaesthetists).
- Optimization of haemoglobin levels antenatally.
- Early recourse to methods such as insertion of a uterine balloon tamponade, uterine artery embolization, stepwise pelvic devascularization or life-saving hysterectomy.

The latter can be life-saving especially in individuals who decline blood products.

In cases of massive antepartum haemorrhage, prompt delivery of the foetus and placenta should be considered to control the bleeding, despite the gestation or viability of the pregnancy.

Thromboembolism

Thrombosis and thromboembolism remain the leading cause of direct maternal death during or up to 6 weeks after the end of pregnancy (MBRRACE 2018–2020). Pregnancy is a prothrombotic state with a four to six times increased relative risk antenatally and a further five times the antenatal risk in the puerperal period. All patients therefore should be educated about signs and symptoms of blood clots, as well as how to seek help. All patients should be risk assessed to identify those who require thromboprophylaxis:

- at booking
- at 28 weeks
- on every antenatal admission
- after delivery

Pulmonary embolism (PE) can present with chest pain, tachycardia, tachypnoea and shortness of breath. Large PEs can, however, cause maternal collapse. Initial management with cardiopulmonary resuscitation, oxygen and anticoagulation should be commenced until the diagnosis can be ruled out. In certain cases thrombolysis may be necessary. See Chapter 22 (Medical disorders in pregnancy) for further details on this topic.

Preeclampsia and eclampsia

Preeclampsia and eclampsia are both discussed in detail in Chapter 21: Hypertension in pregnancy. With regard to the collapsed patient, eclampsia should always be considered a cause of maternal collapse. By definition, eclampsia is seizure-like activity associated with hypertension and proteinuria (>30 g/L).

If an eclamptic fit is suspected, management with magnesium sulphate and antihypertensives should be started. The recognition of the importance of prompt treatment of hypertension, particularly systolic hypertension, is essential to prevent serious complications such as stroke and death. Therefore patients with headache and visual disturbances who have high blood pressure must have urinalysis and blood tests to exclude preeclampsia. There were eight reported deaths due to this in the last MBRRACE (2018–2020) report.

> **HINTS AND TIPS**
>
> It should be emphasized that stabilization of the mother in all cases takes precedence over the foetus.

Sepsis

Sepsis remains one of the leading direct causes of maternal death (second most likely cause of direct death, MBRRACE 2018–2020). Prompt recognition and management is essential when faced with a collapsed patient in whom sepsis is suspected. Septic patients may present with:

- pyrexia/hypothermia
- tachycardia
- tachypnoea
- hypotension
- rigors
- confusion
- collapse

> **RED FLAGS**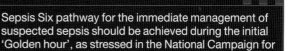
>
> Sepsis Six pathway for the immediate management of suspected sepsis should be achieved during the initial 'Golden hour', as stressed in the National Campaign for Sepsis Management:
> 1. Administer oxygen: maintain saturations > 94%
> 2. Take blood cultures, consider urine microscopy, culture and sensitivity, vaginal swab, sputum, etc. as indicated
> 3. Give broad-spectrum antibiotics (trust specific, taking into account patient's allergies if known)
> 4. Give intravenous fluids
> 5. Check serial lactate, call critical care if >4
> 6. Measure urine output, start fluid balance chart with or without urinary catheter

Shock

Shock is a potentially life-threatening situation where there is a state of cellular and tissue hypoxia resulting from either decreased oxygen delivery, increased oxygen demand, poor oxygen utilization or a combination of these. Shock can be categorized into either hypovolemic, cardiogenic, obstructive or distributive (Fig. 32.4). Prompt recognition and management are essential.

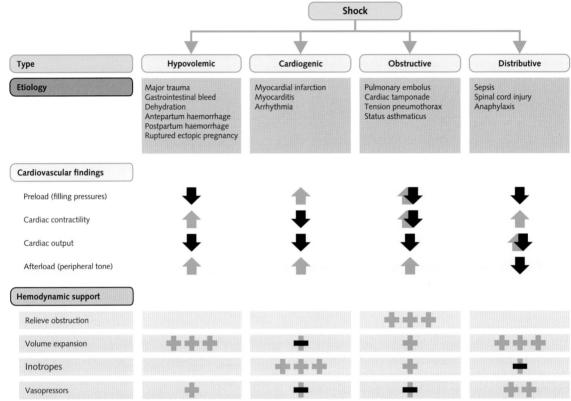

Fig. 32.4 The causes, cardiovascular findings and haemodynamic support for different types of shock. Under cardiovascular findings, bidirectional arrows indicate variation in findings among patients with the particular type. Under haemodynamic support, the number of + signs indicate the importance of therapy. A combined + and – indicates that the intervention could help some patients but must be used with caution. https://www.clinicalkey.com/student/content/book/3-s2.0-B9780323532662000989#3-s2.0-B9780323532662000989-f98-01-9780323532662. Approach to the Patient with Shock - Goldman-Cecil Medicine Angus, Derek C.; Goldman-Cecil Medicine, 98, 641-648.e2

Amniotic fluid embolism

An amniotic fluid embolism (AFE) is a rare but very serious cause of maternal collapse, which carries a high rate of mortality. An AFE is thought to occur when amniotic fluid enters maternal circulation and travels to distant sites such as the lungs and occludes pulmonary vessels. In addition, an anaphylactic-like reaction is thought to occur. These patients then rapidly develop a coagulopathy and haemorrhage can ensue. Sadly the diagnosis is often made retrospectively at postmortem and in patients who do survive, there can be significant morbidity. Patients may present with:

- acute hypotension
- hypoxia
- respiratory distress
- seizures
- cardiac arrest

It should be considered as a diagnosis when patients collapse during labour, caesarean section, manual removal of placenta or within 30 minutes of these.

Management of these patients is largely supportive with maintenance of their airway, breathing and circulation. Cardiopulmonary resuscitation may be necessary and regular blood tests, including clotting studies, to identify any possible coagulopathy should be performed. Close liaison with the anaesthetic and haematology teams is vital, with prompt correction of any coagulopathy and likely ITU admission.

Cardiac disease

Cardiac disease remains the leading cause of indirect maternal death and in the most recent report was responsible for 34 deaths. The exact causes of death included aortic dissection, myocardial infarction and cardiomyopathy.

Cardiac disease must be considered in patients:

- with a history of congenital heart defects
- with a history of previous cardiac surgery
- with a history of rheumatic fever or infective endocarditis
- who smoke
- who have hypertension
- who have a high body mass index

Patients may present collapsed or give a history of chest pain (central crushing), which radiates to the jaw, left arm and/or back. Some may complain of orthopnoea, peripheral oedema and shortness of breath. An electrocardiogram should be performed and medical advice sought as soon as possible. If aortic dissection is suspected, bilateral blood pressures as well as assessing for radial–radial delay and radial–femoral delay is essential.

> **RED FLAGS**
>
> Signs and symptoms that warrant further assessment for cardiac causes of collapse:
> - Central chest pain
> - Interscapular pain
> - Wide pulse pressure
> - New cardiac murmur
> - Orthopnoea

Ectopic pregnancy

An ectopic pregnancy can be defined as implantation of an embryo outside of the uterine cavity (see Chapter 18). However, pregnancies may implant at the site of a previous caesarean section, also referred to as 'scar ectopics'. Most commonly the site of implantation is the fallopian tube and if left untreated, the pregnancy will eventually rupture. The rupture can lead to massive haemoperitoneum and sadly, even death.

The diagnosis must always be considered in patients of childbearing age who present with abdominal pain and or vaginal bleeding. A pregnancy test should be performed and if positive, an ectopic pregnancy should be ruled out by ultrasound scan and blood tests. Education about signs and symptoms of an ectopic should be given to all patients as well as information on how to seek help. Any patient who presents with a positive pregnancy test with an intrauterine device in situ (Mirena or copper coil) should be treated as an ectopic until proven otherwise.

> **HINTS AND TIPS**
>
> Signs and symptoms of haemoperitoneum include:
> - Abdominal pain and distension
> - Guarding
> - Loose stools
> - Shoulder tip pain
> - Presyncope
> - Syncope

Drug toxicity

Drug toxicity can occur due to a number of causes and should be kept in mind when assessing a collapsed patient (Table 32.1). Any history of the following should be considered:

- Recreational drug use.
- Epidural analgesia can cause collapse due to a 'high epidural block' or 'total spinal' anaesthetic.
- Local anaesthetic agents may have had inadvertent IV administration.
- Magnesium toxicity of preeclampsia patients with renal dysfunction (respiratory depression).
- Anaphylaxis.

Table 32.1 Signs, symptoms and management for collapse due to drug toxicity

Drug	Signs and symptoms	Management
Opioids	Pinpoint pupils Respiratory depression 'Track marks' if intravenous drug user	Naloxone
Ecstasy and cocaine	Seizures Hyperthermia Headaches Chest pain +/− cardiac event Bruxism	Benzodiazepines to terminate seizures Supportive management
'High spinal' or 'High epidural block'	Respiratory depression Hypoxia Presyncope Collapse → cardiac arrest	IV fluids Intubation Vasopressors
Magnesium sulphate	Respiratory depression Absent reflexes	10 mL of 10% calcium gluconate by IV injection over 10 minutes

Anaphylaxis

Anaphylaxis is a very serious potentially fatal hypersensitivity reaction that needs prompt recognition and management. Anaphylactic reactions affect a number of systems and cardiac arrest can rapidly occur. Any recent administration of drugs should be noted, especially antibiotics, and any known allergies identified, including latex.

Anaphylaxis is said to be likely when there is rapid onset and progression of symptoms with life-threatening airway, breathing or circulation problems and skin or mucosal changes.

Management of anaphylaxis

- Rapid treatment with oxygen
- IV fluids
- IV Steroids (hydrocortisone)
- IV antihistamines (chlorphenamine)
- IM or IV adrenaline
- Removal of any potentially further triggering factors
- Intensive care may be needed and again, a multidisciplinary approach is advised

Hypoglycaemia or hyperglycaemia

Hypoglycaemia and hyperglycaemia should be considered in pregnancy as patients may have preexisting diabetes or gestational diabetes (see Chapter 22). A finger-prick blood glucose level should be taken for every collapsed patient as part of their assessment and acted on promptly.

Hypoglycaemia as a cause of collapse is likely to be severe and should be treated urgently with IV glucose (50 mL of 50% glucose), which should rapidly correct the situation.

Hyperglycaemia when presenting with a collapse can indicate diabetic ketoacidosis. Blood and urinary ketones should be measured. Prompt treatment with IV fluids and sliding scale insulin is important as well as monitoring of potassium levels and seeking advice from the endocrinologists.

COMMUNICATION

A maternal collapse can be traumatic, not only for the woman but also for her birth partners who may have witnessed the event and the medical staff involved in the care. Debriefing the patient and her family will allow them to understand what occurred and also prevent future complications such as posttraumatic stress disorder, postnatal depression and tocophobia.

MATERNAL DEATH

Maternal mortality rates in the UK have fallen dramatically since the early 1900s. Since 1952, triennial reports have been published to report on the deaths and make recommendations about changes in practice. Maternal deaths, however, still continue to happen and the reporting and learning from these events is essential to further reduce the rates of maternal mortality.

Mothers and Babies: Reducing Risk through Audit and Confidential Enquiries

MBRRACE is an organization whose aim is to improve the care given to mothers by carrying out confidential enquiries into maternal and infant deaths.

The report is published highlighting the main causes of maternal death and trends over the last 3 years. Each report focuses on a particular theme (e.g., mental health or cardiac disease), and then provides recommendations to help reduce the risks. In the most recent report published in November 2022 the maternal mortality rate was 10.9/100,000 maternities.

Definitions

When assessing maternal deaths, various definitions are used to categorize them:

- **Maternal deaths:** Deaths of women while pregnant or within 42 days of the end of the pregnancy from any cause related to or aggravated by the pregnancy or its management, but not from accidental or incidental causes (includes ectopic pregnancy, miscarriage and terminations of pregnancy).
- **Direct maternal death:** Deaths resulting from obstetric complications of the pregnant state (pregnancy, labour and puerperium), from interventions, omissions, incorrect treatment or from a chain of events resulting from any of the above.
- **Indirect maternal death:** Deaths resulting from previous existing disease, or disease that developed during pregnancy and which was not the result of direct obstetric causes, but which was aggravated by the physiological effects of pregnancy.
- **Late maternal death:** Deaths occurring between 42 days and 1 year after abortion, miscarriage or delivery that are the result of direct or indirect maternal causes.
- **Coincidental:** Deaths from unrelated causes, which happen to occur in pregnancy or the puerperium.

Psychiatric illness

The majority of deaths related to psychiatric illness are due to suicide. Good communication with networks between primary care, perinatal mental health services and maternity services is critical to provide the best care for patients with mental health problems. In 2020 however, death by suicide was three times higher during or up to 6 weeks after the end of pregnancy compared to 2017–2019. Psychiatric disorders and cardiovascular disorders are now responsible for the same number of maternal deaths in the UK.

> **RED FLAGS**
>
> The following signs and symptoms should prompt urgent senior psychiatric assessment:
> - Recent significant change in mental state
> - New thoughts or acts of violent self-harm
> - New and persistent expression of incompetency as a mother affecting bonding with child

Race and socioeconomic status

Sadly, there remains a recognized and documented disparity of care between people from lower socioeconomic backgrounds. Rates of maternal death among those from the most deprived areas continues to increase. Black patients were 3.7× more likely to die than White patients (34/100,000 giving birth). Asian patients were 1.8× more likely to die than White patients (16/100,000 giving birth). More needs to be done to address this at a local, national and international level for us to break down these barriers.

Coincidental maternal deaths

This category includes a large number of varied causes of death, with road traffic accidents and murder being the two most common. Domestic violence remains a major cause for concern to all clinicians caring for obstetric patients and should be actively screened for at each contact. Rates of domestic abuse increase significantly in pregnancy.

Patients suffering from domestic violence are likely to be:

- late bookers
- have a poor attendance record
- have repeated admissions for seemingly trivial matters

Partners may appear to be domineering, constantly present during all visits and those who do not let the patient answer questions should raise concerns about domestic violence. Professional interpreters should be used rather than family members and any concerns acted upon. Equally, there are sometimes no outward signs that domestic violence is happening. We must therefore create a safe space for patients to speak alone on at least one occasion throughout their pregnancy.

> **COMMUNICATION**
>
> If there is any disclosure of domestic violence, it is advised to inform the specialist safeguarding team immediately who can provide continuity of care to the woman and also make appropriate referrals to social services to ensure the newborn infant or any existing children are protected.

● Chapter Summary

- Maternal collapse is 'an acute event involving the cardiorespiratory systems and/or brain, resulting in a reduced or absent conscious level (and potentially death), at any stage in pregnancy and up to six weeks after delivery'.
- There are many causes of maternal collapse with haemorrhage being the most common.
- During pregnancy, a left lateral tilt position should be adopted during resuscitation to avoid aortocaval compression, which severely limits cardiac circulation.
- A maternal death is defined as death while pregnant or within 1 year of the end of the pregnancy; it is further categorized into direct, indirect, early, late and coincidental causes.

UKMLA Conditions
Placenta praevia
Placental abruption
Postpartum haemorrhage
Pre-eclampsia
Gestational hypertension
Sepsis

UKMLA Presentations
Bleeding antepartum
Bleeding postpartum
Breathlessness
Chest pain
Fits/seizures
Headache
Hypertension
Mental health problems in pregnancy or postpartum
Shock

FURTHER READING

MBRRACE-UK Mother and Babies: Saving lives, improving mothers care 2018 -20. November 2022. Available at: www.npeu.ox.ac.uk.

Royal College of Obstetricians and Gynaecologists (RCOG), 2019. Maternal collapse in pregnancy and the puerperium. *RCOG green-top guideline No. 56*. Available at: www.rcog.org.uk.

Sepsis Trust Maternity Guidelines. Available at: www.sepsistrust.org.

UKOSS UK Obstetric Surveillance System. Available at: www.npeu.ox.ac.uk.

Self-Assessment

UKMLA High Yield Association Table

Presentations

Key Findings	Diagnoses
Dysmenorrhoea, dyspareunia, dyschezia and dysuria	Endometriosis
'Chocolate cyst'	Endometrioma
Tender, bulky uterus	Adenomyosis
Cervical excitation	PID or ectopic pregnancy
Severe sudden onset lateralized pain with nausea/vomiting	Ovarian torsion or ruptured ovarian cyst
Mid-cycle pain	Mittelschmerz
Vulval swelling with pain and fever	Bartholin's abscess
Loin-to-groin pain	Renal calculi
Multiple sexual partners, unprotected sexual intercourse, change in vaginal discharge and pelvic pain	PID
Strawberry cervix	*Trichomonas vaginalis*
Long-acting reversible contraceptives	LNG-IUS, Cu-IUD, subdermal contraceptive implant, depot progesterone injection
Emergency contraception	Levonorgestrel (up to 72 hours from UPSI) Ella-One (Up to 120 hours from UPSI) Cu-IUD (Up to 120 hours from UPSI or up to 5 days after ovulation)
Measure of degree of prolapse	POP-Q Baden-Walker halfway system
Leaking of urine with urgency, irritability, frequency	Urge incontinence
Leaking of urine with sneezing, coughing and running	Stress incontinence
Bladder filling pain, nocturia and bladder base pain	Bladder pain syndrome
Anosmia	Kalman syndrome
Wide carrying angle, widened spacing of nipples, webbed neck and shield chest	Turner syndrome
Striae, buffalo hump and central obesity	Cushing syndrome
Acne, hirsutism, high BMI, oligomenorrhoea	PCOS
Headache, bitemporal hemianopia, galactorrhoea	Pituitary adenoma
Secondary amenorrhoea following endometrial curettage	Asherman syndrome
Undergoing IVF treatment, abdominal girth increase, abdominal pain, nausea and vomiting	OHSS
Previous chlamydia/gonorrhoea, smoking, cystic fibrosis or PID	Tubal factor subfertility
Hot flushes, brain fog, reduced libido, mood swings and night sweats	Menopause
FSH >30 on two or more occasions 4–6 weeks apart	Diagnosis of menopause
Snowstorm appearance on TVS	Gestational trophoblastic disease

Continued

Vulval itching, pale white plaques in figure-of-eight pattern over vulva, absorption of labia minora, narrowing of introitus	Lichen sclerosus
Partial or total removal of the external female genitalia, or other injury to the female genital organs for nonmedical reasons	Female genital mutilation
Vulval itching, thick white curd-like discharge, immunocompromised state	Vulvovaginal candidiasis
Fishy smelling greyish-white vaginal discharge, presence of 'clue cells'	Bacterial vaginosis
Painful shallow ulcers, dysuria, bilateral tender inguinal lymphadenopathy	Genital herpes
Single painless indurated ulcer with rolled edges caused by a spirochete bacterium	Chancre in primary syphilis
Benign cyst containing hair, teeth and fat	Dermoid cyst
Ultrasound score (U) × Menopausal status (M) × CA-125 (IU/mL)	RMI (risk of malignancy index)
NT (nuchal translucency), βHCG, pregnancy-associated plasma protein A	Combined screening test
α-feto-protein, oestriol and βHCG	Triple test
α-feto-protein, oestriol and βHCG, inhibin	Quadruple test
First-trimester diagnostic test for chromosomal abnormalities	CVS
Second-trimester diagnostic test for chromosomal abnormalities	Amniocentesis
Pregnant, painless PV bleeding, +/- previous caesarean	Placenta praevia
Pregnant, PV bleeding, abdominal pain, +/- high blood pressure	Placental abruption
Hypertension after 20 weeks, NO proteinuria	Gestational or pregnancy-induced hypertension (PIH)
Hypertension after 20 weeks, headaches, visual disturbance, epigastric pain, pedal oedema with proteinuria	Preeclampsia
Known hypertensive at booking, poor blood pressure control after 20 weeks with +/- headaches, visual disturbance, epigastric pain, pedal oedema with proteinuria, low PIGF	Superimposed preeclampsia
Deranged liver enzymes, raised LDH, low platelets	HELLP syndrome
Low haemoglobin, normal ferritin levels, Mediterranean origin	Haemoglobinopathies
High BMI, long haul flight, sudden onset shortness of breath	Pulmonary embolism
Postnatal headaches, seizures, vomiting, photophobia, reduced consciousness, +/- focal neurology	Cerebral vein thrombosis
Itching after 20 weeks of gestation, NO rash, increased bile acids	Intrahepatic cholestasis of pregnancy
Nausea, vomiting, anorexia, malaise, abdominal pain or polyuria in the third trimester	Acute fatty liver of pregnancy
Symphysis pubis hight measures 3 cm less than weeks of pregnancy, +/- reduced foetal movements	Growth restriction/small for gestational age
Large for gestational age, polyhydramnios, glucosuria	Gestational diabetes
Lambda sign	Dichorionic diamniotic pregnancy
T sign	Monochorionic diamniotic pregnancy.

278

Foetus 1: growth restricted, oligohydramnios; foetus 2: polyhydramnios, foetal weight larger than foetus 1	Twin-to-twin transfusion syndrome
Cervical cerclage at 11–14 weeks of pregnancy, history of three preterm births	History-indicated cerclage
Cervical cerclage at second trimester, cervical dilatation + exposed foetal membranes	Emergency cerclage
Intermittent abdominal pain, <34 weeks, +/- cervical dilatation, +/- raised foetal fibronectin levels	Threatened preterm labour
>37 weeks of gestation, regular contractions 4 in every 10 minutes, cervical dilatation >4 cm	Established labour
Previously well foetus, uterine contractions 7 in 10 minutes, palpation of the uterus shows no resting tone, decelerations and increased baseline rate on CTG	Uterine hyperstimulation
Previous CS, in established labour, previously well baby, foetal bradycardia on CTG	Uterine rupture
Rupture of membranes, foetal bradycardia	Cord prolapse

UKMLA Single Best Answer (SBA) Questions

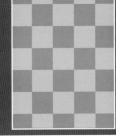

Chapter 1 Basic anatomy and examination

1. A woman has an appointment in the antenatal clinic. She is 34 weeks' pregnant. Which of the following cannot be determined by abdominal palpation alone?
   A Gestation
   B Foetal lie
   C Engagement
   D Presentation
   E Foetal heart rate

2. A woman who is at 36 weeks' gestation should have a symphysial-fundal height (SFH) of approximately?
   A 36 cm
   B 33–36 cm
   C 34–38 cm
   D 35–37 cm
   E 36–39 cm

3. A 50-year-old presents with a lump in the vagina and urinary leakage during coughing. What is the most appropriate initial assessment?
   A Urodynamics
   B Assessment with Cusco's speculum
   C Assessment with Sims' speculum
   D Physiotherapy assessment
   E Pelvic ultrasound

4. When examining a woman with singleton pregnancy, the foetal pole is palpated in the iliac fossa. The foetal lie is therefore:
   A Longitudinal
   B Oblique
   C Transverse
   D Uncertain
   E Superior

5. The ovarian arteries are a direct branch of which of the following:
   A Abdominal aorta
   B Inferior mesenteric artery
   C Renal artery
   D Uterine artery
   E Internal iliac artery

6. To avoid postural hypotension and syncope, obstetric patients should be examined in the ____ position:
   A Supine
   B Prone
   C Semirecumbent
   D Right lateral
   E Sitting

7. The presence of thickening of vaginal nodules in the Pouch of Douglas is suggestive of:
   A Bartholin's cyst
   B Lymph nodes
   C Endometriosis
   D Fibroids
   E Nabothian follicles

Chapter 3 Common investigations

1. The current UK national screening in cervical cytology programme invites women aged 25–49 to attend for their smear test once every:
   A One year
   B Two years
   C Three years
   D Four years
   E Five years

2. Smear tests are used to detect the presence of which virus:
   A Human parainfluenza virus
   B Human parvovirus
   C Herpes simplex virus type 1
   D Human papillomavirus
   E Herpes simplex virus type 2

3. The first line imaging modality of choice for detecting ovarian pathology is:
   A Transvaginal ultrasound
   B MRI pelvis
   C CT abdomen-pelvis
   D Abdominal X-ray
   E Transabdominal ultrasound

4. Which of the following statements about open surgery versus laparoscopy are true:

A Open surgery is associated with better visualization of the pelvic organs compared with laparoscopy

B Open surgery is associated with a shorter postoperative length of stay compared with laparoscopy

C Open surgery is associated with a lower rate of postoperative adhesions compared with laparoscopy

D Open surgery is associated with less blood loss than laparoscopy

E Open surgery is associated with more postoperative pain than laparoscopy

Chapter 4 Abnormal uterine bleeding

1. Which of the following is not a recognized cause of abnormal menstrual bleeding?

A Coagulopathy

B Fibroids

C Malignancy

D Systemic lupus erythematosus (SLE)

E Adenomyosis

2. A 45-year-old woman presents with heavy regular periods. She requests appropriate management and has tried hormonal treatment in the past with no success. Her husband has had a vasectomy. Which should be offered next?

A Tranexamic acid

B Levonorgestrel intrauterine system (LNG-IUS; e.g., Mirena)

C Abdominal hysterectomy

D Endometrial ablation

E Uterine artery embolization (UAE)

3. A 55-year-old woman presents with postmenopausal bleeding. An ultrasound demonstrates an endometrial thickness of 8 mm. What is the most appropriate next form of management?

A Pipelle biopsy

B Hysteroscopy and biopsy

C Laparoscopy

D Repeat ultrasound in 4 months

E Hysterectomy

4. A 47-year-old woman opts to have a hysterectomy. What complications must she be warned of?

A Haemorrhage

B Pain

C Injury to viscera

D Postoperative fever

E All of the above

5. A 65-year-old woman presents with two episodes of postmenopausal bleeding. What is the most likely cause?

A Atrophic vaginitis

B Endometrial fibroid

C Anovulatory cycle

D Endometrial adenocarcinoma

E Endometrial polyp

6. A 45-year-old woman presents with heavy menstrual bleeding. She has tried medical therapy and ablation, but has been unsuccessful. She would like definitive management. Which of the following is most appropriate:

A Abdominal hysterectomy

B Laparoscopic hysterectomy

C Uterine artery embolization (UAE)

D Myomectomy

E Transcervical resection of endometrium

7. A 21-year-old woman presents with heavy painful menstrual bleeding. She has had one termination of pregnancy (TOP) in the past. Which of the following is most appropriate:

A Levonorgestrel intrauterine system (LNG-IUS; e.g., Mirena)

B Tranexamic acid

C Combined oral contraceptive pill

D Uterine artery embolization (UAE)

E Transcervical resection of endometrium

8. A 47-year-old woman with heavy regular periods who has tried medical therapy. She has been sterilized in the past. Which of the following is most appropriate?

A Hysterectomy

B Copper intrauterine contraceptive device (IUCD; or 'copper coil')

C Endometrial ablation

D Uterine artery embolization (UAE)

E Hysteroscopy

9. A 21-year-old woman presents with heavy periods but is hoping to conceive in the next year. Which of the following is most appropriate?

A Tranexamic acid

B Combined oral contraceptive pill

C Levonorgestrel intrauterine system (LNG-IUS; e.g., Mirena)

D Uterine artery embolization (UAE)

E Hysteroscopy

10. A 35-year-old with intermenstrual bleeding has a pelvic ultrasound scan which identified a 2 × 1 cm endometrial lesion with a feeding vessel. Which of the following is most appropriate?

    A Tranexamic acid
    B Hysterectomy
    C Levonorgestrel intrauterine system (LNG-IUS; e.g., Mirena)
    D Hysteroscopy with resection of endometrial polyp
    E Uterine artery embolization (UAE)

Chapter 5 Fibroids

1. Which type of fibroid projects into and can distort the endometrial cavity?

    A Intramural
    B Subserosal
    C Submucosal
    D Cervical
    E Pedunculated

2. With regard to the prevalence of fibroids, which is untrue?

    A They are more common in Afro-Caribbeans
    B Can grow in pregnancy
    C Decrease in size in the postmenopausal period
    D Can become malignant in 1:100 cases
    E Occur in around a quarter of women of reproductive age

3. A 40-year-old woman presents with menorrhagia and a palpable pelvic mass measuring 14 weeks in size. You suspect uterine fibroids. What would be the most appropriate initial investigation in this instance?

    A Magnetic resonance imaging
    B Computer tomography scan
    C Hysteroscopy
    D Pelvic ultrasound
    E Hysteroscopy and pelvic ultrasound

4. A 49-year-old woman with heavy periods and a large fibroid uterus does not want surgical intervention, but would like her fibroids to reduce in size and to have less heavy bleeding. What would be the appropriate management for her?

    A Hysterectomy
    B Endometrial ablation
    C Uterine artery embolization (UAE)
    D Mirena coil
    E Iron supplementation

5. A 28-year-old woman with subfertility has heavy periods. Pelvic ultrasound reveals a submucosal fibroid. Which of the following is most appropriate?

    A Transcervical resection of fibroids
    B Myomectomy
    C Tranexamic acid
    D Hysteroscopy and biopsy
    E GnRH analogues

6. A 40-year-old has known fibroids approximately 30 weeks in size, with hydronephrosis diagnosed on scan. She would like to conceive. Which of the following is most appropriate?

    A Hysterectomy
    B Uterine artery embolization (UAE)
    C Myomectomy
    D Ureteric re-implantation
    E GnRH analogues

7. A 50-year-old postmenopausal woman with a 28-week fibroid uterus has hydronephrosis diagnosed on scan. Which of the following is most appropriate?

    A Repeat magnetic resonance imaging (MRI) in 6 months
    B Myomectomy
    C Hysterectomy
    D Urethroscopy
    E Uterine artery embolization (UAE)

8. A 47-year-old woman has heavy periods, increased urinary frequency and a large fibroid uterus diagnosed on scan. She declines to have surgery. Which of the following is most appropriate?

    A Endometrial ablation
    B Tranexamic acid
    C Mirena coil
    D Repeat magnetic resonance imaging (MRI) in 6 months
    E Uterine artery embolization (UAE)

9. A 35-year-old woman has a pedunculated fibroid diagnosed incidentally on scan measuring 3 cm. Which of the following is most appropriate?

    A Repeat ultrasound scan in 6 months
    B Repeat magnetic resonance imaging (MRI) in 6 months
    C Transcervical resection of fibroids
    D Myomectomy
    E Hysteroscopy and biopsy

Chapter 6 Endometriosis

1. Which of the following is not a commonly recognized symptom of endometriosis:
   A Dysmenorrhoea
   B Dyspareunia
   C Dyschaezia
   D Dystonia
   E Dysuria

2. The incidence of endometriosis in female patients is thought to be:
   A 1%
   B 5%
   C 10%
   D 20%
   E 33%

3. Which of the following is not a recognized sign associated with ultrasound findings of endometriosis:
   A Pain experienced during scanning
   B Thickened endometrium
   C 'Kissing ovaries'
   D Thickening of the uterosacral ligaments
   E Presence of an ovarian endometrioma

4. Which of the following is an absolute contraindication to prescribing the combined oral contraceptive pill for the management of endometriosis:
   A Migraine with aura
   B BMI <16
   C Varicose veins
   D Epilepsy
   E Family history of breast cancer

5. Sampson's theory for the aetiology of endometriosis is:
   A Lymphatic and venous embolization of endometrial tissue
   B Coelomic metaplasia and differentiation
   C Immunological and genetic factors affecting predisposition to endometriosis
   D Seeding from previous surgery
   E Retrograde menstruation and implantation

Chapter 7 Pelvic pain and dyspareunia

1. Which of the following is a cause of superficial dyspareunia?
   A Vulvovaginitis
   B Uterine fibroids
   C Endometriosis
   D Large ovarian cyst
   E Pelvic inflammatory disease

2. A 24-year-old nulliparous patient attends A+E with severe sudden onset left iliac fossa pain associated with nausea and vomiting. HR 106, BP 90/65, RR 18, T 37.2, Sats 98% OA. What is the first investigation that needs to be performed?
   A Full blood count
   B CT abdomen pelvis
   C Urine pregnancy test
   D Transvaginal ultrasound scan
   E 'Triple swabs' – High vaginal, low vaginal and endocervical

3. A 19-year-old patient attends A+E with gradually worsening diffuse lower abdominal pain associated with foul-smelling discharge and fever. Which clinical sign would you expect to elicit upon examination?
   A Rovsing's sign positive
   B Shifting dullness
   C Fixed retroverted uterus
   D Bladder base tenderness
   E Cervical excitation

4. Which of the following is **not** a risk factor for future ectopic pregnancy?
   A Previous ectopic pregnancy
   B Smoking
   C Previous twin pregnancy
   D Pelvic inflammatory disease
   E Conceiving with an intrauterine system in situ

5. Clinical signs and symptoms of haemoperitoneum include all **except**:
   A Confusion
   B Presyncope
   C Shoulder tip pain
   D Vaginal bleeding
   E Diarrhoea

Chapter 8 Vaginal discharge and sexually transmitted infections

1. Which of the following is not a pathological cause of vaginal discharge?
   A Cervical carcinoma
   B Cervical ectropion
   C *Candida albic*ans
   D *Chlamydia trachomatis*
   E Fistula

2. A patient has been diagnosed with candida infection. Which of the following supports this diagnosis?
   A Grey, fishy-smelling discharge

B Thick, itchy, white discharge
C Dysuria
D Urinary frequency
E Lower abdominal pain

3. A patient presents with abnormal vaginal discharge. Which aspect of her history is more helpful to rule out an infective cause?

A Age
B Weight loss
C Irregular vaginal bleeding
D Anorexia
E Sexual history

4. Which of the following in a patient's history is known to predispose them to pelvic inflammatory disease (PID)?

A Monogamous relationship
B >25 years of age
C History of sexually transmitted infection (STI)
D Later onset of sexual activity
E Use of the Mirena intrauterine system

5. A patient is diagnosed with acute pelvic inflammatory disease (PID). Which of the following signs does not support that diagnosis?

A Raised temperature >37.5°C
B Tachycardia
C Vulval pruritus
D Abdominal tenderness
E Adnexal mass

6. A 20-year-old woman who is 8 weeks pregnant presents with a 2-week history of fishy-smelling PV discharge. It is nonitchy and cream coloured. She has had previous episodes outside of pregnancy which resolved spontaneously. She is in a monogamous relationship with the same partner for 5 years. On speculum examination, there is a small amount of smooth grey discharge seen coating the vaginal walls. Which is the most likely diagnosis?

A Bacterial vaginosis (BV)
B *Trichomonas vaginalis* (TV)
C *Chlamydia trachomatis*
D *Neisseria gonorrhoea*
E Foreign body

7. A 14-year-old presented to the Accident and Emergency department with her mother. She has been feeling unwell with abdominal pain, high temperature, rigors, nausea and vomiting and an offensive PV discharge. She has been busy and stressed with examinations at school. Her period started 4 days ago and she has been using tampons. Which is the most likely diagnosis?

A Foreign body
B *Candida albicans*
C *Chlamydia trachomatis*
D Retained tampon
E Toxic shock syndrome

8. A 35-year-old lady has been referred by her GP to colposcopy clinic. She has recently arrived in the UK from Sub-Saharan Africa and the GP was concerned that she never had a smear and has been complaining of an offensive blood-stained PV discharge. On speculum examination, there is a fungating, bleeding cervical mass that was biopsied. Which is the most likely diagnosis?

A Cervical carcinoma
B Foreign body
C Retained tampon
D *Trichomonas vaginalis* (TV)
E *Neisseria gonorrhoea*

9. A 26-year-old woman presents to gynaecology clinic with a history of postcoital PV bleeding mixed with discharge. She is up to date with her cervical smears, which have been normal. She is in a new relationship and is using the combined oral contraceptive (COCP) for contraception. She recalls feeling unwell 3 days ago with right upper quadrant discomfort which has now resolved. Speculum examination showed an inflamed cervix with contact bleeding, consistent with cervicitis. An endocervical swab was taken. Which is the most likely diagnosis?

A *Trichomonas vaginalis* (TV)
B *Chlamydia trachomatis*
C *Neisseria gonorrhoea*
D Retained tampon
E Toxic shock syndrome

10. A 6-year-old girl is seen in general outpatients with her parents. She has been having persistent vaginal discharge on her underwear and the GP has not found a cause. An abdominal ultrasound scan has been unremarkable. She is an only child and has a good relationship with both her parents and is especially close to her mother who she wants to be like 'when she grows up'. There is no suspicion of abuse. The parents comment that she is usually very talkative and inquisitive and likes exploring the house. However, she recently has not been herself and appears to be in intermittent discomfort in the suprapubic region. She has been booked on an elective list for an examination under anaesthetic. Which is the most likely diagnosis?

A Toxic shock syndrome
B Foreign body
C Bacterial vaginosis
D *Candida albicans*
E *Chlamydia trachomatis*

Chapter 9 Pelvic inflammatory disease

1. The name of the disease associated with perihepatitis secondary to PID is called:

   A Fergerson-Harris-Carling syndrome
   B Field-Headon-Cramer syndrome
   C Fleming-Hill-Cruzon syndrome
   D Fitz-Hugh-Curtis syndrome
   E Filby-Howard-Calnan syndrome

2. Which of the following organisms are most commonly responsible for PID:

   A *Chlamydia trachomatis* and *Neisseria gonorrhoeae*
   B *Gardnerella vaginalis*
   C *Mycoplasma genitalium*
   D *Mycobacterium tuberculosis*
   E *Trichomonas vaginalis*

3. Which of the following is not part of the outpatient management for mild to moderate PID:

   A Oral antibiotics for 2 weeks
   B Contact tracing of sexual partners
   C Repeat ultrasound examination in 6–8 weeks
   D Follow up in 72 hours after discharge
   E Safety netting advice to attend if worsening symptoms

4. Which of the following is not a recognized long-term complication of PID?

   A Subfertility
   B Endometriosis
   C Chronic pelvic pain
   D Psychological disturbances
   E Ectopic pregnancy

Chapter 10 Contraception and TOP

1. Which of the following is an example of a long-acting reversible contraceptive?

   A Progesterone-only pill
   B Combined oral contraceptive pill
   C Levonorgestrel-intrauterine system (LNG-IUS)
   D Contraceptive transdermal patch
   E Condoms

2. Which of the following has the highest perfect use success for preventing unwanted pregnancies?

   A Copper intrauterine device (Cu-IUD)
   B Oral contraceptives
   C Levonorgestrel-intrauterine system (LNG-IUS)
   D Progesterone-only implant
   E Female sterilization

3. Which of the following is the definition for the UK Medical Eligibility Criteria for contraceptive use (UK-MEC) category 3?

   A A condition where the theoretical or proven risks usually outweigh the advantages of using the method
   B A condition for which there is no restriction for the use of the method
   C A condition that represents an unacceptable health risk if the method is used
   D A condition where the advantages of using the method generally outweigh the theoretical or proven risks
   E A condition where expert opinion in that field must be sought to determine the theoretical or proven risks in using the method

4. Which of the following is a contraindication to prescribing Ella-One (ulipristal acetate 30 mg) as emergency contraction?

   A Age <18
   B Concurrent use of warfarin
   C Unprotected sexual intercourse 3 days prior
   D Migraine with aura
   E Severe asthma

5. Which of the following is a recognized serious risk associated with surgical termination of pregnancy?

   A Infertility
   B Uterine perforation
   C Retained products of conception
   D Urinary retention
   E Increased risk of ectopic pregnancy in subsequent pregnancies

Chapter 11 Benign gynaecological tumours

1. A 44-year-old woman presents with abdominal pain and a palpable pelvic mass. Useful initial investigations are performed. Which of the following is not recommended as an initial investigation?

   A Urine human chorionic gonadotrophin (HCG)
   B Haemoglobin (Hb)
   C Pelvic ultrasound scan
   D White cell count (WCC) and C-reactive protein (CRP)
   E CA-125

2. A woman is diagnosed with a dermoid ovarian cyst. Which of the following statements about dermoid cysts is correct?
   A Are never bilateral
   B Mainly occur in the 30s age group
   C Are usually malignant
   D Have an over 50% chance of torting
   E Usually present with cyst rupture

3. What is the most appropriate initial action if a 21-year-old woman presents to the emergency department with a 7 cm left-sided ovarian cyst seen on scan, severe pain and vomiting?
   A CA-125 blood test
   B Computed tomography scan
   C Discussion with an oncology multidisciplinary team
   D Laparoscopy with or without ovarian cystectomy
   E Magnetic resonance imaging (MRI)

4. Common presenting symptoms of benign ovarian cysts include the following, except:
   A Abnormal uterine bleeding
   B Hirsutism
   C Clitoromegaly
   D Hoarse voice
   E Constipation

5. Simple cysts are associated with the following features on ultrasound, except:
   A A round or oval shape
   B Thin or imperceptible wall
   C Posterior acoustic enhancement
   D Anechoic fluid
   E Solid nodules

6. A 23-year-old woman presents with right-sided pelvic pain. Her beta-HCG test is negative. The most appropriate course of management is:
   A Emergency laparotomy
   B Emergency laparoscopy
   C Transvaginal/transabdominal ultrasound
   D White cell count (WCC) and C-reactive protein (CRP)
   E Magnetic resonance imaging (MRI)

7. A 55-year-old woman with a right-sided 6 cm ovarian cyst presents with acute pelvic pain and vomiting. The most appropriate course of management is:
   A CA-125
   B Laparoscopy and bilateral salpingo-oophorectomy
   C Computed tomography abdomen/pelvis
   D Magnetic resonance imaging (MRI)
   E Emergency laparotomy

8. A 30-year-old woman presents with right-sided pelvic pain. Ultrasound reveals an 8 cm ovarian cyst with free fluid. She feels faint and is slightly tachycardic. The most appropriate course of management is:
   A Emergency laparotomy
   B Emergency laparoscopy
   C Haemoglobin (Hb)
   D Computed tomography abdomen/pelvis
   E Magnetic resonance imaging (MRI)

9. A 55-year-old postmenopausal woman presents with left iliac fossa pain that is troublesome for her. Ultrasound revealed a 3 cm simple cyst. Her risk of malignancy index is very low. The most appropriate course of management is:
   A Laparoscopy and bilateral salpingo-oophorectomy
   B Emergency laparotomy
   C Emergency laparoscopy
   D White cell count (WCC) and C-reactive protein (CRP)
   E Haemoglobin (Hb)

10. A 60-year-old woman had an incidental finding of a 4 cm ovarian cyst identified on ultrasound. The most appropriate course of management is:
    A CA-125
    B Haemoglobin (Hb)
    C White cell count (WCC) and C-reactive protein (CRP)
    D Computed tomography abdomen/pelvis
    E Magnetic resonance imaging (MRI)

Chapter 12 Gynaecological malignancies

1. Which of the following is not a risk factor for cervical cancer?
   A Human papillomavirus (HPV)
   B Smoking
   C Multiple sexual partners
   D Early age of first intercourse
   E History of endometriosis

2. Sarah is a 65-year-old and has not had a period for 14 years. She attended the general practitioner as she has noted abdominal bloating and nausea. An ultrasound scan showed a multiloculated right-sided ovarian cyst, and her CA-125 is 90. What is her risk of malignancy index?
   A 270
   B 720
   C 90
   D 810
   E 320

3. Regarding the risk of malignancy index (RMI), which of the following is untrue?

   A CA-125 IU/mL is used in the score
   B The premenopausal score is 1
   C The postmenopausal score is 3
   D The ultrasound score when 1 characteristic is present is 1
   E Any RMI greater than 100 is associated with a higher risk of malignancy

4. A 73-year-old woman noted a few episodes of vaginal spotting and her transvaginal ultrasound showed an endometrial thickness of 9 mm. What is the next most important investigation she should undergo?

   A Computed tomography scan of the abdomen and pelvis
   B Magnetic resonance imaging (MRI)
   C Hysterosalpingogram
   D Endometrial biopsy
   E Cervical cytology

5. Which of the following is not a risk factor for developing vulval cancer?

   A Lichen sclerosus
   B Vulval intraepithelial neoplasia (VIN)
   C Lichen planus
   D Human papillomavirus (HPV)
   E Paget abscess

6. Which of the following most accurately confirms endometrial pathology?

   A Hysteroscopy and biopsy
   B Pipelle biopsy
   C Magnetic resonance imaging (MRI) of the pelvis
   D Laparoscopy
   E Transvaginal ultrasound scan

7. A 46-year-old premenopausal woman presents with abdominal bloating and a unilateral loculated ovarian cyst. Her CA-125 is 29. Her most likely diagnosis is:

   A Polycystic ovarian syndrome (PCOS)
   B Ovarian cancer
   C Haemorrhagic ovarian cyst
   D Endometrial cancer
   E Endometrial hyperplasia

8. A 65-year-old woman has a pipelle biopsy result showing 'proliferation of endometrial glands with an increase in the gland-to-stroma ratio compared to proliferative endometrium'. Her most likely diagnosis is:

   A Endometrial hyperplasia
   B Endometrial cancer

C Endometriosis
D Leiomyosarcoma
E Chronic endometritis

9. A 25-year-old woman presents with heavy, irregular bleeding patterns since menarche and weight gain. She has no family history of endometrial cancer. Her most likely diagnosis is:

   A Polycystic ovarian syndrome (PCOS)
   B Endometrial hyperplasia
   C Paget disease of the vulva
   D Endometriosis
   E Haemorrhagic ovarian cyst

10. A 93-year-old is noted to have a vaginal lesion. She is known to have breast cancer. Her most likely diagnosis is:

    A Cervical intraepithelial neoplasia (CIN)
    B Vulval intraepithelial neoplasia (VIN)
    C Paget disease of the vulva
    D Paget abscess
    E Human papillomavirus (HPV)

11. The following are risk factors for vaginal cancer, except:

    A Coexisting cervical intraepithelial neoplasia (CIN)
    B History of another gynaecological malignancy
    C Vaginal intraepithelial neoplasia (VAIN).
    D Persistent infection with human parainfluenza virus
    E In utero exposure to diethylstilboestrol

12. The factors increasing a woman's risk of ovarian cancer include the following, except:

    A Increasing age
    B Multiparity
    C Late motherhood (>35 years)
    D Early menarche
    E Late menopause

Chapter 13 Benign vulval disease

1. A 45-year-old woman presents with pruritus vulvae. Which of the following is suggestive of an infective cause:

   A Progressively worsening symptoms over 6 months
   B Menorrhagia
   C A thick creamy white discharge
   D Red plaques in the vulva area
   E Fused labia

2. Which of the following are important in the management of a woman with pruritus vulvae:

   A Administering antibiotics
   B A speculum examination of the cervix and smear test

C   All women should be seen in colposcopy clinic

D   Excision of the area of the discomfort

E   An abdominal X-ray

3. Which of the following is a possible method of investigation of vulva disease?

    A   C-reactive protein (CRP)

    B   Biopsy of the vulva

    C   Ultrasound scan

    D   Hysteroscopy

    E   Endocervical swabs

4. Which of the following is correct about lichen sclerosus?

    A   The vulval skin always appears white

    B   Skin biopsy shows thinning of the epidermis

    C   A biopsy is not necessary as the diagnosis is usually obvious

    D   Surgical excision is first-line treatment

    E   A short course of antibiotic treatment is usually required

5. A 20-year-old woman from Sudan presents with dysuria and dyspareunia. On examination, there is a narrowed vaginal introitus and the labia minora was not identifiable. Which type of female genital mutilation (FGM) is this?

    A   Type 1

    B   Type 2

    C   Type 3

    D   Type 4

    E   Normal

6. A 65-year-old presents with pruritus vulvae. She has noticed a lump growing on the vulva for the last six months. Examination confirms an ulcerated, hard, raised lesion 1 cm in diameter. The most likely diagnosis is:

    A   Lichen sclerosus

    B   Carcinoma of the vulva

    C   Herpetic lesion

    D   Psoriasis

    E   Contact dermatitis

7. A 16-year-old has recently become sexually active. She complains of intense pruritus vulvae associated with an offensive discharge with a fishy odour. On examination, she has a marked vulvovaginitis and a frothy green vaginal discharge. The most likely diagnosis is:

    A   Contact dermatitis

    B   Behcet syndrome

    C   *Candida* infection

    D   Herpetic lesion

    E   *Trichomonas vaginalis*

8. A 60-year-old presents with intermittent episodes of pruritus vulvae. On examination, the labia have fused, the tissues are thin and leucoplakia is present. The most likely diagnosis is:

    A   *Candida* infection

    B   Psoriasis

    C   Vulval intraepithelial neoplasia

    D   Lichen sclerosus

    E   Behcet syndrome

9. A 35-year-old has developed pruritus vulvae since changing her soap and bubble bath. Examination reveals vulvitis with no discrete lesion visible. The most likely diagnosis is:

    A   Contact dermatitis

    B   Lichen sclerosus

    C   Psoriasis

    D   Enterobius

    E   Behcet syndrome

10. A 42-year-old develops an itchy lesion of the left vulva. Examination reveals an erythematous plaque on the left labium majora and scaly plaques on her elbows. The most likely diagnosis is:

    A   Contact dermatitis

    B   Lichen sclerosus

    C   Psoriasis

    D   Enterobius

    E   Behcet syndrome

Chapter 14 Urogynaecology

1. What is a complete procidentia?

    A   Complete descent beyond the vaginal opening of the bladder

    B   Complete descent beyond the vaginal opening of the bowel

    C   Complete descent beyond the vaginal opening of the cervix

    D   Complete descent beyond the vaginal opening of the vagina

    E   Complete descent beyond the vaginal opening of the uterus

2. Which of the following do **not** form part of the pelvic floor musculature?

    A   Coccygeus

    B   Obturator internus

    C   Levator Ani

    D   Obturator externus

    E   Piriformis

3. A 65-year-old patient presents with a history of urinary leaking when coughing, sneezing and running. What is the most likely diagnosis?
   - A Stress urinary incontinence
   - B Detrusor instability
   - C Over active bladder syndrome
   - D Urge incontinence
   - E Mixed urinary incontinence

4. Which of the following **is not** a recognized conservative management option for prolapse?
   - A Weight loss if BMI >30
   - B Pelvic floor repair
   - C Optimizing asthma control
   - D Avoiding constipation
   - E Treating vaginal atrophy

5. Which of the following is true for the diagnosis of bladder pain syndrome?
   - A A cystoscopy should be performed
   - B Incontinence is a key feature of its diagnosis
   - C It is a diagnosis of exclusion
   - D Concurrent urinary infection supports its diagnosis
   - E Bladder emptying pain is a key feature of its diagnosis

Chapter 15 Gynaecological endocrinology

1. A 16 year old presents with primary amenorrhoea. She describes having cyclical pelvic pain and breast tenderness for the last 6 months. External inspection of the vagina reveals a blue bulge in the vagina. What is the diagnosis?
   - A Turner syndrome
   - B Rokitansky-Kustner-Hauser syndrome
   - C Constitutional delay
   - D Androgen insensitivity syndrome
   - E Haematocolpos

2. Which of the following would warrant investigation for alternate causes of hyperandrogenism other than PCOS?
   - A Longstanding hirsutism
   - B Testosterone levels >5 nmol/L
   - C More than 12 follicles seen on ultrasound scan in at least one ovary
   - D Oligomenorrhoea
   - E Subfertility

3. A 33-year-old patient presents with secondary amenorrhoea 8 months after giving birth to her first child. She had an uncomplicated pregnancy except for a postpartum haemorrhage of 1.5 L. What is the most likely diagnosis?
   - A Sheehan syndrome
   - B Asherman syndrome
   - C Premature ovarian insufficiency
   - D Cervical stenosis
   - E Hyperprolactinaemia

4. A 25 year-old-patient presents with secondary amenorrhoea for 6 months. She has a BMI of 19 and is vegan. She is nulliparous and has had three early miscarriages and one termination. What is the most likely diagnosis?
   - A Sheehan syndrome
   - B Asherman syndrome
   - C Premature ovarian insufficiency
   - D Cervical stenosis
   - E Hyperprolactinaemia

5. A 16-year-old is brought to the GP by her mother who is concerned that she has not yet started her periods. Her mother tells you she started her periods at 13 years of age. The patient is short in stature, has a webbed neck and a wide carrying angle. What is the most likely diagnosis?
   - A Constitutional delay
   - B Rokitansky-Kustner-Hauser syndrome
   - C Turner syndrome
   - D Androgen insensitivity syndrome
   - E Fragile-X syndrome

Chapter 16 Subfertility

1. What percentage of couples will conceive naturally by 2 years of trying, who are under the age of 40 and having regular unprotected sexual intercourse?
   - A 10%
   - B 25%
   - C 50%
   - D 75%
   - E 90%

2. What percentage of couples trying to conceive have no clear cause for subfertility identified (unexplained subfertility)?
   - A 10%
   - B 25%
   - C 50%
   - D 75%
   - E 90%

3. A patient presents to A+E following ovarian stimulation for IVF with clinical ascites, oliguria, vomiting and abdominal pain. Which of the following is the most important medical treatment?

A IV fluids
B Furosemide
C Low-molecular-weight heparin
D Antiemetics
E Aspirin

4. A 36-year-old male presents to the fertility clinic as he and his partner have been trying to conceive for 2 years. The patient's total sperm number was 5x106 per ejaculate with a total semen volume of 1 mL. The patient is tall, and does not suffer from erectile dysfunction but does have anosmia. What is the most likely diagnosis?
A Prada-Willi syndrome
B Kleinfelter syndrome
C XX male syndrome
D Kallman syndrome
E Noonan syndrome

5. A 28 year old presents with primary subfertility. Her partner's sperm test is normal. She phenotypically appears female and has regular menstrual cycles with normal secondary sexual characteristics. She has a history of Crohn disease and PID. What is the most likely cause for her subfertility?
A Tubal factor
B Male factor
C Coital dysfunction
D Ovulatory dysfunction
E Congenital anomaly

Chapter 17 Menopause

1. Which of the following hormonal changes are what you would expect to see with the menopause?
A FSH↑ LH↑ Oestradiol↑ Progesterone↓
B FSH↑ LH↑ Oestradiol↓ Progesterone↓
C FSH↑ LH↓ Oestradiol↑ Progesterone↔
D FSH↓ LH↑ Oestradiol↔ Progesterone↓
E FSH↓ LH↑ Oestradiol↓ Progesterone↓

2. An FSH level of what level or higher can be used in patients aged 40–45 with menopausal symptoms or change in menstrual cycle to diagnose the menopause or those <40 with suspected menopause?
A 10
B 20
C 30
D 40
E 50

3. Which of the following would be a correct preparation of hormonal replacement therapy (HRT) to offer a patient who still have their uterus and ovaries to manage menopausal symptoms. The patient has no other contraindications to using hormones:
A LNG-IUS with oestrogen patch
B Copper-IUD with oestrogen gel
C Oestrogen patch alone
D Oestrogen gel alone
E LNG-IUS with oral progestogen

4. A 33-year-old patient presents with secondary amenorrhoea for 9 months. She has no past medical or past surgical history. Her bloods show a high FSH levels on two separate occasions 4 weeks apart. She has a low oestradiol levels and high LH levels. What is the most likely diagnosis?
A Pregnancy
B PCOS
C Anorexia
D Primary ovarian insufficiency
E Hypothyroidism

Chapter 18 Early pregnancy complications

1. A 26-year-old woman attends Accident and Emergency with mild lower abdominal pain and vaginal spotting with mild lower abdominal pain and vaginal spotting. Her β-human chorionic gonadotrophin is positive and her last menstrual period was 6 weeks ago. Her observations are stable and haemoglobin 134. How would you proceed?
A Admit to hospital and consider laparoscopy
B Admit to hospital for observation
C Arrange an ultrasound scan (USS) at the earliest opportunity
D Reassure and discharge without follow-up
E Reassure and discharge with USS booked in 2 weeks

2. A 34-year-old woman attends early pregnancy unit with mild abdominal pain, no bleeding and a positive pregnancy test. She is clinically well and observations are stable. She has transvaginal ultrasound scan but no pregnancy is seen either intrauterine or extrauterine. How can this be described?
A She has a confirmed ectopic pregnancy
B She has a confirmed intrauterine pregnancy
C It is possible to rule out ectopic pregnancy
D She has had a miscarriage
E It is not yet possible to rule out ectopic pregnancy

3. A 25-year-old is being seen in early pregnancy unit with a pregnancy of unknown location. No pregnancy can be seen on scan. Her serial serum β-human chorionic gonadotrophin levels are as follows:

   Day 1: 258 IU/L
   Day 3: 490 IU/L
   How can we describe this scenario?
   a   Normal rise, conclusive of intrauterine pregnancy
   b   Normal rise, can exclude ectopic pregnancy
   c   Normal rise, cannot exclude ectopic pregnancy
   d   Suboptimal rise suggestive of miscarriage
   e   Suboptimal rise suggestive of ectopic pregnancy

4. The following are possible clinical presentations of an ectopic pregnancy except:
   A   Abdominal pain without vaginal bleeding
   B   Shoulder tip pain
   C   Fingertip pain
   D   Syncope and dizziness
   E   Diarrhoea and vomiting

5. A 35-year-old woman presents with pelvic pain in early pregnancy. Ultrasound diagnoses a right-sided tubal ectopic pregnancy. At laparoscopy, her left fallopian tube appears entirely normal. What procedure would you perform to manage the ectopic pregnancy?
   A   Transvaginal ultrasound (TVUS)
   B   Laparotomy
   C   Laparoscopic salpingostomy
   D   Laparoscopic salpingectomy
   E   Laparoscopy hysterectomy

6. A 26-year-old woman presents in early pregnancy with pain and PV bleeding. She is 8 weeks' pregnant by dates. Speculum examination reveals an open cervical os. What is the outcome of this pregnancy?
   A   Ectopic pregnancy
   B   Inevitable miscarriage
   C   Placenta praevia
   D   Complete miscarriage
   E   Incomplete miscarriage

7. A 25-year-old woman presents with pelvic pain and some PV spotting. She is 9 weeks by dates and human chorionic gonadotrophin level 2000. Ultrasound reveals an empty uterus, with a mass measuring 2 × 3 cm adjacent to the left ovary. What is the likely diagnosis?
   A   Ectopic pregnancy
   B   Complete miscarriage
   C   Complete molar pregnancy
   D   Partial molar pregnancy
   E   Ovarian cancer

Chapter 19 Antenatal booking and prenatal diagnosis

1. A 24-year-old Mediterranean primiparous woman had her booking appointment. Which of the following test result needs to be reviewed if microcytic anaemia is detected at this appointment?
   A   Serum electrophoresis
   B   Serum antibody screen
   C   Group and screen
   D   Toxoplasmosis immunity
   E   Urea and electrolytes

2. A 33-year-old woman with type I diabetes presented for the booking appointment. Which of the following test should be performed at this appointment to identify the risk of congenital malformations?
   A   Blood glucose level
   B   Serum electrophoresis
   C   Glycosylated haemoglobin
   D   Oral glucose tolerance test
   E   Serum electrophoresis

3. Which one of the following is a routine test performed on every pregnant woman that identifies the need for anti-D prophylaxis?
   A   Crossmatch blood
   B   Group and screen
   C   Serum electrophoresis
   D   Full blood count
   E   Urea and electrolytes

4. Which one of the following screening tests detects a condition where intervention can reduce the risk of vertical transmission from 25% to <1%?
   A   Screening for toxoplasmosis
   B   Screening for Hepatitis A
   C   Screening for Hepatitis B
   D   Screening for Hepatitis C
   E   Screening for human immunodeficiency virus (HIV)

5. At 41 weeks' gestation, a primiparous woman is seen in antenatal clinic. Her pregnancy has been straightforward and she is keen to avoid induction of labour. Which one of the following is the most appropriate intervention?
   A   Cardiotocograph
   B   Speculum examination
   C   Membrane sweep
   D   Cervical cerclage
   E   External cephalic version

6. At 30 weeks' gestation, a primiparous woman complains of a 4-hour history of a clear watery vaginal loss. She has no abdominal pain. Which one of the following is the most appropriate next step?
   A Cervical cerclage
   B Speculum examination
   C Membrane sweep
   D Foetocide
   E External cephalic version

7. A multiparous woman is diagnosed with a breech presentation at 37 weeks. Her pregnancy is uncomplicated. She is keen on vaginal delivery. Which one of the following is the most appropriate next step?
   A Wait for the foetus to turn to cephalic position as she is multiparous
   B Speculum examination
   C Membrane sweep
   D Cardiotocograph
   E External cephalic version

8. A 38-year-old woman has an increased risk of trisomy 21 on serum screening testing at 16 weeks. Which one of the following is the most appropriate diagnostic test for her?
   A NIPT (noninvasive prenatal test)
   B Chorionic villus sampling
   C Amniodrainage
   D Amniocentesis
   E Umbilical artery Doppler

9. At 34 weeks' gestation, ultrasound scan shows a slowing of the foetal growth rate with a reduction in the liquor volume. There is no evidence of spontaneous rupture of membranes. Which one of the following should be done next when managing this patient?
   A Membrane sweep
   B Speculum examination
   C Umbilical artery Doppler
   D Ductus venosus Doppler
   E Delivery

10. A 21-year-old who works as a nursery nurse presents for antenatal booking at 8 weeks and has never had chicken pox. She reports contact with a child with chickenpox. She is currently clinically well. Which one of the following is the single most appropriate test investigation for her?
    A Routine booking investigations
    B Toxoplasmosis IgG
    C Varicella zoster IgM
    D Full blood count
    E Chorionic villous sampling

11. A 43-year-old presents to antenatal clinic at 13 weeks to discuss her combined screening result which shows a risk of 1:90. Which one of the following is the single most appropriate screening test for her?
    A NIPT (noninvasive prenatal test)
    B Chorionic villus sampling
    C Amniodrainage
    D Amniocentesis
    E Umbilical artery Doppler

12. A 25 year old with a history of intravenous drug use attends at 11 weeks for booking. Which one of the following should be performed in addition to routine booking investigations?
    A Screening for human immunodeficiency virus (HIV)
    B Screening for Hepatitis A
    C Screening for Hepatitis B
    D Screening for Hepatitis C
    E Screening for toxoplasmosis

13. A 37-year-old solicitor in her first pregnancy attends for booking at 9 weeks, she has a normal body mass index and no past medical history of note apart from anxiety. Which one of the following should be performed?
    A NIPT (noninvasive prenatal test)
    B Chorionic villus sampling
    C Amniocentesis
    D Routine booking investigations
    E Referral to consultant-led care

14. A 32-year-old Indian lady, 20 weeks pregnant, was seen in the clinic. Her booking bloods were unremarkable. A combined screening test showed low chance. Her body mass index was 36 kg/m². Her mother has type II diabetes. Which one of the following should be organized in this pregnancy?
    A Detailed cardiac ultrasound
    B Glucose tolerance test
    C Detailed eye examination
    D Renal function
    E Serum ferritin, vitamin B12 and folate

Chapter 20 Antepartum haemorrhage

1. A 35-year-old woman has had two previous caesarean sections presents with vaginal spotting and a transverse lie at 35 weeks. She does not have any medical conditions, and is up to date with her smear tests. She does not report any abdominal pain and foetal movements are normal. Which one of the following is the most likely diagnosis for her?

A Molar pregnancy
B Cervical cancer
C Placenta praevia
D Placental abruption
E Heavy show

2. A 22-year-old woman has artificial rupture of membranes (ARM) during labour. Following ARM there is heavy vaginal bleeding in association with an abnormal cardiotocography (CTG). The uterus is soft and nontender. Which one of the following is the single most likely diagnosis for her?
   A Trauma to cervix
   B Vasa praevia
   C Placenta praevia
   D Placental abruption
   E Heavy show

3. A 28-year-old woman has a history of 16 weeks' amenorrhoea. She has severe nausea and vomiting. On abdominal palpation the uterus is 24 weeks in size. No intrauterine sac can be seen on ultrasound scan. Which one of the following is the most likely diagnosis?
   A Fibroid uterus
   B Twin pregnancy
   C Ectopic pregnancy
   D Molar pregnancy
   E Retained placenta

4. A 32-year-old woman is 28 weeks' pregnant. She has a 2-hour history of vaginal bleeding. She also complains of a headache and constant abdominal pain. On examination, the uterus is firm and tender. Which one of the following is the most likely diagnosis?
   A Molar pregnancy
   B Braxton-Hicks contractions
   C Placenta praevia
   D Placental abruption
   E Heavy show

5. A 30-year-old woman presents with a light postcoital bleed at 22 weeks gestation. She does not have abdominal pain. Her smear tests are up to date and have been normal. Which one of the following is the single most likely diagnosis?
   A Placenta praevia
   B Cervical cancer
   C Vaginal candidiasis
   D Cervical ectropion
   E Vaginal tear

Chapter 21 Hypertension in pregnancy

1. 19-year-old primigravida booked with a blood pressure of 90/60 mmHg at 12 weeks. She is asthmatic and on regular inhalers. Asthma is well controlled and she does not have any other medical conditions. She had an uneventful pregnancy until 38 weeks of gestation when she presented with swelling of the lower legs. Her blood pressure (BP) was noted to be 160/95 mmHg and urinalysis revealed ++ proteinuria. Which one of the following is considered a first-line treatment agent to control BP?
   A Enalapril
   B Nifedipine
   C Methyldopa
   D Labetalol
   E Hydralazine

2. A 42-year-old primigravida books at 13 weeks' gestation. Her blood pressure was 150/90 mmHg at booking and there was no proteinuria. She was started on methyldopa 500 mg t.d.s. which maintained her BP within the normal range for the rest of the pregnancy. Which one of the following is the single most likely diagnosis?
   A Pregnancy-induced hypertension
   B Preeclampsia
   C Hypertension secondary to renal disease
   D Essential hypertension
   E Essential hypertension with superimposed preeclampsia

3. A 25-year-old primigravida books at 16 weeks' gestation with a BP of 155/95 mmHg. She has a history or ureteric reflux and recurrent urinary tract infections as a child requiring ureteric reimplantation surgery. Her creatinine was slightly raised.
   A Pregnancy-induced hypertension
   B Preeclampsia
   C Hypertension secondary to renal disease
   D Essential hypertension
   E Essential hypertension with superimposed preeclampsia

4. A 41-year-old primigravida booked with a BP of 140/95 mmHg at 10 weeks' gestation. She is a known essential hypertensive with proteinuria. She was commenced on labetalol and had an uneventful pregnancy until 34 weeks when she was noted to have developed oedema and worsening blood pressure control. Which one of the following is the most helpful test for diagnosis?
   A Urine albumin level
   B Urine dip

C   Renal ultrasound
D   Placental growth factor (PIGF)
E   Placental-associated plasma protein A (PAPP-A)

5. A 37-year-old woman booked at 12 weeks' gestation with a BP of 95/60 mmHg. She had an uneventful pregnancy until 24 weeks' gestation when she was found to be hypertensive with oedema but normal biochemistry. She was managed conservatively with methyldopa. At 29 weeks she felt unwell and blood tests revealed a haemoglobin concentration of 8.5 g/dL with evidence of haemolysis on blood film. Her platelet concentration was 85×10^9 and her alanine aminotransferase concentration was raised. Which one of the following is the single most likely diagnosis for her?
   A   Pregnancy-induced hypertension
   B   Preeclampsia
   C   Hypertension secondary to renal disease
   D   Severe fulminating preeclampsia
   E   HELLP syndrome (*h*aemolysis, *e*levated *l*iver enzymes and *l*ow *p*latelets)

6. An 18-year-old patient who is 33 weeks' pregnant is brought in by ambulance fitting with a BP of 205/120 mmHg. She has been fit and well before this episode. Which one of the following is considered the first-line treatment?
   A   Diazepam.
   B   Methyldopa.
   C   Labetalol.
   D   Hydralazine.
   E   Magnesium sulphate.

7. A 38-year-old woman with a history of essential hypertension attends the antenatal clinic following her booking appointment at 14 weeks. Her general practitioner has already changed her regular antihypertensives to labetalol 200 mg twice a day. Which of the following medication should be offered to reduce the risk of preeclampsia?
   A   Folic acid 400 mcg.
   B   Nifedipine 10 mg.
   C   Aspirin 150 mg.
   D   Vitamin D 10 mcg.
   E   Enalapril 5 mg.

Chapter 22 Medical disorders in pregnancy

1. Which of the following is **NOT** a risk factor for gestational diabetes?
   A   Body mass index >30 kg/m^2.
   B   South Asian origin.

C   Family history of type 2 diabetes in a first-degree relative.
D   Previous gestational diabetes.
E   Partner with type 2 diabetes.

2. Which of the following is **NOT** a known risk factor for venous thromboembolism in pregnancy?
   A   Thrombophilia (factor V Leiden, protein C deficiency, antiphospholipid syndrome).
   B   Age >35 years.
   C   Body mass index >30 kg/m^2.
   D   Parity >3.
   E   Age <20 years.

3. A 26-year-old primiparous woman presents to the labour ward at 33 weeks' gestation with a 2-day history of feeling increasingly unwell with nausea and vomiting. On admission, she has mildly raised blood pressure. She has blood investigations which show a raised alanine aminotransferase, a very high uric acid level and low blood glucose. What is the most likely diagnosis?
   A   Fulminating preeclampsia.
   B   Acute fatty liver of pregnancy.
   C   Obstetric cholestasis.
   D   Pregnancy-induced hypertension.
   E   Cholelithiasis.

4. A 32-year-old patient is referred to the obstetrician at 16 weeks' gestation because of a history of previous gestational diabetes. Which one of the following is the most appropriate management plan?
   A   Take folic acid 5 mg daily
   B   Book a glucose tolerance test
   C   Check the peak expiratory flow rate
   D   Start on a low-calorie diet
   E   Start aspirin 150 mg daily

5. A 40-year-old woman with a body mass index (BMI) of 51 kg/m^2 presents to A&E at 18 weeks of gestation with unilateral calf swelling. Which one of the following is the single most likely diagnosis?
   A   Cardiac failure
   B   Normal physiological changes in pregnancy
   C   Deep vein thrombosis
   D   Iron-deficiency anaemia
   E   Intrahepatic cholestasis of pregnancy

6. Ultrasound scan shows a macrosomic foetus with polyhydramnios. Which one of the following maternal conditions is the single most likely cause?
   A   Intrahepatic cholestasis of pregnancy
   B   Gestational diabetes

C   Iron-deficiency anaemia
D   Hypothyroidism
E   Ulcerative colitis

7. At 28 weeks gestation, a multiparous patient presents with severe abdominal pain. On abdominal examination, there are palpable uterine contractions; vaginal examination shows cervical effacement. Which one of the following is the single most likely diagnosis?
    A   Symphysis pubis dysfunction
    B   Placental abruption
    C   Intrauterine growth restriction
    D   Pyelonephritis
    E   Preterm labour

8. A 25-year-old woman with a 10-year history of epilepsy sees her GP because she is planning to stop the oral contraceptive pill. Which one of the following is the single most appropriate management plan?
    A   Take folic acid 5 mg daily
    B   Book a glucose tolerance test
    C   Arrange urgent investigations including coagulation screen and glucose level
    D   Start aspirin 150 mg daily
    E   Check the body mass index

9. A primiparous patient presents to the labour ward at 34 weeks' gestation with a 24-hour history of nausea, vomiting and abdominal pain. Which one of the following is the single most appropriate management plan?
    A   Take folic acid 5 mg daily
    B   Book a glucose tolerance test
    C   Arrange urgent investigations including coagulation screen and glucose level
    D   Start aspirin 75 mg daily
    E   Check the body mass index

10. A 40-year-old multiparous woman with a body mass index of 38 kg/m^2 at booking attends A&E at 18 weeks' gestation with a 48-hour history of breathlessness and chest pain. Which one of the following is the most appropriate next step?
    A   Organize leg venous Doppler scan
    B   Organize CT pulmonary angiogram
    C   Organize ventilation perfusion scan
    D   Organize a chest X-ray
    E   Check the peak expiratory flow rate

11. A 33-year-old primiparous woman with a body mass index of 46 kg/m^2 attends antenatal clinic as she is having shared care (consultant and midwife). Which one of the following is not a known risk factor for this patient?

A   Gestational diabetes (GDM)
B   Preeclampsia
C   Foetal abnormalities
D   Caesarean birth
E   Vitamin D deficiency

12. About 2 weeks postnatally, a 36-year-old multiparous woman starts to worry that her partner is spying on her as she cares for her baby. She begins to think she can hear someone telling her she is doing tasks incorrectly. Her partner calls the health visitor who suspects that the most likely diagnosis is:
    A   Baby blues.
    B   Bipolar disorder.
    C   Schizophrenia.
    D   Postnatal depression.
    E   Puerperal psychosis.

Chapter 23 Common presentations in pregnancy

1. A 29-year-old woman in her first pregnancy presented with abdominal pain at 26 weeks of gestation. Her vital signs are normal. On examination, the uterus palpates large with a symphysis pubis height of 29 weeks. There is tenderness elicited over a specific site. Which one of the following is the most likely diagnosis?
    A   Fibroid degeneration
    B   Gastroenteritis
    C   Symphysis pubis dysfunction
    D   Placental abruption
    E   Acute appendicitis

2. A 41-year-old pregnant woman presented to a routine antenatal appointment at 30 weeks. In the first trimester she had high chance for trisomy 21 and she declined further diagnostic tests as she is committed to the pregnancy. Her abdomen palpates large for dates with a suspicion of increased amniotic fluid. Which one of the following is the most likely cause?
    A   Placental insufficiency
    B   Oesophageal atresia
    C   Renal agenesis
    D   Uterine fibroid
    E   Ibuprofen use

3. A 36-year-old woman in her third pregnancy at 36 weeks presents with central lower abdominal pain and difficulty walking. She has no urinary or bowel symptoms. Pain is constant and gets worse when climbing the stairs. What is the likely diagnosis?
    A   Urinary tract infection.
    B   Appendicitis.

C Early labour.
D Symphysis pubis dysfunction.
E Gallstones.

4. A 39-year-old woman of Indian origin measures large for dates at her 28th-week antenatal appointment and her midwife arranges a growth ultrasound scan. The ultrasound scan shows a macrosomic baby with polyhydramnios. Her combined screening test shows low chance for chromosomal abnormalities and the anomaly scan is normal. Which is the most important investigation to perform next?

A TORCH screen.
B Glucose tolerance test.
C Rhesus status.
D Full blood count.
E Amniocentesis.

5. A 26-year-old woman presented with reduced foetal movements and she is measuring small for dates at 36 weeks. She is in her second pregnancy, first child had growth restriction and she had an induction of labour. Her combined screening test shows low chance for chromosomal abnormalities and the anomaly scan is normal. She has normal blood pressure, no protein in her urine. She is fit and well, she does not report any concerns. What is the most likely diagnosis?

A Gestational diabetes
B Gestational trophoblastic disease
C Placental insufficiency
D Pregnancy
E Uterine fibroid

Chapter 24 Multiple pregnancy

1. A 39-year-old woman in her first pregnancy had a viability scan and found out that she is having a twin pregnancy. This is the third attempt of an in vitro fertilization (IVF) and she is 8 weeks pregnant. Which one of the following is the most important factor in defining risks in multiple pregnancies?

A Maternal age
B Chorionicity
C Zygosity
D Primiparity
E Conceived via artificial reproductive techniques

2. A 33-year-old woman has a monochorionic twin pregnancy. Ultrasound scan at 22 weeks shows discrepant growth and liquor volumes. Which is the most likely diagnosis?

A Gestational diabetes.
B Preeclampsia.

C Foetal infection.
D Maternal anaemia.
E Twin-to-twin transfusion syndrome.

3. A 25-year-old woman in her second pregnancy is induced at 37 weeks with a twin pregnancy. The labour progresses at a normal rate and both babies are delivered normally. However, she has a heavy blood loss after delivery of approximately 900 mL. Which is the most likely cause?

A Uterine atony.
B Second-degree tear.
C Placental abruption.
D Retained placenta.
E Maternal infection.

4. A 29-year-old woman has an ultrasound scan at 13 weeks which shows she is expecting twins. It is a spontaneous conception. The scan shows a lambda sign looking at the membranes, one placental mass and two male foetuses. Which of the following statements is true?

A The pregnancy is a monochorionic pregnancy.
B The twins must be identical.
C The pregnancy must be dizygotic.
D The pregnancy is a dichorionic pregnancy.
E There is a placenta praevia.

Chapter 25 Preterm labour

1. A 19-year-old woman attends the labour ward at 28 weeks' gestation with increasingly regular tightenings every 10 minutes. On cervical assessment, there is cervical effacement and dilatation of 1 cm. Which is your first line of management?

A Urinalysis.
B Administration of steroids.
C Liaising with the paediatric team.
D Tocolysis.
E Caesarean section.

2. A 32-year-old woman presents to labour ward at 33 weeks with regular uterine contractions. She had a history of large loop excision of the transformation zone (LLETZ) before the pregnancy, otherwise fit and well. Her examination findings showed a cervical dilatation of 8 cm. Which of the following is **NOT** appropriate in managing this patient?

A Caesarean section
B Continuous CTG monitoring
C Forceps delivery
D Ventouse delivery
E Giving prophylactic antibiotics

3. Which of the following is **NOT** a risk factor for preterm labour?

A Bacterial vaginosis.
B Previous preterm delivery.
C Previous caesarean section at full dilatation.
D Lack of social support.
E Previous miscarriage at 8 weeks.

4. Which one of the following cases can be managed with a cervical cerclage?

A G1P0, 23 weeks of gestation, incidental finding of cervical length of 27 mm
B G2P1, 8 weeks of gestation, previous history of delivery at 25 weeks
C G8P0, 13 weeks of gestation, previous seven miscarriages between 6 and 8 weeks of gestation
D G1P0, 19 weeks of gestation, incidental finding of a cervical dilatation of 2 cm with bulging membranes
E G1P0, 20 weeks of gestation, previous large loop excision of the transformation zone (LLETZ), cervical length 31 mm

5. A 31-year-old woman in her first pregnancy has been diagnosed with preterm prelabour rupture of membranes at 33 weeks. You are called to assess her on the antenatal ward. Which feature of your history and examination makes you most concerned for the wellbeing of the woman and her baby?

A Maternal tachypnoea.
B Vaginal swab confirms candida infection.
C Small amount of mucoid vaginal bleeding.
D White blood cell count of 15×10^9/L.
E Pain on passing urine (dysuria).

Chapter 26 Labour

1. During the course of labour, abdominal palpation is the most appropriate method of assessing which of the following parameters?

A To exclude obstructing fibroids.
B Strength of uterine contractions.
C Presence of moulding.
D Presence of caput.
E Baseline variability of the foetal heart rate.

2. Which of the following describes the mechanism for delivery of the foetal head in the correct order?

A Internal rotation-external rotation-flexion-extension
B Internal rotation-flexion-external rotation-extension.
C Flexion-internal rotation-external rotation-extension.
D Flexion-internal rotation-extension-external rotation.
E Internal rotation-flexion-extension-external rotation.

3. In obstetric palpation, which factor is the most important for assessing progress in labour?

A Symphysis-fundal height.
B Foetal presentation.
C Engagement.
D Foetal position.
E Liquor volume.

4. Which one of the following terms is used to define the relationship between the denominator of the presenting part and the maternal pelvis?

A Foetal presentation
B Foetal lie
C Position of the presenting part of the foetus
D Station of the presenting part of the foetus
E Foetal attitude

Chapter 27 Foetal monitoring in labour

1. In a low-risk primiparous woman, which of the following indications necessitates continuous foetal monitoring in labour?

A Irregular contractions.
B Mucoid show.
C Second stage of labour.
D Pethidine analgesia.
E Meconium-stained liquor.

2. With regard to cardiotocograph monitoring, what is the definition of acceleration?

A Increase in the foetal heart rate (FHR) of 5 bpm above the baseline rate lasting for 15 seconds.
B Increase in the FHR of 15 bpm above the baseline rate lasting for 15 seconds.
C Decrease in the FHR of 15 bpm below the baseline for 15 seconds.
D Increase in the FHR of 5 bpm above the baseline rate lasting for 5 seconds.
E Increase in the FHR of 15 bpm above the baseline rate lasting for 5 seconds.

3. A 29-year-old woman in her second pregnancy presents to labour ward in active labour. Her booking body mass index is 40 kg/m^2. This pregnancy has been uneventful and regular growth scans have been normal. On examination, cervix is 5 cm dilated and she is regularly contracting, membranes are spontaneously ruptured, liquor is clear. During labour, there is difficulty monitoring the foetal heart rate with CTG due to maternal habitus. Which one of the following is the most appropriate next step in the managing this labour?

A Foetal blood sample

B Foetal scalp electrode
C Caesarean section
D Epidural anaesthesia
E Artificial rupture of membranes

4. A 24-year-old primiparous woman, 40 weeks plus 5 days pregnant, transferred to labour ward from midwife-led unit due to meconium-stained labour. She is fit and well and pregnancy has been uneventful. On vaginal examination, cervix is 2 cm dilated, presenting part is at −2, no caput or no moulding noted. Below is the CTG trace following admission to labour ward. Which one of the following is not a feature of the trace?

A Baseline appropriate for the gestation
B Stable baseline
C Normal variability (between 5 and 25)
D Accelerations present
E Decelerations present

Chapter 28 Operative interventions in labour

1. Which one of the following is the advantage of mediolateral episiotomy compared to midline episiotomy?

A Less postpartum pain
B Technically easier to repair
C Better cosmetic results
D Less infection
E Less third- and fourth-degree tears

2. Which one of the following is not true for the postpartum care following a third-degree tear?

A Patients should be debriefed regarding the extent of the tear
B Antibiotics should be taken following the repair
C Routine laxatives should be taken for the first 2 weeks
D Referral to physiotherapy
E Patients should be counselled that in the next pregnancy vaginal delivery will be contraindicated

3. A 31-year-old Asian-origin primiparous woman has a forceps delivery and perineal trauma involving the perineal muscles and external anal sphincter muscle? What is the correct classification for the perineal trauma described?

A Midline episiotomy.
B First-degree perineal tear.
C Fourth-degree perineal tear.
D Third-degree perineal tear.
E Second-degree perineal tear.

4. A woman has been started on syntocinon for augmentation of labour as meconium-stained liquor was noted when her membranes ruptured spontaneously. She

is 4 cm dilated and is contracting 6 in 10 and the cardiotocograph shows atypical decelerations. What is the immediate management?

A Deliver the baby by caesarean section.
B Reduce/stop the syntocinon infusion.
C Start oxygen therapy.
D Start intravenous fluids.
E Give terbutaline.

5. A 28-year-old P1 woman presented to labour ward in spontaneous labour at 39 weeks of gestation. Previous delivery was an emergency caesarean section at a cervical dilatation of 8 cm due to foetal stress. Caesarean section was uncomplicated and patient recovered well. She is aiming for a vaginal delivery in this pregnancy. Which one of the following is not appropriate when managing this patient?

A Intravenous cannula
B Full blood count and group-and-save sample available in laboratory
C Intermittent auscultation until second stage of labour
D Monitor vaginal loss to exclude bleeding
E Monitor abdominal pain

Chapter 29 Complications of labour

1. A 26-year-old woman who has been an insulin-dependent diabetic since the age of 10 years. Booking body mass index (BMI) is 32 kg/m². She is being induced at 37 weeks as the glucose levels are high and uncontrolled. She has been on syntocinon for 10 hours and contracting 4 in 10 minutes. For the last 12 hours there is 2 cm progress in dilatation. On the most recent examination cervix is 5 cm dilated, vulva is oedematous. What is the most likely explanation for lack of progress?

A Frequency of the uterine contractions is not sufficient
B Occiputo posterior position
C High BMI
D Foetal macrosomia
E Maternal exhaustion

2. A 38-year-old African woman is in her fifth pregnancy with a diagnosis of preterm labour at 35 weeks. The membranes rupture whilst she is being assessed for signs of labour. There is a prolonged foetal bradycardia which is not recovering. Which is the most likely diagnosis?

A Foetal infection.
B Uterine rupture.
C Amniotic fluid embolism.
D Umbilical cord prolapse.
E Hyperstimulation of the uterus.

3. Which of the following is NOT a contraindication to external cephalic version (ECV)?
   A Ruptured membranes.
   B Multiparity.
   C Placenta praevia.
   D Severe preeclampsia.
   E Multiple pregnancy.

4. A patient who has previously had a caesarean section is having a vaginal delivery in this pregnancy. At 8-cm dilatation, the cardiotocography (CTG) suddenly shows a prolonged foetal bradycardia. Which one of the following is the most likely diagnosis?
   A Cord prolapse
   B Ruptured uterus
   C Uterine hyperstimulation
   D Maternal hypotension
   E Placental abruption

5. A 39-year-old woman who had previous five vaginal deliveries with a body mass index of 35 kg/m^2 has a ventouse delivery for a prolonged second stage. The foetal head shows the turtle-neck sign as it delivers and there is difficulty delivering the baby. Which one of the following options has the most likely three complications?
   A Postpartum haemorrhage/shoulder dystocia/postpartum deep vein thrombosis
   B Shoulder dystocia/cord prolapse/postpartum haemorrhage
   C Cord prolapse/sepsis/postpartum deep vein thrombosis
   D Sepsis/shoulder dystocia/postpartum haemorrhage
   E Sepsis/postpartum haemorrhage/postpartum deep vein thrombosis

6. A 30-year-old P2 at 39 weeks of gestation in early labour. On examination, cervical dilatation is 3 cm and membranes are intact. Foetus is in breech position, mother is keen to have vaginal delivery and aware of the risks to the baby. In established labour with the CTG suddenly shows a prolonged foetal bradycardia. Which one of the following is the most likely explanation?
   A Meconium-stained liquor
   B Placental abruption
   C Cord prolapse
   D Ruptured uterus
   E Uterine hyperstimulation

7. A patient who has been diagnosed with severe preeclampsia is having labour induced at 37 weeks. She starts to complain of constant sharp abdominal pain. The uterus is tender and hard on palpation. The CTG has become suspicious. Which one of the following is the most likely explanation?
   A Meconium-stained liquor
   B Placental abruption
   C Cord prolapse
   D Ruptured uterus
   E Uterine hyperstimulation

8. A 36-year-old P3, who had previous three vaginal deliveries, has been induced for intrahepatic cholestasis. Following rupture of membranes intravenous syntocinon is started. She is contracting 6 in 10. The CTG shows variable decelerations with a rise in the baseline heart rate. Which one of the following is the most likely explanation?
   A Meconium-stained liquor
   B Placental abruption
   C Cord prolapse
   D Ruptured uterus
   E Uterine hyperstimulation

Chapter 30 Stillbirth

1. The definition of a stillbirth is …
   A A baby born with no signs of life at or after 20 completed weeks of pregnancy.
   B A foetus in utero greater than 24 completed weeks of pregnancy found to have no cardiac activity.
   C A baby born with no signs of life at or after 28 completed weeks of pregnancy.
   D A foetus in utero greater than 22 completed weeks of pregnancy found to have no cardiac activity.
   E A baby that is born with no signs of life at or after 24 completed weeks of pregnancy.

2. As part of the investigations of a stillbirth a TORCH screen for infections is performed. Which of the following infections is NOT tested for?
   A Toxoplasmosis.
   B Parvovirus B19.
   C Malaria.
   D Cytomegalovirus.
   E Rubella.

3. Which one of the following test is not routine following a stillbirth?
   A Random blood sugar and HbA1c
   B Kleihauer-Bethke
   C Full blood count, C-reactive protein
   D Parental karyotype
   E Liver function

Chapter 31 Postnatal complications

1. Management of postpartum haemorrhage must start with:
   A Identifying the cause of bleeding
   B Multidisciplinary team approach
   C Basic resuscitation (Airway, Breathing, Circulation (ABC))
   D Contacting haematology and anaesthetic specialists
   E Making an accurate estimation of blood loss

2. The definition of secondary postpartum haemorrhage (PPH) is as follows:
   A >500 mL vaginal bleeding 24 hours after delivery, within 6 weeks
   B >1000 mL vaginal bleeding after delivery up to 6 weeks
   C >2000 mL vaginal bleeding post delivery
   D >500 mL vaginal bleeding within 24 hours of delivery
   E <2000 mL vaginal bleeding within 24 hours of delivery

3. A 29-year-old primiparous woman, known to have fibroids, has just delivered a baby weighing 4.1 kg, after being induced and having a long first stage of labour. As the placenta delivers, she suddenly feels faint and passes 700 mL of blood and clot vaginally. What is the most likely cause of the postpartum haemorrhage?
   A Genital tract trauma
   B Retained placental cotyledon
   C Cervical ectropion
   D Placenta accreta
   E Uterine atony

4. A 33-year-old woman who delivered 3 days previously by normal vaginal delivery has called her community midwife as she feels increasingly unwell with lower abdominal pain and a fever. Her 7-year-old son is off school with a sore throat. The most likely possible cause of sepsis in this patient is:
   A Urinary tract infection
   B Mastitis
   C Pneumonia
   D Endometritis
   E Group A streptococcus

5. The following are risk factors of postpartum (puerperal) psychosis, except:
   A Personal history of bipolar affective disorder
   B Personal history of postpartum psychosis
   C Personal history of psychotic illness
   D Family history of bipolar affective disorder
   E Family history of baby blues

6. A patient has had a forceps delivery with an episiotomy after a prolonged labour. On examination, the episiotomy has extended into the external anal sphincter and the patient is bleeding heavily from the area. The most likely diagnosis is:
   A Second-degree tear
   B Third-degree tear
   C Uterine rupture
   D Uterine inversion
   E Haemorrhoids

7. A patient has just had a normal vaginal delivery of a twin pregnancy. She is bleeding heavily. On examination, the uterine fundus is above the umbilicus and poorly contracted. The most likely diagnosis is:
   A Retained products of conception
   B Endometritis
   C Uterine atony
   D Uterine rupture
   E Placenta accreta

8. A woman has previously had two caesarean sections. At the time of caesarean section in this pregnancy, the placenta was morbidly adherent to the uterine wall. The most likely diagnosis is:
   A Placenta accreta
   B Placenta praevia
   C Placental abruption
   D Vasa praevia
   E Uterine inversion

9. Within the first 24 hours of delivery of her baby, a woman has lost more than 500 mL of blood. The most likely diagnosis is:
   A Primary postpartum haemorrhage (PPH)
   B Secondary PPH
   C Sheehan syndrome
   D Grand multiparity
   E High body mass index (BMI)

10. At the time of controlled cord traction in the third stage of labour, the patient suddenly complains of severe abdominal pain and bleeding. The uterine fundus cannot be palpated on abdominal examination. The most likely diagnosis is:
   A Uterine atony
   B Endometritis
   C Uterine rupture
   D Retained products of conception
   E Uterine inversion

Chapter 32 Maternal collapse and maternal death

1. What do the 4 Hs for reversible causes of maternal collapse stand for?
   A Hypoxia, Hypo/hyperkalaemia, Hypovolaemia, Hypotension
   B Hypoxia, Hypo/hyperkalaemia, Hypotension, Hypothermia
   C Hypoxia, Hypo/hypermagnesaemia, Hypotension, Hypothermia
   D Hypoxia, Hypo/hypermagnesaemia, Hypovolaemia, Hypothermia
   E Hypoxia, Hypo/hyperkalaemia, Hypovolaemia, Hypothermia

2. What do the 4 Ts for reversible causes of maternal collapse stand for?
   A Toxicity, Thromboembolism, Tension pneumothorax, Tetany
   B Toxicity, Thromboembolism, Trauma, Tamponade
   C Toxicity, Thromboembolism, Tension pneumothorax, Tamponade
   D Thromboembolism, Trauma, Tension pneumothorax, Tamponade
   E Thromboembolism, Tension pneumothorax, Tamponade, Tetany

3. Which of the following is not one of the 'Ts' for causes of postpartum haemorrhage?
   A Tocophobia
   B Tone
   C Trauma
   D Thrombin
   E Tissue

4. During CPR for pregnant women >20 week's gestation. Which of the following manoeuvre should be performed alongside the DR ABC approach?
   A Supine tilt
   B Head-down tilt
   C Head-up tilt
   D Right lateral tilt
   E Left lateral tilt

5. Which of the following is the correct statement for physiological changes by the third trimester during pregnancy ?
   A Plasma volume↑ Uterine blood flow↑ Respiratory rate↓ Heart rate↑
   B Plasma volume ↑ Uterine blood flow ↑ Respiratory rate ↓ Heart rate↓
   C Plasma volume ↑ Uterine blood flow↑ Respiratory rate↑ Heart rate↑
   D Plasma volume ↓ Uterine blood flow ↑ Respiratory rate↑ Heart rate↑
   E Plasma volume ↓ Uterine blood flow ↑ Respiratory rate ↓ Heart rate↓

UKMLA SBA Answers

Chapter 1 Basic anatomy and examination

1. E. Foetal heart rate
2. C. 34–38 cm. The SFH measurement ± 2 cm should equal the gestation (e.g., at 36 weeks' gestation the SFH should be between 34 and 38 cm). Whilst SFH is a crude measurement technique and varies in precision between measurers, it can be used to identify patients measuring large- or small-for-dates (e.g., growth-restricted babies).
3. C. Assessment with Sims' speculum. All may be required, but the history suggests a cystocele with stress incontinence. The best assessment for prolapse is an examination with a Sims' speculum.
4. B. Oblique. The foetal 'lie' is the relationship between the long axis of the foetus and the long axis of the uterus. In an oblique lie, the foetus is lying at 45 degrees to the long axis of the uterus, and one of the foetal poles will be palpable in the iliac fossa.
5. A. Abdominal aorta
6. C. Semirecumbent
7. C. Endometriosis

Chapter 3 Common investigations

1. C. Three years. The UK National Screening in Cervical Cytology Programme invites people aged 25–49 years to have one smear every 3 years and those aged 50 – 64 years once every 5 years.
2. D. Human papillomavirus (HPV). HPV has been linked to >95% of cervical cancers.
3. A. Transvaginal ultrasound scan. Transvaginal ultrasound scans allow for the clearest imaging of the ovaries. This scan can not only detect the presence of cysts or tubal pathology but can also be used in the acute setting when assessing for ovarian cyst accident.
4. E. Open surgery is associated with more postoperative pain than laparoscopy. Laparoscopy, when compared with open surgery, is associated with less pain and blood loss, better visualization of organs and pathology, a shorter hospital stay and better cosmetic results.

Chapter 4 Abnormal uterine bleeding

1. D. SLE. Abnormal uterine bleeding has multiple causative factors, but lupus is not known to be one of them.
2. D. Endometrial ablation. A and B are not appropriate as although it was not stated, tranexamic acid is likely to have been tried. C and E are still options, but the quickest and least invasive will be an endometrial ablation which can be performed as an outpatient procedure. Permanent contraception is advised for this (which is fine as her husband has had a vasectomy).
3. B. Outpatient hysteroscopy and biopsy. The next appropriate form of management is to obtain an endometrial biopsy. This can be performed with blind biopsy, but if there is a polyp for instance, this may be missed. A hysteroscopy is more appropriate. This is more quickly performed as an outpatient.
4. E. All of the above. There are several risks of a hysterectomy which need to be explained to women before they consent to a procedure. All the above are important as well as others.
5. A. Atrophic vaginitis. Initially, an ultrasound and hysteroscopy with biopsy is likely to be required (if endometrial thickness is abnormal). However, statistically atrophic vaginitis is the most likely cause.
6. B. Laparoscopic hysterectomy. If medical therapy and ablation have failed, the options include UAE and hysterectomy. As she would like definitive treatment, hysterectomy is the only option and laparoscopic is less invasive than open.
7. A. Levonorgestrel intrauterine system (LNG-IUS; e.g., Mirena). As she has had a TOP, she would benefit from long-term contraception. Therefore, the Mirena coil would help her symptoms and act as contraception.
8. C. Endometrial ablation. As she has been sterilized, she would be a candidate for endometrial ablation. Other options such as UAE or hysterectomy are possible, but ablation is the safest and least invasive. If it does not work, she can try the other two options.

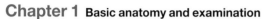

9. A. Tranexamic acid. If someone is trying to conceive and has heavy periods, only tranexamic acid or conservative measures are appropriate.
10. D. Hysteroscopy with resection of endometrial polyp. It is likely this woman has an endometrial polyp. So, removal of the polyp via hysteroscopy should alleviate her symptoms.

Chapter 5 Fibroids

1. C. Submucosal. These fibroids are located close to the endometrium. Growth extending into the endometrial cavity results in distortion of the endometrium.
2. D. Can become malignant in 1:100 cases. Malignant change is rare (1:1000 cases or less).
3. E. Hysteroscopy and pelvic ultrasound. All can provide information for fibroids. But inevitably a pelvic ultrasound and hysteroscopy are likely. An ultrasound can measure the size and location of the fibroid and a hysteroscopy is used to assess if there is a submucosal fibroid causing bleeding and whether it can be resected via hysteroscopy (if so, it can also be performed at the same time).
4. C. UAE. A and B are both surgical options so they are not appropriate. The Mirena coil will not shrink the size of the fibroids. She may require iron, but UAE is likely to improve her symptoms and hopefully reduce the size of the fibroids.
5. A. Transcervical resection of fibroids. This will help with conceiving and improve her symptoms.
6. C. Myomectomy. As she would like to conceive, a myomectomy is the most appropriate to immediately improve her hydronephrosis.
7. C. Hysterectomy. As childbearing is not an option here, hysterectomy would be preferred to myomectomy.
8. E. UAE. Uterine artery embolization will help her symptoms if she does not want surgery.
9. A. Repeat ultrasound scan in 6 months. If there are no symptoms, the fibroid can be monitored to ensure it does not rapidly increase in size. Ultrasound is more appropriate to monitor the size compared with MRI which is more expensive.

Chapter 6 Endometriosis

1. D. Dystonia. The 4 Ds of pain associated with endometriosis are: Dysmenorrhoea (Painful periods), Dyspareunia (Pain having sex – often deep), Dyschaezia (Pain opening bowels) and Dysuria (Bladder pain/pain passing urine).
2. C. 10%. Endometriosis is thought to affect 1:10 women, and this number may be an underestimate due to the challenges with definitive endometriosis diagnosis.

3. B. Thickened endometrium. Thickened endometrium implies endometrial pathology, e.g., endometrial polyp, endometrial hyperplasia or endometrial cancer. Typical ultrasound features for deep infiltrating endometriosis include a retroverted uterus, kissing ovaries with or without endometriomas, thickening of the uterosacral ligaments and pain experienced during the scan.
4. A. Migraine with aura. Absolute contraindications to the combined oral contraceptive pill include: <6 weeks postpartum, smoker over the age of 35 (>15 cigarettes per day), hypertension (systolic >160 mmHg or diastolic >100 mmHg), current or past history of venous thromboembolism (VTE), ischemic heart disease, history of cerebrovascular accident, complicated valvular heart disease, migraine with focal neurological symptoms, breast cancer (current), diabetes with retinopathy/nephropathy/neuropathy, severe cirrhosis and liver tumour.
5. E. Retrograde menstruation and implantation

Chapter 7 Pelvic pain

1. A. Vulvovaginitis. Superficial dyspareunia causes include congenital pathologies, infection, postsurgical or postvaginal delivery, vulval disease, atrophic changes or psychosexual issues.
2. C. Urine pregnancy test. A positive urine pregnancy test immediately narrows down your differential diagnoses and therefore management plan. This test is essential for all female patients of childbearing age presenting to hospital.
3. E. Cervical excitation. Cervical excitation is the sensation of pain when palpating the cervix at the time of a bimanual examination. This sign is often present in cases of PID and ectopic pregnancy.
4. C. Previous twin pregnancy. Risk factors for ectopic pregnancies include any pathology that might have caused damage to the fallopian tubes, e.g., PID, previous ectopic pregnancy, smoking (reduced motility of cilia) or in cases of concurrent pregnancy with IUD in situ.
5. D. Vaginal bleeding. Patients presenting with haemoperitoneum will often complain of shoulder-tip pain due to diaphragmatic irritation, diarrhoea from bowel irritation and presyncope or collapse.

Chapter 8 Vaginal discharge and sexually transmitted infections

1. B. Cervical ectropion. An ectropion is not pathological. It is simply an extension of endocervical columnar epithelium, which bleeds easily. On the ectocervix and is common in pregnancy due to the influence of oestrogen. No treatment is necessary unless a coexisting infection is proven.

2. B. Thick, itchy, white discharge. The thick, white discharge of candida infection has a typical appearance of cottage cheese noted on speculum examination. It is treated easily with clotrimazole pessary or cream.

3. E. Sexual history. A detailed sexual history is imperative to exclude sexually transmitted infections.

4. C. History of STI. Most common organisms held responsible for PID are *Chlamydia* and *Neisseria gonorrhoeae*, both sexually transmitted infections. Hence, any history of previous STI would predispose a patient to PID.

5. C. Vulval pruritus is not characteristically associated with PID.

6. A. Bacterial vaginosis (BV). BV is not a sexually transmitted infection. There is a change in the natural flora of the vagina. Its clinical significance is that it has been linked to second-trimester miscarriage.

7. E. Toxic shock syndrome. This girl has been distracted with examinations and has forgotten to change her tampon. Her symptoms and clinical signs are in keeping with toxic shock syndrome.

8. A. Cervical carcinoma. There is no cervical screening in this patient's country of origin. It would be prudent to check her human immunodeficiency virus (HIV) status which is a known risk factor for cervical cancer.

9. B. *Chlamydia trachomatis.* The COCP does not protect against sexually transmitted infections.

10. B. Foreign body. This is the most likely option in this scenario. Foreign body insertion into the vagina is not uncommon in this age group and should be suspected if child abuse has been ruled out.

Chapter 9 Pelvic inflammatory disease

1. D. Fitz-Hugh-Curtis syndrome. Peri-hepatic adhesions may be visualized at the time of laparoscopy in cases of severe PID.

2. A. *Chlamydia trachomatis* and *Neisseria gonorrhoeae.* These organisms are by far the most common culprits for PID; 10% of women diagnosed with *Chlamydia*, develop PID within 1 year of infection.

3. C. Repeat ultrasound examination in 6–8 weeks. Patients with mild-moderate PID do not require repeat ultrasound scan. In cases of tubo-ovarian abscess, all patients should have follow-up imaging to ensure abscess resolution.

4. B. Endometriosis. PID is not a cause for endometriosis, however women with endometriosis may be more likely to suffer from recurrent episodes of PID, especially when they have concurrent endometriomas.

Chapter 10 Contraception and TOP

1. C. Levonorgestrel-intrauterine system (LNG-IUS). Long-acting reversible contraceptives are reliable forms of contraception with low rates of failure. They do not require remembering to take daily medication and do not have long-term impact on fertility rates.

2. C. Levonorgestrel-intrauterine system (LNG-IUS). The LNG-IUS is more than 99% effective against preventing unwanted pregnancies.

3. A. A condition that represents an unacceptable health risk if the method is used. KMEC 1: A condition for which there is no restriction for the use of the method, UKMEC 2: A condition where the advantages of using the method generally outweigh the theoretical or proven risks, UKMEC 3: A condition where the theoretical or proven risks usually outweigh the advantages of using the method and UKMEC 4: A condition that represents an unacceptable health risk if the method is used.

4. E. Severe asthma. Contraindications to prescribing Ella-One (ulipristal acetate 30 mg) are Severe asthma on steroids, antiepileptic drugs and proton pump inhibitors/antacids.

5. B. Uterine perforation. Uterine perforation occurs on average in 1/1000 women with surgical termination. This risk increases however as gestation of pregnancy increases.

Chapter 11 Benign gynaecological tumours

1. E. CA-125. Urine HCG is important to rule out pregnancy. Hb can indicate if there has been an ovarian cyst accident, such as a haemorrhagic ovarian cyst. WCC and CRP are useful to rule out an inflammatory/infective process and ultrasound to diagnose an ovarian cyst. CA-125 should only be reserved if a malignancy is suspected with other investigations, otherwise it may lead to false positives.

2. B. Mainly present in the 30s age group. Dermoid cysts can present bilaterally, malignancy can occur but is rare. Only a small percentage tort (10%), and although some can rupture at presentation, this is uncommon.

3. D. Laparoscopy with or without ovarian cystectomy. This is clearly an acute ovarian torsion and so the answer is to immediately detort the ovary and remove the ovarian cyst if feasible. Performing investigations in this instance will lead to delay and the ovary possibly becoming necrotic.

4. D. Hoarse voice. Androgen-secreting tumours may present with symptoms of virilization such as deepening of the voice, hirsutism and clitoromegaly.

5. E. Solid nodule. The fifth ultrasound feature of simple cysts is unilocular – absence of septations or nodules.

6. C. Transvaginal/transabdominal ultrasound. It is important that a pelvic scan is performed to identify if an ovarian cyst exists, as the other alternative diagnosis is appendicitis.

7. B. Laparoscopy and bilateral salpingo-oophorectomy. This scenario is likely to represent an acute torsion. In a likely postmenopausal woman, the most appropriate management would be a bilateral salpingo-oophorectomy.

8. C. Haemoglobin (Hb). This is likely to represent a ruptured haemorrhagic cyst. This may resolve spontaneously but one must check the haemoglobin and ensure that a blood transfusion is not required.

9. A. Laparoscopy and bilateral salpingo-oophorectomy. Even though this is not likely to be malignant, as she is having symptoms she would benefit from both her ovaries and tubes being removed. If she was premenopausal, she would only require the symptomatic side to be removed.

10. A. CA-125. Any ovarian cyst in a postmenopausal woman must have a risk of malignancy index calculated. A CA-125 blood test is required to calculate this.

Chapter 12 Gynaecological malignancies

1. E. History of endometriosis. There is no known link between endometriosis and cervical cancer. HPV has shown to be present in up to 100% of cases of cervical cancer.

2. A. 270. With a unilateral loculated cyst her ultrasound score is 1 × postmenopausal score 3 × CA-125.

3. E. An RMI ≥200 (not 100) is associated with a higher risk of malignancy.

4. D. Endometrial biopsy. This patient requires endometrial sampling to assess for endometrial hyperplasia or endometrial cancer as the underlying cause for her postmenopausal bleeding. This can now be done as an outpatient with hysteroscopy. She may go on to require further imaging.

5. E. Paget disease of the vulva (not Paget abscess) and the other options listed (including lichen planus) are risk factors for developing vulval cancer.

6. A. Hysteroscopy and biopsy. A biopsy must be taken to confirm endometrial pathology. Conditions such as endometrial hyperplasia would not be seen on imaging. Biopsy at hysteroscopy has a higher specificity than a pipelle biopsy.

7. C. Haemorrhagic ovarian cyst. This woman has a low risk of malignancy index score so the pathology is most likely benign.

8. A. Endometrial hyperplasia.

9. A. Polycystic ovarian syndrome (PCOS). As the patient is premenopausal and has had this pattern of her periods since menarche, it is unlikely to be due to malignant pathology. A diagnosis of PCOS is more likely and can be confirmed with a transvaginal ultrasound scan and hormone profile blood tests.

10. C. Paget disease of the vulva is associated with primary cancer in 20% of cases. It is possible, however, that this lesion could be benign.

11. D. Persistent infection with high-risk human papillomavirus (HPV) is a risk factor for vaginal cancer.

12. B. Nulliparity, rather than multiparity, is a risk factor for ovarian cancer.

Chapter 13 Benign vulval disease

1. C. A thick creamy white discharge. This supports a diagnosis of infection, possibly *Candida.* An acute onset, rather than progressively worsening symptoms over 6 months suggests infection. There is no association between menorrhagia and pruritus vulvae. Red plaques in the vulval areas suggest psoriasis or eczema. Fused labia suggest lichen sclerosus.

2. B. A speculum examination of the cervix and smear test. Cervical intraepithelial neoplasia is often associated with vulval intraepithelial neoplasia. Antibiotics should only be prescribed where infection is found. Women should be referred to colposcopy only where clinically indicated. Surgical intervention is not common practice. Abdominal X-ray is not a usual part of routine work-up for pruritus vulvae.

3. B. Biopsy of the vulva. Biopsy of the vulva enables histological diagnosis. CRP does not identify a cause, but provides a marker for infective causes only. Ultrasound is not commonly used to investigate vulval disease; computed tomography and magnetic resonance imaging are more sensitive when considering vulval malignancy. Hysteroscopy alone does not identify vulval pathology, but an examination under anaesthetic may. Endocervical swabs will exclude endocervical infection only.

4. B. Skin biopsy shows thinning of the epidermis. The epidermis is usually thin and hyalinized. Lichen sclerosus can appear as white or reddish plaques. A skin biopsy is mandatory to exclude malignant change. About 50% of symptoms of pruritus vulvae can recur following surgical excision. A long course of steroids is often required.

5. C. Type 3. The FGM in this patient corresponds to type 3 (infibulation) defined as: Narrowing of the vaginal introitus through the creation of a covering seal by cutting and appositioning the labia minora and/or the labia majora, sometimes through stitching, with or without removal of the clitoris and prepuce/clitoral hood.

6. B. Carcinoma of the vulva. Any lesion that is raised, growing in size and ulcerated is suspicious of carcinoma.

7. E. *Trichomonas vaginalis.* An offensive fishy green discharge is characteristic of *Trichomonas.*

8. D. Lichen sclerosus. Fused labia in this age group with leucoplakia is characteristic of lichen sclerosus. The treatment being steroids.
9. A. Contact dermatitis. The clue is in the history as in a lot of these cases where changes in cleansing products can result in contact dermatitis.
10. C. Psoriasis. Erythema with plaques in other areas, particularly flexor surfaces, are characteristics of psoriasis, which is quite common. Treatment is usually topical steroids.

Chapter 14 Urogynaecology

1. E. Complete descent beyond the vaginal opening of the uterus.
2. D. Obturator externus. The pelvic floor muscles consist of the coccygeus, obturator internus, piriformis and levator ani muscles.
3. A. Stress urinary incontinence. Stress urinary incontinence is involuntary urine leakage on effort or exertion such as with sneezing, coughing or laughing and accounts for 50% of incontinence.
4. B. Pelvic floor repair. Pelvic floor repair is a surgical procedure performed to restore the normal anatomy of the vagina. An anterior repair refers to the repair of a cystocoele, whilst a posterior repair is the repair of a rectocoele.
5. C. It is a diagnosis of exclusion. Bladder pain syndrome can only be diagnosed once all other causes of urinary symptoms have been excluded. The triad of signs and symptoms are; nocturia, bladder filling pain and bladder base tenderness on vaginal examination.

Chapter 15 Gynaecological endocrinology

1. E. Haematocolpos. Haematocolpos can be visualized on speculum as a blue bulge in the vagina. Treatment involves incision and drainage of the transverse septum to release the old menstrual blood which has collected proximal to this.
2. B. Testosterone levels >5 nmol/L. Very high testosterone levels are linked with malignancies which can cause rapid virilization. Levels such as this should always prompt further investigation.
3. A. Sheehan syndrome. Sheehan syndrome is a unique condition resulting from postpartum infarction of the pituitary gland, triggered due to massive obstetric haemorrhage.
4. B. Asherman syndrome. Asherman syndrome is the presence of endometrial adhesions usually secondary to

instrumentation of the uterus, e.g., Surgical termination of pregnancy or surgical management of miscarriage. This condition may present as secondary amenorrhoea or subfertility.
5. C. Turner syndrome. Constitutional delay, Rokitansky-Kustner-Hauser syndrome, androgen insensitivity syndrome and Fragile-X syndrome would not present with these physical attributes.

Chapter 16 Subfertility

1. E. 90%. The vast majority of couples will conceive unassisted within 2 years of regular unprotected sexual intercourse under the age of 40.
2. B. 25%. Unexplained subfertility accounts for approximately one-quarter of cases of fertility issues. This diagnosis can sometimes be disheartening to couples who are looking for a 'cause' to identify the issue stopping them from being able to conceive.
3. C. Low-molecular-weight heparin (LMWH). Whilst the other options may play a role in the management of OHSS, prescribing LMWH is imperative given the extremely hypercoagulable state these patients are in.
4. D. Kallmann syndrome. The other answers may result in infertility, however it is the 'anosmia' which is the key to the answer to this question – none of the other conditions affect the olfactory centre.
5. A. Tubal factor. The answer is tubal factors because of the history of PID. Infertility is a major long-term complication of PID, especially in severe or recurrent cases.

Chapter 17 Menopause

1. B. FSH ↑ LH ↑ Oestradiol ↓ Progesterone ↓
2. C. 30. An FSH level of 30 or higher on two separate occasions 4–6 weeks apart can be used to diagnose menopause in patients aged 40–45 with menopausal symptoms or change in menstrual cycle or those <40 years of age with suspected menopause.
3. A. LNG-IUS with oestrogen patch. For patients without hysterectomy requiring HRT, oestrogen AND progesterone must be given in order to prevent unopposed oestrogenic effects on the endometrium which could result in endometrial hyperplasia or cancer. None of the answers provide this.
4. D. Primary ovarian insufficiency. The other answers will likely alter this patient's hormonal profile, however a raised FSH (>30) with low oestradiol levels and high LH is indicative of premature ovarian insufficiency.

Chapter 18 Early pregnancy complications

1. C. Arrange a USS at the earliest opportunity. Spotting may be normal in early pregnancy, but an ectopic pregnancy cannot be ruled out until an ultrasound scan is performed.
2. E. It is not yet possible to rule out ectopic pregnancy. This patient is in early pregnancy and has a pregnancy of unknown location.
3. C. Normal rise, cannot exclude ectopic pregnancy. Until an ultrasound scan confirms an intrauterine pregnancy, an ectopic cannot be ruled out. An ultrasound should therefore be performed in a weeks' time to see if an intrauterine pregnancy is viable.
4. C. All other options except C are possible symptoms of ectopic pregnancy. In cases of a ruptured ectopic, irritation of the inferior diaphragm from blood can cause referred shoulder tip pain (not fingertip).
5. D. Salpingectomy. An ectopic tubal pregnancy requires surgical treatment; if the contralateral tube appears normal, the best course of action is a salpingectomy.
6. B. Inevitable miscarriage.
7. A. Ectopic pregnancy. An empty uterus with an adnexal mass is generally an ectopic pregnancy until proven otherwise.

Chapter 19 Antenatal booking

1. A. serum electrophoresis to rule out beta-thalassaemia as a cause.
2. C. Glycosylated haemoglobin. The HbA1c level indicates how well-controlled the diabetes has been.
3. B. Group and screen. Women who are rhesus negative will require anti-D prophylaxis at 28 weeks and if there are any other sensitizing events.
4. E. HIV. Vertical transmission of HIV is reduced with the use of highly active antiretroviral therapy, planning the mode of delivery based on the viral load and by not breastfeeding.
5. C. Membrane sweep. This encourages spontaneous labour as examining the cervix releases labour-inducing prostaglandins.
6. B. Speculum examination. To assess if she has ruptured her membranes. If the watery loss is identified as liquor, then steroids and antibiotics should be administered.
7. E. External cephalic version should be offered to try and turn the baby to a cephalic position so that a vaginal delivery can be achieved.
8. D. Amniocentesis. Foetal cells from the amniotic fluid can be karyotyped to determine if the foetus has trisomy 21.
9. C. Umbilical artery Dopplers. Allows the resistance within the umbilical cord to be assessed and helps in planning the timing and mode of delivery.

10. D. Varicella zoster IgG. To assess if she has had a past exposure and hence immunity to chicken pox.
11. A. NIPT (noninvasive prenatal test). As the chance is <1 in 150, further testing should be offered. NIPT has a high sensitivity for detecting trisomy 21 and is still a screening test. Invasive tests such as chorionic villus sampling and amniocentesis are diagnostic tests however there is a risk of miscarriage.
12. D. Hepatitis C. Intravenous drug users are at higher risk of having Hepatitis C and they may present a risk to the unborn foetus that would need to be managed during the pregnancy. HIV and Hepatitis B status are routinely screened for all pregnant patients.
13. D. Routine booking investigations. No additional risk factors have been identified and this is a routine investigation performed at the booking appointment.
14. B. Glucose tolerance test. Risk factors for developing gestational diabetes have been identified: these are Indian origin, raised body mass index and family history. Therefore, gestational diabetes mellitus screening should be performed in pregnancy with a glucose tolerance test.

Chapter 20 Antepartum haemorrhage

1. C. Placenta praevia. A low-lying placenta can cause foetal malpresentation as it blocks the cervical os and does not allow the foetal head to engage.
2. B. Vasa praevia. Bleeding comes from the foetal circulation and therefore is associated with CTG abnormalities. The treatment is prompt delivery with the neonatal team present for assessment of foetal blood transfusion after delivery. Trauma to the cervix during ARM does not cause CTG abnormalities.
3. D. Molar pregnancy. In a molar pregnancy, there are elevated human chorionic gonadotropin levels causing the symptoms of nausea and vomiting.
4. D. Placental abruption. This woman has preeclampsia which is associated with placental abruption.
5. D. Cervical ectropion. Can cause bleeding on contact.

Chapter 21 Hypertension in pregnancy

1. B. Preeclampsia is defined as hypertension (>140/90 mmHg) and proteinuria (>0.3 g in 24 hours) that develops after 20 weeks' gestation. In nonasthmatic patients first-line treatment for PET is labetalol. In this case, the patient is asthmatic therefore first-line treatment to control blood pressure is nifedipine. In nonasthmatic patients first-line treatment is labetalol if there are no other contraindications.

2. D. Essential hypertension. Diagnosed at booking with a raised booking BP (>140/90 mmHg) and no proteinuria. Blood pressure is usually low in the first trimester due to the physiological changes of pregnancy therefore it is more likely to be essential.

3. C. Hypertension secondary to renal disease is the likely diagnosis in view of her previous renal history. There is likely to have been damage to the renal tract causing raised blood pressure.

4. D. As this patient is already hypertensive with proteinuria the differential diagnosis will include essential hypertension with superimposed preeclampsia (PET) and worsening essential hypertension. If pregnant women with chronic hypertension are suspected of developing preeclampsia, placental growth factor (PIGF) could be offered to rule out PET.

5. E. HELLP syndrome is defined by evidence of haemolysis, elevated liver enzymes and a low platelet count.

6. E. Magnesium sulphate is the first-line treatment in the management of eclamptic fits.

7. C. Aspirin 150 mg is recommended for patients who have hypertensive disorders to reduce the risk of superimposed preeclampsia.

Chapter 22 Medical disorders in pregnancy

1. E. Partner with type 2 diabetes. The partner's medical history is not relevant to risk of gestational diabetes.

2. E. Age <20 years. Older age, rather than younger age, is associated with an increased risk of venous thromboembolism in pregnancy.

3. B. Acute fatty liver of pregnancy. The history and the investigations, with the very high uric acid and hypoglycaemia, are in keeping with a diagnosis of acute fatty liver of pregnancy.

4. B. Book a glucose tolerance test. A previous history of gestational diabetes mellitus (GDM) is a risk factor for developing GDM in the current pregnancy.

5. C. Deep vein thrombosis. Pregnancy is a prothrombotic state and so there is an increased risk of thrombosis.

6. B. Gestational diabetes. If not controlled, can cause foetal macrosomia and polyhydramnios.

7. E. Preterm labour. Labour is defined as regular uterine contractions associated with cervical change, in this case the woman is also preterm.

8. A. Take folic acid 5 mg daily. Neural tube defects are increased in those taking antiepileptic medications; high-dose folic acid can reduce this risk.

9. C. Arrange urgent investigations including coagulation screen and glucose level as a diagnosis of acute fatty liver needs to be excluded.

10. D. Organize a chest X-ray in the first instance. If this is normal, then further investigations to rule out a pulmonary embolism are needed.

11. C. Obesity increases the risk of gestational diabetes (GDM), preeclampsia, foetal macrosomia, caesarean birth rates and vitamin D deficiency. It does not increase the risk of abnormality for the foetus however patients need to be counselled; all forms of structural anomaly screening will be limited due to obesity.

12. E. Puerperal psychosis. The history fits with a diagnosis of puerperal psychosis. Treatment should involve admission to a mother and baby unit and antipsychotic medication, as well as social support.

Chapter 23 Common presentations in pregnancy

1. A. Fibroid degeneration. Fibroids can enlarge during pregnancy due to the hormonal changes that occur. They can become so large that they outgrow their blood supply, which causes degeneration of the fibroid and this is painful for the woman. Symphysis pubis height is bigger than expected due to fibroid size and pain is localized as it is related to the fibroid.

2. B. This patient had an increased chance for trisomy 21. Foetuses with trisomy 21 are at increased risk for duodenal atresia and they may present with polyhydramnios usually in the early third trimester. All the other options are causes for oligohydramnios.

3. D. Symphysis pubis dysfunction. Symphysis pubis dysfunction can progressively get worse throughout the pregnancy causing increasing difficulty with mobility, as progesterone affects bony joints. Women can be referred to physiotherapy where they can be assessed for crutches or even a wheelchair. Appendicitis usually presents with localized tenderness in the right iliac fossa and pyrexia. Gallstones present with right upper quadrant pain. Ligament pain is bilateral and worse on movement.

4. B. Glucose tolerance test. As the woman has risk factors for diabetes (Asian origin, LGA) GDM needs to be ruled out first as it is the most likely cause of foetal macrosomia and polyhydramnios. If the glucose tolerance test was negative, then a recent seroconversion for infections would have to be ruled out with TORCH screen testing for toxoplasmosis, cytomegalovirus and rubella. Rh status needs to be checked to assess the risk for foetal anaemia. Normal anatomy scan and a combined screening test indicate less likely to have genetic or chromosomal abnormalities as the cause for polyhydramnios.

5. C. Placental insufficiency. The abdomen is measuring small for dates. The patient has high risk for growth restriction in view of the previous pregnancy. On this

presentation she comes with reduced movements therefore most likely cause is placental insufficiency as a cause for measuring small for dates. An ultrasound scan needs to be requested. Gestational diabetes and fibroids would cause increased symphysis fundal height measurements.

Chapter 24 Multiple pregnancy

Antenatal care of multiple pregnancies

1. B. Chorionicity. This relates to the placentation. If the placentae are separate, with separate amnions and chorions (dichorionic diamniotic), the blood supply to each foetus during the pregnancy is independent. If there are blood vessel anastomoses between the placentae (monochorionic diamniotic/monochorionic monoamniotic), then there is a risk of uneven distribution of blood. Determining zygosity is not important clinically – however, a dichorionic pregnancy could be dizygotic or it could be a monozygotic pregnancy that splits before day 3 after fertilization.

2. E. Twin-to-twin transfusion syndrome. Twin-to-twin transfusion syndrome complicates 15% of monochorionic twin pregnancies. In monochorionic pregnancies there are blood vessel anastomoses between the placenta causing uneven distribution of blood. This can lead to one twin being the donor and one the recipient. The donor twin will be growth restricted and have oligohydramnios whilst the recipient twin will be larger and have polyhydramnios. Therefore scans should be performed every 2 weeks from 16 weeks. Stage 1 disease presents with discrepant liquor volumes.

3. A. Uterine atony. Because of the larger placental site in a multiple pregnancy, postpartum haemorrhage is more common and therefore a prophylactic syntocinon infusion should be used for the third stage, regardless of the mode of delivery.

4. D. The pregnancy is a dichorionic pregnancy. A lambda sign seen on scan at 11–14 weeks indicates that this pregnancy must be dichorionic, and not monochorionic. Determining zygosity is not important clinically – however, a dichorionic pregnancy could be dizygotic or it could be a monozygotic pregnancy that splits before day 3 after fertilization.

Chapter 25 Preterm labour

1. B. Administration of steroids. Although A–D are all part of the management plan, steroids should be given first because the woman already appears to be in labour.

2. D. Ventouse delivery. This is contraindicated in preterm labour in view of the risk of intracranial bleeding.

3. E. Previous miscarriage at 8 weeks. First-trimester miscarriages do not predispose to preterm delivery in concurrent pregnancies. All the other options are correct.

4. C. If there is no sign of infection a rescue cerclage can be considered for a patient with cervical dilatation of 2 cm. Option A not an indication as cervical length of more than 25 mm is normal; option B – only one preterm birth is not an indication unless there is cervical shortening; option C – this patient has first trimester miscarriages therefore a cervical cerclage is not a management option; option E – following one LLETZ operation with normal cervical length is also do not fulfil the criteria for cervical cerclage.

5. A. Maternal tachypnoea. With preterm prelabour ruptured membranes, infection must be excluded, and the most sensitive sign for this is maternal tachypnoea. Candida infection is common in pregnancy and is of no concern to the foetus. Mucoid vaginal bleeding may simply be the show, or mucus plug coming from the cervix. This can be passed if contractions commence. In pregnancy, the white blood cell count shown is within the normal range.

Chapter 26 Labour

1. B. Strength of uterine contractions. The strength of contractions is best determined by abdominal palpation rather than electronic monitoring. The latter can be used to assess the frequency of contractions, as well as the foetal heart rate. The presence and proximity to the cervix of the fibroids are best determined with an ultrasound scan. The position, station and presence of caput and moulding on the presenting part are part of the vaginal examination.

2. D.

3. C. Engagement. Assessment of whether the widest diameter of the presenting part has entered the pelvic brim is essential in monitoring the progress of labour (i.e., assessing the engagement of the head).

4. C. Position of the presenting part of the foetus.

5. D. Station of the presenting part of the foetus.

6. B. Submentobregmatic diameter. From the centre of the bregma to the angle of the mandible, measuring 9.5 cm. This is the presenting diameter in face presentation where the neck is hyperextended.

Chapter 27 Foetal monitoring in labour

1. E. Meconium-stained liquor. Provided the course of the pregnancy antenatally and during delivery has been normal, meconium-stained liquor is the only indication given for continuous foetal monitoring. It can occur postterm as the foetus is more mature, or it can be associated with foetal hypoxia.

2. B. Increase in the FHR of 15 bpm above the baseline rate lasting for 15 seconds. An acceleration is an increase in the FHR of 15 bpm above the baseline rate lasting for 15 seconds. This is a feature of a normal cardiotocograph.
3. BD foetal scalp electrode. This will attach to the baby's head and detect the foetal heart rate by direct contact. This should not be applied if the mother has human immunodeficiency virus or Hepatitis B.
4. E. Decelerations. This CTG trace is normal and options A to D are the features of a normal CTG trace.

Chapter 28 Operative interventions in labour

1. E. Less third- and fourth-degree tear. Midline episiotomy is widely used in the USA and, although it is easier to repair and likely to result in less postpartum pain, it is more likely to involve the anal sphincter if it extends.
2. E. In the following pregnancy if the patient is asymptomatic for incontinence they can have vaginal delivery or caesarean section. The decision will be based on patient's preferences.
3. D. Third-degree perineal tear. A third-degree tear involves the anal sphincter and may also involve the internal anal sphincter. It is further classified as 3A, 3B or 3C, depending on how much of the external anal sphincter is torn, and whether the internal anal sphincter is involved as well. A fourth-degree tear goes through to the anal mucosa.
4. B. Reduce/stop the syntocinon infusion. The immediate management is to stop the syntocinon infusion as there is evidence of hyperstimulation. This should reduce the frequency of contractions, which may in turn correct the cardiotocograph. You may want to start intravenous fluids and give terbutaline, but these would be second-line management options.
5. E. Patients in labour with previous caesarean section should have continuous CTG monitoring. Foetal CTG concerns can be the first sign of a scar rupture. Abdominal pain should also be monitored as scar rupture can present with continuous pain, as opposed to intermittent contractions.

Chapter 29 Complications of labour

1. D. Foetal macrosomia. Poorly controlled diabetes in pregnancy can cause foetal macrosomia as the excess sugar in the maternal bloodstream crosses to the foetus. Labour dystocia can be seen in foetal macrosomia.
2. D. Umbilical cord prolapse. An abnormal lie is more common in a grand multiparous woman, and also in preterm labour, with either an oblique lie or a transverse lie. Therefore at the time of ruptured membranes, there is a risk of cord prolapse because the head is not engaged in the maternal pelvis. If it occurs, it results in a foetal bradycardia as the blood vessels in the cord spasm.
3. B. Multiparity. External cephalic version is more likely to be successful in a multiparous patient because the maternal abdominal wall muscles are usually more relaxed. The other factors are all considered contraindications for ECV.
4. B. Ruptured uterus. One of the first signs of scar rupture is foetal distress. Other signs and symptoms include tachycardia, pain along the scar, haematuria and vaginal bleeding.
5. A. Postpartum haemorrhage/shoulder dystocia/ postpartum deep vein thrombosis. Shoulder dystocia occurs when the anterior shoulder does not deliver due to being lodged behind the symphysis pubis. The baby can become hypoxic and various manoeuvres are applied to attempt delivery of the baby. Turtle sign indicates shoulder dystocia. See Box 29.12. Prolonged labour, parity >3 and high BMI are risk factors for postpartum haemorrhage. Maternal age >35, parity >3 are risk factors for venous thrombosis. Cord prolapse not expected as the head is already delivered. Patient's temperature has been normal and no other signs of infections mentioned in the text for the risk of sepsis.
6. B. Placental abruption. Preeclampsia is associated with placental abruption. This can present with vaginal bleeding in a revealed abruption and no bleeding in a concealed abruption. The examination findings include a 'woody' hard uterus that does not relax and it can be associated with foetal distress.
7. B. Placental abruption. Preeclampsia is associated with placental abruption. This can present with vaginal bleeding in a revealed abruption and no bleeding in a concealed abruption. The examination findings include a 'woody' hard uterus that does not relax and it can be associated with foetal distress.
8. E. Uterine hyperstimulation. Occurs when there are more than 5 in 10 contractions and is associated with foetal distress. This is different from tachysystole where there are more than 5 in 10 contractions and no foetal distress. Risk of hyperstimulation is higher in patients with multiple previous deliveries.

Chapter 30 Stillbirth

1. E. A baby that is born with no signs of life at or after 24 completed weeks of pregnancy.
2. C. Malaria. TORCH is an acronym of the five infections covered in the screening:
   - toxoplasmosis
   - other diseases, including human immunodeficiency virus, syphilis and measles
   - rubella (German measles)

- cytomegalovirus
- herpes simplex

If the patient has a history of recent travel to a country affected by malaria, then investigations with blood films are required.

3. D. Parental karyotype. It is indicated if foetal karyotype indicates an unbalanced translocation or if foetal karyotyping is not possible and features indicate a chromosomal cause.

Chapter 31 Postnatal complications

1. C. Basic resuscitation ABC. Although all the options are required to manage postpartum haemorrhage, the first, most important step is to ensure that the woman's airway (A), breathing (B) and circulation (C) are intact and maintained. Make sure you are well acquainted with the ABC of resuscitation – the essential first response in every emergency situation.
2. A. >500 mL vaginal bleeding 24 hours after delivery, within 6 weeks. Secondary PPH occurs from 24 hours after delivery until 6 weeks. Maintain a high index of clinical suspicion for secondary PPH if a woman presents several weeks postpartum with heavy prolonged vaginal bleeding. Causes include retained products of conception or endometritis.
3. E. Uterine atony. The history is in keeping with uterine atony with the risk factors including a fibroid uterus, prolonged labour and a large baby. This primary postpartum haemorrhage needs urgent assessment of airway, breathing, circulation and then treatment to improve the uterine contractility.
4. E. Group A streptococcus. The key to diagnosis in this patient is the history of her unwell son – the patient should have a throat swab sent to exclude Group A streptococcus infection and appropriate antibiotics. Depending on her clinical signs, she may be advised admission to hospital for treatment and monitoring. Sepsis, including postnatally, remains a leading cause of maternal mortality.
5. E. The options A–D are risk factors for postpartum psychosis. A family history of bipolar affective disorder or postpartum psychosis confers a 25% risk.

6. B. Third-degree tear. Perineal tears involving the anal sphincter complex are classified as a third-degree tear. It is a fourth-degree tear if the anal mucosa has been involved.
7. C. Uterine atony. This occurs when the uterus does not contract after delivery. There can be ongoing bleeding. Treatment is with uterogenic drugs including oxytocin, ergometrine and prostaglandins.
8. A. Placenta accreta. An abnormal attachment of the placenta to the uterine myometrium. A history of previous caesarean sections increases the risk.
9. A. Primary PPH. The commonest causes are uterine atony and genital tract trauma. Option C is a complication of PPH. Options D and E are two of the maternal risk factors of PPH.
10. E. Uterine inversion. During the third stage of labour if controlled cord traction is applied before the placenta has delivered, uterine inversion can occur. This causes severe pain if the woman does not have any anaesthesia and brisk bleeding. The treatment is to replace the uterus manually.

Chapter 32 Maternal collapse and maternal death

1. E. Hypoxia, Hypo/hyperkalaemia, Hypovolaemia, Hypothermia
2. C. Toxicity, Thromboembolism, Tension pneumothorax, Tamponade
3. A. Tocophobia. The '4 Ts' which cause postpartum haemorrhage are: Tone (uterine atony), Trauma (vaginal or cervical lacerations with vaginal deliveries or uterine angle extensions at the time of caesarean section), Thrombin (patients with clotting disorders or in severe cases of massive obstetric haemorrhage when disseminated intravascular coagulation can ensue) or with Tissue (retained placenta or retained products of conception). Tocophobia is the name given to a pathological fear of childbirth/pregnancy.
4. E. Left lateral tilt. None of the other answers will displace the uterus to allow for improved aorto-caval circulation.
5. C. Plasma volume↑ Uterine blood flow↑ Respiratory rate↑ Heart rate↑

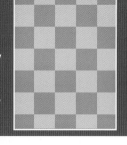

Obstetrics & Gynaecology OSCEs

OBSTETRICS OSCES

1. Antepartum haemorrhage

Candidate instructions
You have been asked to take a history from Mrs SS who is 36 weeks in her first pregnancy and has presented with vaginal bleeding. After you have completed your history, please summarize your findings and then you will be asked five questions with regard to this case.

Patient details
Name: Samantha Smith

Age: 34 years

Presenting complaint (PC): Vaginal bleeding

History of presenting complaint (HPC): This is your first pregnancy and so far you have attended all your antenatal appointments and scans and have had no problems in the pregnancy. You are rhesus negative and all other booking blood tests were normal. You are a smoker.

Your anomaly ultrasound scan showed that your placenta was not low lying. At 28 weeks you were found to be anaemic and have been commenced on ferrous sulphate.

You are now 36 weeks' pregnant. This morning you woke up with intermittent abdominal pain and noticed some vaginal bleeding. Your abdomen feels tense. Foetal movements are reduced since this morning.

Obstetric history: G1P0

Gynaecology history: Last smear was taken 3.5 years ago and results were normal. Regular menstrual cycle prepregnancy with periods lasting 5 days and occurring every 28 days with normal flow.

Medical history (MH): Nil

Drug history (DH): Ferrous sulphate

Allergies: Nil

Smoking history (SH): Smoker – cut down to five a day in pregnancy

Family history (FH): Mother had preeclampsia in first pregnancy

Checklist
- Introduces self and gains consent to take a history.
- Identifies patient.
- Starts with an open question to establish PC.
- Identifies salient points in the HPC (i.e., vaginal bleeding associated with abdominal pain).
- Enquires about foetal wellbeing by asking about foetal movements.
- Enquires about the history of this pregnancy (i.e., booked at correct gestation, attended all the antenatal ultrasound scans, blood test results).
- Identifies that the patient is rhesus negative.
- Identifies that the placenta was not low lying at the 20-week anomaly ultrasound scan.
- Identifies risk factors for abruption such as SH.
- Enquires about smear history and establishes that she is due a smear test.
- Completes the history by asking about MH, DH, allergies, SH and FH.

Questions
1. What is the most likely diagnosis?
   - Antepartum haemorrhage secondary to placental abruption – because the vaginal bleeding is associated with abdominal pain, as opposed to the painless vaginal bleeding that typically occurs with a placenta praevia.
2. What are the risk factors for placental abruption?
   - Previous abruption.
   - Advanced maternal age.
   - Multiparity.
   - Maternal hypertension or preeclampsia.
   - Abdominal trauma (e.g., assault, road traffic accident).
   - Cigarette smoking.
   - Lower socioeconomic group.
   - External cephalic version.
3. Explain the difference between a concealed and revealed haemorrhage.
   - A revealed haemorrhage is when maternal blood escapes from the placental sinuses and tracks down between the membranes and the uterus and runs through the cervix into the vagina.
   - A concealed haemorrhage is when the blood remains sealed within the uterine cavity; in this case the degree of hypovolemic shock can be out of proportion to the vaginal loss that is visualized.
4. This woman is rhesus negative; what investigations and management are required for this?
   - The patient should receive anti-D as she has had an antepartum haemorrhage, which is a sensitizing event.
   - A Kleihauer test should be performed to diagnose foetomaternal haemorrhage. This test of maternal

blood allows quantification of the degree of haemorrhage and therefore guides the dose of anti-D that is needed.

5. What are the complications of a placental abruption?
   - This depends on the volume of the antepartum haemorrhage, and your assessment of the maternal and foetal health. With major blood loss, maternal observations must be checked and airway, breathing, circulation resuscitation started urgently if necessary. The foetal heart rate must be auscultated and electronic monitoring started as this woman is more than 28 weeks' pregnant.
   - Once the woman is stable, delivery may be indicated if the foetal heart rate monitoring is abnormal. The neonatal team must be informed as well as the rest of the multidisciplinary team, including the anaesthetist, so that delivery can be expedited. The haematology team must also be informed as blood and blood products may be needed. There is a risk of developing disseminated intravascular coagulation and the urine output must be monitored carefully to exclude renal failure.

2. Postnatal sepsis

Candidate instructions

You have been asked to take a history from Mrs RD. She has presented to hospital 5 days following an emergency caesarean section for delivery of her third child for failure to progress in labour. She attended her GP surgery today complaining of feeling generally unwell. Her temperature at the GP surgery was 38.3°C. Once you have completed your history please summarize your findings. You will then be asked five questions with regard to this case.

Patient details

Name: Rachel Dean

Age: 37 years

Presenting complaint: Generally unwell

History of presenting complaint: This morning you woke up with abdominal pain that was worse than the postoperative pain you have been having. You have noticed that your vaginal loss has increased and you have passed some small clots. The loss is offensive. The wound appears clean and dry. Your temperature was raised at the GP surgery. You do not have any other symptoms.

This was your third pregnancy. This pregnancy has been uncomplicated and you had consultant-led care as you had had a previous caesarean section. At 40^{+10} weeks' gestation, you had an induction of labour, with artificial rupture of your membranes and intravenous syntocinon was commenced after 4 hours because you had not

started contracting. After 12 hours of labour, the doctors recommended a caesarean section as you had not progressed past a cervical dilatation of 4 cm.

The caesarean was complicated by scar tissue from your previous caesarean section. You lost 700 mL of blood and did not require a blood transfusion. Your postoperative recovery was uncomplicated and you were able to go home on day 2.

You are breastfeeding your new baby and that is going well.

Obstetric history: You delivered your first child 8 years ago; the pregnancy was uncomplicated and you had a normal vaginal delivery. Your second child was delivered 5 years ago by elective caesarean section for breech presentation.

Gynaecology history: Your smear tests are up to date and have always been normal. You have had normal regular periods since age 14 years.

Medical history (MH): Mild asthma

Drug history (DH): Blue (salbutamol) and brown (beclomethasone) inhaler

Allergies: Penicillin

Smoking history (SH): Nonsmoker, occasionally drinks alcohol. Lives with husband and three children.

Family history (FH): Nil

During the consultation you get irritated as you need to get home to your children and you are concerned about the new baby as you only left a small amount of expressed milk at home and will need to feed him soon.

Checklist

- Introduces self and gains consent to take a history.
- Explains why it is important to take a clear history and perform an examination, sepsis is an important cause of maternal morbidity and mortality.
- Identifies patient.
- Starts with an open question to establish presenting complaint.
- Performs a systems enquiry to establish the cause of sepsis, including headache, sore throat, breast pain, shortness of breath, chest pain, cough, abdominal pain, gastrointestinal symptoms, nature of vaginal loss, urinary symptoms and calf tenderness.
- Clarifies previous obstetric history.
- Asks about the details of this pregnancy.
- Asks about the details of the labour.
- Enquires about complications at caesarean section.
- Enquires about any postnatal problems.
- Establishes if she is breastfeeding.
- Completes the history by asking about PGH, MH, DH, allergies, SH and FH.
- Addresses the patient's concerns about being away from her newborn baby and two other children.

Questions

1. What are the differential diagnoses in this case?
   - Endometritis.
   - Pelvic collection.
   - Wound infection.
   - Mastitis.
2. What investigations need to be performed?
   - Full blood count to check the white cell count.
   - C-reactive protein level to assess inflammation.
   - Blood cultures to attempt to colonize the causative organism.
   - Lactate level.
   - High vaginal swab.
   - Wound swab.
   - Urine dipstick and midstream urine sample if there are any positive findings.
3. What are the steps in the Sepsis Six pathway for the immediate management of suspected sepsis?
   - Administer oxygen – maintain saturations >94%.
   - Take blood cultures, consider urine microscopy, culture and sensitivity; vaginal swab; sputum, etc. as indicated.
   - Give broad-spectrum antibiotics.
   - Give intravenous fluids.
   - Check serial lactate; call critical care if >4.
   - Measure urine output, start fluid balance chart with or without urinary catheter.
4. What is the most common causative organism of postnatal sepsis?
   - Group A streptococcus.
5. What are the five most common causes of direct maternal deaths in the most recent national confidential enquiry?
   - Thrombosis.
   - Haemorrhage.
   - Sepsis.
   - Ectopic pregnancy.
   - Amniotic fluid embolism.

3. Shoulder dystocia and postpartum haemorrhage

Candidate instructions

Your fellow medical student was unwell yesterday and missed a tutorial on shoulder dystocia. They have asked you to help, by teaching them about the relevance and management of shoulder dystocia. You may use a doll and model pelvis if available.

Checklist

- Check with the medical student about their current knowledge on shoulder dystocia.
- Explain that shoulder dystocia is a problem of the pelvic inlet, preventing the shoulders from delivering once the head is out. It is not a problem of the pelvic outlet.
- Excessive traction on the foetal head to facilitate the delivery of the shoulders can cause damage to the brachial plexus nerve roots in the neck (i.e., Erb palsy).
- There is a risk of increasing hypoxia as the foetus is lodged in the vagina with pressure on the umbilical cord.
- Explain the manoeuvres to aid delivery using the HELPERR pneumonic:
   - *H* – Call for help (i.e., obstetrician, labour ward coordinator, anaesthetist, paediatrician).
   - *E* – Evaluate for episiotomy – this is not to aid delivery of the shoulders but to allow adequate space to perform the internal procedures that help delivery.
   - *L* – Legs into McRoberts position – the hips are flexed in knee–chest position to widen the anteroposterior diameter of the maternal pelvis.
   - *P* – Suprapubic pressure – can be continuous or intermittent and is applied on the maternal abdomen suprapubically on the posterior aspect of the foetal shoulder to enable delivery.
   - *E* – Enter manoeuvres – internal rotation techniques, where the operator puts hands inside the vagina to try and rotate the anterior shoulder from under the pubic symphysis.
   - *R* – Remove (i.e., deliver the posterior arm so that there is more space for the shoulders to deliver).
   - *R* – Roll the patient onto all fours and repeat all the steps above.
- Ask the medical students to demonstrate what they have learnt.

Questions

1. What are the risk factors for a shoulder dystocia?
   Antenatal and intrapartum:
   - gestational diabetes
   - macrosomia
   - previous shoulder dystocia
   - raised maternal body mass index
   - postdates
   - instrumental delivery
2. What are the common complications following shoulder dystocia?
   - Postpartum haemorrhage (PPH).
   - Third-degree tear.
3. What are the common reasons for PPH?
   - Uterine atony
   - Trauma (cervical, vaginal and perineal)
   - Coagulation disorders
   - Retained placental tissue
4. What are the risk factors for uterine atony?
   - Multiple pregnancy
   - Grand multiparity
   - Foetal macrosomia

- Polyhydramnios
- Fibroid uterus
- Prolonged labour
- Previous PPH

5. How do you manage PPH due to uterine atony?
   - Start with basic resuscitation (ABC)
   - Estimate blood loss
   - IV access large bore cannulas ×2
   - Send full blood count, cross-match, clotting and urea and electrolytes.
   - Massage uterine fundus
   - Uterotonic agents such as oxytocin, ergometrine, carbetocin
   - Tranexamic acid
   - Prostaglandins such as misoprostol
   - Consider surgical options or uterine artery embolization if needed
   - Debrief the patient and team following the event
   - Incident report

GYNAECOLOGY OSCES

4. Emergency contraception

Candidate instructions
You are working in accident and emergency and a 21-year-old female patient attends requesting emergency contraception.

Please take a relevant history from her, advise her about options for emergency contraception and advise on future contraceptive options.

OSCE patient instructions
Personal details: Rebecca Jones, 21 years old, university student (studying law)

Presenting complaint: You have a new boyfriend of 1 month and during vaginal intercourse last night the condom split. You have no other casual partners and you believe your boyfriend also does not. He is your first sexual partner in over a year and you have had a negative sexually transmitted infection (STI) screen a few months ago.

Medical/surgical history: Nil of note – no migraines, venous thromboembolism (VTE), stroke. No regular medications. No allergies.

Obstetrics and gynaecology history: No pregnancies. No history of STI. Never used hormonal or intrauterine contraception – condoms only. Not yet had a smear. Regular 30-day cycle with heavy flow for 3 days and lighter flow for a further 3. Last menstrual period 3 weeks ago. No intermenstrual bleeding, no postcoital bleeding, no vaginal discharge.

Social history/Family history (FH): Body mass index 24 kg/m^2. Smoker (10/day). Lives in university accommodation. No FH of VTE/stroke/migraine.

Mark scheme
Introduces self and establishes rapport.

Identifies patient name and personal details.

Open questions regarding presenting complaint.

Addresses patient concern.

Establishes time of unprotected intercourse and number of occasions.

Inquires STI risk:
    Regular or casual partners, number of casual partners in the past year, any previous STI.

Obstetrics and gynaecology history including:
    Last menstrual period, menstrual history, contraceptive history, smear history, any previous pregnancies.
    Medical history including:
    Any history of migraine, VTE, stroke.

Social history and FH.

Drug history.

Explains the emergency contraceptive options:
    Levonorgestrel (Levonelle) – single-dose 1.5-mg tablet which must be used within 72 hours of unprotected sexual intercourse. It can only be used once per cycle.
    Ulipristal acetate (EllaOne) – single dose 30-mg tablet which must be used within 120 hours of unprotected sexual intercourse. It can be used as many times as needed per cycle.
    Copper intrauterine device can be inserted up to 120 hours (5 days) following unprotected sexual intercourse or more, if not more than 5 days after the earliest predicted date of ovulation.

Explains to take the contraception immediately.

Explains what to do if vomiting or diarrhoea occurs after taking contraceptive.

Explains may have a heavy period.

Discusses future contraception options.

Advises STI screening.

Explores that ideas, concerns and expectations are met.

Questions
1. What are common side effects of emergency contraception?
   Side effects include dizziness, nausea, headaches, breast tenderness or abdominal pain. Vomiting is a common side effect and if within 2 hours of ingestion, the treatment should be repeated.

2. What are absolute contraindications for combined hormonal contraception?
   Contraindications to combined hormonal contraception include:

- 15 cigarettes a day
- ischaemic heart disease, atrial fibrillation, stroke or severe hypertension
- previous or current personal history of VTE or known thrombogenic mutations
- migraine with aura
- current breast cancer

All women can use emergency contraception safely and effectively – no medical conditions are contraindicated as it is a one-off dose.

3. How does the copper intrauterine device work?

It is a T-shaped plastic and copper device that works by both spermicidal action and thickening cervical mucus. The copper has a toxic effect on the sperm and ovum, which prevents fertilization. It can remain in place for up to 10 years.

4. If a woman is already taking hormonal contraception but misses a dose, can she still take emergency contraception?

Yes, the additional hormone dose is small and only taken as a one-off.

5. Can emergency contraceptives be used more than once?

Emergency contraception can be repeated safely, even within the same menstrual cycle. However, it is important to counsel women about more suitable long-acting contraceptive options.

5. Smear test

Candidate instructions

You are working at a genitourinary medicine clinic and a 25-year-old woman attends for her first smear test. She is anxious about the procedure.

Please explain the procedure and then perform a cervical smear.

OSCE patient instructions

Personal details: Phillipa Lake, 25 years old, shop assistant

Presenting complaint: You have attended for your first cervical smear as part of the screening programme. You have had one previous speculum with a sexually transmitted infection (STI) test. You have had three previous regular sexual partners. You feel very nervous because your friend recently had a smear text and said it was very painful.

Medical/surgical history: Nil of note.

Obstetrics and gynaecology history: No pregnancies. No history of STI. Regular 30-day menstrual cycle. Last menstrual period 2 weeks ago. No intermenstrual bleeding, no postcoital bleeding, no vaginal discharge.

Social/family history: Maternal aunt has had abnormal smear tests in the past.

Mark scheme

Introduce self and establish rapport.
Identify patient name and personal details.
Address patient concern.
Explain the basis of screening programme to identify precancerous changes to treat appropriately.
Explain how smear is performed:
  Explain the need for chaperone; the procedure may feel uncomfortable but should not hurt. Advise that you can stop if the patient wishes.
  Ask if the patient would like to empty their bladder first.
  Explain the position that the patient will need to be in for the smear.
  Check understanding and gain consent prior to the procedure.
Perform the smear test:
  Wash hands and put on gloves.
  Inspect vulva.
  Warn the patient you are about to insert the speculum – gently insert the speculum sideways and once inserted rotate 90 degrees so the handle is upwards.
  Open the speculum blades to achieve a full view of the cervix and lock the position of the speculum.
  Inspect the vaginal tissue and cervix.
  Insert the endocervical brush into the endocervical canal through the open speculum.
  Rotate the brush five times, a full 360 degrees.
  Remove the endocervical brush and deposit it in the liquid-based cytology container.
  Gently remove the speculum and dispose of it.
  Re-cover the patient and wash hands.
Label the sample and the cytology form.
Summarize the findings to the patient.
Explain how results will be received by the patient.
Explore that ideas, concerns and expectations are met.

Questions

1. When are cervical smears performed?

As part of the screening programme cervical smears are performed on a 3-yearly basis between the ages of 25 and 49 years and on a 5-yearly basis from the ages of 50 to 64 years.

2. What are known risk factors for cervical cancer?
- Human papilloma virus.
- Smoking.
- Young age/first intercourse/pregnancy.
- Smoking.
- Oral contraceptive pill.
- Human immunodeficiency virus.

3. What types of human papillomavirus (HPV) are associated with development of cervical cancer?

HPV types 16, 18, 6 and 11 are all known to cause cervical cancer with 16 and 18 known as 'high-risk subtypes'.

4. Dyskaryosis is found at the time of cervical smear. What is the next step for investigations and diagnosis?

Women with abnormal smear test results and positive HPV should be referred for colposcopy. Cervical intraepithelial neoplasia is diagnosed from histology, therefore a biopsy should be performed in order for the diagnosis to be made.

5. An abnormality is noted on the cervix during an examination in pregnancy – what should be done about this?

Colposcopy procedure can be safely performed in pregnancy if there is any concern about cervical lesions. It will not cause any risk to the pregnancy. However, routine smear tests can be temporarily delayed until after pregnancy.

6. Fertility investigations

Candidate instructions

You are working at a GP surgery and a 34-year-old woman and her partner attends for an appointment. They have been trying to conceive a pregnancy for 18 months without success.

Please take a relevant history from the couple and discuss the first-line investigations that you will request.

OSCE patient instructions

Personal details – female: Emma Bennett, 34 years old, caterer, body mass index (BMI) 23 kg/m^2.

Presenting complaint: 18 months of subfertility, no previous pregnancies. She and her partner have regular, unprotected vaginal intercourse without difficulty.

Medical/surgical history: Nil of note, no regular medications, no allergies.

Obstetrics and gynaecology history: No known gynaecological diagnosis. Regular 28-day menstrual cycle, last menstrual period 3 weeks ago. Heavy flow for 3 days then light for 2. Associated with moderate pain for the first days of her period. No intermenstrual or postcoital bleeding. No pain on intercourse. Had chlamydia aged 19 years, which was treated. Smears up to date and normal. Previously had Implanon removed 2 years ago.

Social/family history: Nil of note. Smokes two to three cigarettes a day. Drinks approximately eight units a week socially.

Personal details – male: Simon Bennett, 35 years old, builder, BMI 28 kg/m^2.

Presenting complaint: Has never fathered any pregnancies.

Medical/surgical history: No regular medications, no allergies. No previous injury or operations on the groin or testicles. No chronic medical conditions or childhood infections. No sexually transmitted infection (STI) history.

Social/family history: Nonsmoker. Drinks approximately 15 units a week socially. Previously used anabolic steroids approximately 2 years ago when working out in the gym.

Mark scheme

Introduces self and establishes rapport.

Identifies patient name and personal details of female and male partners.

Addresses their concerns.

Establishes time of subfertility and regularity of intercourse.

Establishes whether either partner has conceived a pregnancy.

Obstetrics and gynaecology history including:

Last menstrual period, menstrual history, contraceptive history, smear history, STI history, signs of polycystic ovarian syndrome.

Medical and surgical history from female including:

Chronic conditions, regular medications, over-the-counter medication, allergies.

Medical and surgical history from male including:

Chronic conditions, regular medications, over-the-counter medication, allergies

Groin or testicular infections or operations

Social and family history of both:

Alcohol, smoking and drug history

Discuss initial investigations to perform:

Examination – BMI, abdominal, vaginal and testicular

Transvaginal ultrasound – to identify structural abnormalities of the pelvic organs

Blood tests – hormone profile

Semen analysis – to assess for male factor infertility

Suggest referral to fertility clinic after results of the investigations are reviewed.

Explore that ideas, concerns and expectations are met.

Questions

1. What are possible underlying causes for their primary infertility and what highlights this in the history?

Female factor:

- Previous history of chlamydia – previous STIs can cause tubal pathology.
- Moderate pain during periods – this could suggest an underlying diagnosis of endometriosis, although her history is otherwise suggestive of this.

Male factor:

- Previous use of anabolic steroids – these drugs are known to reduce sperm quality and quantity, which can be permanent.

2. What are the fertility rates amongst the general population trying to conceive?

Over 80% of couples conceive successfully within 1 year if the woman is aged under 40 years and they are having regular unprotected vaginal sexual intercourse. Of the remaining who do not conceive in the first year, half will go on to conceive within a second year.

3. What conservative measures can Emma and Simon do to help their chances of conception?

Conservative measures to be suggested include:
- Optimize BMI through diet and exercise
- Stop smoking
- Reduce alcohol intake

4. Their investigation results come back. Emma has a normal ultrasound and hormone profile. Simon has a semen analysis which shows <5 million spermatozoa per mL with 1% normal forms – what do you advise they do next?

This semen analysis is abnormal showing oligozoospermia and decreased normal forms. A repeat test should be performed in 3 months' time to confirm these results.

In the meantime, Simon should perform conservative measures to improve semen production, such as male supplements, loose-fitting underwear and reduction of alcohol intake to additionally help.

5. Simon's repeat semen analysis shows similar results – what options are available to the couple?

It would be advisable to refer Simon to see a urologist, in case of any potential reversible pathology, such as a varicocele.

If this is not successful, options include in-vitro fertilization, intracytoplasmic sperm injection or donor sperm insemination.

Alanine transaminase A blood test that measures the amount of a liver enzyme.

Alkaline phosphatase A liver enzyme which normally can be raised level in pregnancy as it is produced by the placenta.

Amenorrhoea Absence of menstrual period in a woman of reproductive age.

Amniotic fluid The fluid that surrounds a foetus in the uterus.

Antepartum haemorrhage Bleeding in pregnancy occurring after 24 weeks.

Artificial rupture of membranes Midwife or doctor breaks the bag of waters around the baby.

Body mass index (BMI) Measure of weight and height, formula: weight (kg) divided by height in meters squared.

Blood pressure Measure of the pressure needed to pump blood around the body.

Booking bloods Routine standard blood tests performed when a woman books for antenatal care. These include screening for human immunodeficiency virus, haemoglobinopathies, hepatitis B, syphilis and full blood count, group and save and random blood glucose level.

Breech The baby is presenting bottom first.

Cardiotocograph Recording on paper of the baby's heartbeat.

Cephalic/ceph The head of the baby is presenting into the maternal pelvis.

Cervix The opening to the uterus.

Clonus An examination for cerebral irritability. A clonus of three beats or over is considered significant.

Colposcopy A diagnostic procedure to examine a magnified view of the cervix.

C-reactive protein Blood test done to see if there is inflammation or infection in the body.

Cryoprecipitate A source of fibrinogen, vital to blood clotting.

Cusco's A bivalve speculum.

Cystocele Prolapse of the bladder into the anterior vaginal wall.

Cystoscopy Endoscopy (camera investigation) of the urinary bladder via the urethra.

Dyschezia Pain and difficulty in defecating.

Dyskaryosis Abnormal cytological changes of the cervical cells.

Dysmenorrhoea Pain during the menstrual period.

Dyspareunia Pain during sexual intercourse – can be deep or superficial.

Dysuria Pain during urination.

Fitz–Hugh–Curtis syndrome Liver capsule adhesion as a complication of pelvic inflammatory disease.

Foetal blood sample Blood test from baby's scalp taken during labour to check on baby's condition.

Foetal fibronectin test A swab taken to see if preterm delivery is likely to happen.

Foetal heart rate Baby's heart rate.

Foetal lie The direction of the long axis of the foetus compared with the mother.

Foetal scalp electrode Clip put on baby's head to allow the heartbeat to be monitored.

Fresh frozen plasma Liquid portion of the blood that has been frozen and preserved.

Full blood count Measure of the white blood cell, red blood cell and platelet levels in the blood.

General anaesthetic Giving medication to induce a controlled state of unconsciousness.

Gravid A pregnant uterus.

Group and save To find out the blood group as well as antibodies and save a sample.

Haematuria The presence of blood in the urine.

Haemoglobin Measure of the oxygen-carrying protein in the red blood cells.

Haemolysis Rupture of the red blood cells, elevated liver enzymes (showing damage to the liver) and low platelets (cells vital to help the blood to clot).

Hysteroscopy Endoscopy (camera investigation) of the uterine cavity via the cervical canal.

Intensive therapy unit Specialized ward that provides care for severe and life-threatening illnesses.

Intrahepatic cholestasis Liver problem in pregnancy that causes itching.

Intramuscular An injection of medication administered into a muscle.

Intravenous An injection of medication administered into a vein.

Laparoscopy Minimally invasive laparoscopic camera investigation of the abdomen or pelvis.

Leiomyoma Uterine fibroid.

Leucocytes White cells found in blood or urine.

Linea nigra Pigmented vertical line that appears on the abdomen during pregnancy.

Liver function test A blood test to measure how the liver is working.

Major obstetric haemorrhage Bleeding during pregnancy or after delivery of more than 1.5 L.

Maternity triage An assessment area for pregnant women.

Meconium Baby's first bowel motion, green in colour (sometimes seen when the bag of waters around the baby breaks before birth).

Menarche The first menstrual period.

Menopause When menstrual periods cease (defined as for over 1 year).

Menorrhagia Menstrual prior with excessively heavy flow.

Midstream urine A urine sample sent to laboratory to look for infection.

Miscarriage Spontaneous abortion or pregnancy loss before 24 weeks' gestation.

Multidisciplinary team Doctors, anaesthetists and midwives working together.

Neonatal unit A specialized unit for looking after babies.

Postpartum haemorrhage Bleeding of more than 500 mL after delivery of the baby.

Preeclampsia A disorder of pregnancy with high blood pressure and protein in the urine.

Procidentia Complete prolapse of the uterus beyond the level of the introitus.

Protein creatinine ratio A urine specimen to measure the amount of protein in the urine.

Rectocoele Prolapse of the bowel into the posterior vaginal wall.

Sims A U-shaped speculum.

Spontaneous rupture of membranes When the bag of waters around the baby breaks.

Striae gravidarum Atrophic linear stretch marks of pregnancy.

Urea and electrolytes A blood test to look at the function of the kidneys.

Vaginal examination An internal examination of the vagina.

Virgo intacta A person who has never had sexual intercourse.

Index